The Effectiveness of Methadone Maintenance Treatment

John C. Ball   Alan Ross

The Effectiveness of Methadone Maintenance Treatment

Patients, Programs, Services, and Outcome

Foreword by Vincent P. Dole

With 11 Illustrations

Springer-Verlag
New York Berlin Heidelberg London
Paris Tokyo Hong Kong Barcelona

John C. Ball
National Institute on Drug Abuse-
Addiction Research Center
and University of Maryland
School of Medicine
Baltimore, Maryland 21224
USA

Alan Ross
Johns Hopkins School of Hygiene
Department of Biostatistics
Baltimore Maryland 21205
USA

Library of Congress Cataloging-in-Publication Data
Ball, John C.
The effectiveness of methadone maintenance treatment : patients, programs, services, and outcome / John C. Ball, Alan Ross.
p. cm.
Includes bibliographical references.
Includes index.
ISBN-13:978-1-4613-9091-6
1. Methadone maintenance. 2. Methadone maintenance—Evaluation.
I. Ross, Alan, 1926– . II. Title.
[DNLM: 1. Methadone—therapeutic use. 2. Outcome and Process Assessment (Health Care)—trends. 3. Prognosis. 4. Substance Dependence—rehabilitation. WM 270 B187ea]
RC568.M4B35 1991
616.86'32061—dc20
DNLM/DLC 90-10299
for Library of Congress

Printed on acid-free paper.

Typeset by Asco Trade Typesetting Ltd., Hong Kong.

9 8 7 6 5 4 3 2 1

ISBN-13:978-1-4613-9091-6 e-ISBN-13:978-1-4613-9089-3
DOI: 10.1007/978-1-4613-9089-3

In collaboration with:

Bridge Plaza Treatment and Rehabilitation Clinic—New York
Fort Greene Treatment Center, ARTC—New York
John F. Kennedy Community Mental Health/Mental Retardation Center—Philadelphia
Achievement Through Counceling and Treatment—Philadelphia
Glenwood Life Counseling Center—Baltimore
Man Alive Research Inc.—Baltimore
Drug Dependence Treatment Unit, Veterans Administration Hospital—Philadelphia
Institute for Survey Research—Philadelphia

This study is dedicated to the staff of methadone maintenance treatment programs throughout the United States.

Foreword

Legislators, journalists and concerned citizens in general, when considering what to do about the plague of heroin addiction in large cities, ask an obvious question: "Is methadone treatment effective?" This question is a critical one since maintenance with methadone is at present the only practical alternative to leaving tens of thousands (in New York City, hundreds of thousands) of untreated addicts on the streets. Other treatments, although effective for limited groups, could not conceivably be expanded to stop heroin use in as much as 10% of the addicted population.

The present study, sponsored by the National Institute on Drug Abuse, was undertaken to provide an authoritative answer to this question. Under the direction of a distinguished expert, the evaluation team made an intensive examination of techniques and outcomes in six different methadone programs located in New York, Philadelphia, and Baltimore, and followed this by two yhears of data analysis and literature review. The present report is the product of this work.

The primary conclusion—namely that methadone treatment is substantially effective in reducing heroin use and associated criminal behavior—is consistent with the findings of several previous independent evaluations. Although no surprise, this further endorsement of maintenance treatment by a prestigious independent group is very welcome. However, what gives a unique importance to the study is that it moves beyond the overbroad question of general effectiveness of "methadone programs" to the specifics of the treatment process. All of the programs, by definition, utilize methadone—and therefore are usually lumped together in public discussion—but in fact, as this study well shows, they differ markedly in treatment philosophy, techniques, and resources. In the present study the evaluators selected a set of programs with considerable variance in treatment techniques, and therefore for the first time in evaluation history were able to join a statistical analysis of process to an analysis of outcome.

The evaluators' success in opening the "black box" of treatment process is a tribute to the unique position of the senior investigator in the evaluation field. Probably no other examiner could have persuaded the beleaguered programs to cooperate in a detailed scrutiny by outside observers. Their trust was well placed. Confidentiality of the sources has been protected, while the variance in treatment techniques has been defined for statistical analyses. Chapter 4 ("Candid Descriptions of Six Programs") is without parallel in the evaluation literature. It should be required reading for serious students of treatment policy. The "black boxes" have quite different contents.

Analyses of treatment outcome are also presented, but the difficult task of relating specific components of treatment process to outcome has only begun. In the opinion of this reviewer, this analysis could have been facilitated by greater emphasis on the inverse relation between dose of methadone and success in terminating use of heroin. In this regard, the findings provided in appendix B which show the frequency of heroin use by all patients in the six programs are worthy of further comment. Note that the dose-response relation is essentially independent of the marked differences in rehabilitation services in the six programs. At methadone dose levels below 71 mg/day a significant fraction of patients in the programs continued to use heroin (although at a lower rate than with no methadone); at doses of 71 mg/day or above no patient in this survey was positive. This finding suggests that the administration of sub-optional doses of methadone in a treatment program unnecessarily handicaps the rehabilitation work and confounds analysis of other process variables. Patients who continue to experience recurrent craving for heroin are poor subjects for counseling, and are likely to drop out early in treatment.

The AIDS epidemic has added a compelling reason for adequate dosage: A single exposure to a contaminated needle and syringe is capable of transmitting a lethal disease. Effective interdiction of viral spread requires that intravenous drug use be not merely reduced, but terminated as quickly as possible in as many addicts as possible. For this, a full blocking dose of methadone is often essential; the blood level of methadone needs to be maintained at all times above 200 ng/ml to suppress narcotic craving. While about half of the patients may respond to lower doses, certainly the daily dose of methadone should be increased if a patient continues to use heroin while in treatment. With adequate dosage of methadone, taken daily, heroin use should be completely eliminated in 95% of all patients.

I wish to join the members of the evaluation team in saluting the dedicated persons working in methadone maintenance programs. They serve under stress with little recognition, underfunded, over-regulated, misunderstood in their communities, often vilified by special interest groups—and yet they persist in their work of saving lives. They already have the gratitude of informed witnesses. One of the great merits of the present study is that it increases the number of informed witnesses.

Vincent P. Dole
The Rockefeller University

Acknowledgments

The collection of data at the programs was made possible by colleagues, treatment staff and researchers. The core project staff were Dr. Eric Corty, Henrietta Bond, Anthony Tommasello, S. Paul Petroski, C. Patrick Myers and Theresa Hancock. Eric Corty and C. Patrick Myers were also co-authors of Chapter 9.

The directors of the methadone maintenance program who collaborated with this study were Dr. George E. Woody, Mr. Richard Lane, Dr. Ronald Brady, Mr. Frank Satterfield, Dr. Beny J. Primm, Barbara G. Goldsmith, Mr. Gene F. Tomlinson, Mr. Steve Richman, Dr. Winston Collins, and Dr. Robert P. Bass, Jr.

The senior staff and interviewers at the Institute for Survey Research who were involved in this project were Dr. Leonard LoSciuto, Mary Ann Ausetts, Sharon Lustig, B. Millhouse, F. Berlin, R. Jacobs, H. VanHorn, M. Farmer, S. Roberts, F. Boyce, B. Schlenger, C. Gorman, L. Basarab, O. Johnson, and T. Williams.

Analysis of the findings during the past several years and preparation of this volume have been supported by the Addiction Research Center. In this regard, I wish to thank Dr. Jerome H. Jaffe for his encouragement; also to be recognized are Dr. Roy W. Pickens, Dr. Barry S. Brown and Dr. David A. Gorelick.

Others who assisted in the project at various times were Linda Rebstock, Diane Erdlen, Nancy Rogers, Carol Beglan, Joanne Golden, Christopher Pick, and Dr. Daniel Levinson.

Theresa Hancock superintended both the compilation of voluminous data sets and the preparation of the final manuscript.

Throughout the study, Dr. A. Thomas McLellan provided continual advice and intellectual support.

Dr. Vincent P. Dole provided both inspiration and invaluable advice during the entire course of this study.

Contents

1
Status of Methadone Maintenance Treatment and Research in the United States

Methadone maintenance treatment was established in New York City in 1964 by Drs. Vincent Dole and Marie Nyswander.[1,2] The original treatment regimen implemented by Drs. Dole and Nyswander with their staff provided comprehensive medical and rehabilitative services to intravenous heroin addicts. Criteria for admission included: 4 years of heroin addiction, a history of prior treatment failure, voluntary desire for treatment, age over 19, primary dependence upon opiates, and absence of psychosis or major medical complications. In the initial studies, addicts were evaluated and stabilized on a daily oral dose of methadone on an inpatient service before transfer to an outpatient clinic for continued treatment. With further experience, it was found feasible to eliminate the inpatient phase of treatment and start with the outpatient clinic.

Outcome studies from these first years of methadone maintenance treatment reported favorable results.[3–5] There were high rates of patient retention, reduced criminality, and improved social rehabilitation.[6] These early programs, then, were found to be effective in rehabilitating intravenous heroin addicts who remained in outpatient treatment on a long-term basis. In this regard, it should be noted that the treatment staff in these first clinics were highly qualified and, in particular, that a high standard of medical treatment and supervision was provided.

During the 1970s methadone maintenance treatment was greatly expanded in New York City[7] and established in large cities throughout much of the United States. As this expansion occurred, a number of programmatic changes took place. One change of pervasive significance was that federal, state, and local governments became involved in the operation of the new or expanded clinics.[8] Thus in 1972 the Food and Drug Administration promulgated regulations which specified the types and amount of treatment services to be provided.* At the same time, state or local juris-

*By 1980 there were 12 pages of regulations pertaining to mandated services at methadone programs (*Federal Register*, September 19, 1980, pp 1–12).

dictions established bureaucracies to administer, fund, and audit these treatment facilities. As a consequence of this expansion, methadone maintenance changed from a medically supervised treatment for a designated population of heroin addicts to a more diversified form of treatment and rehabilitation provided to unselected addict patients. The extent of change that occurred from the Dole-Nyswander methadone maintenance model varied by locale, city, state, and other considerations. In this last regard, methadone maintenance programs were also established by the federal government, e.g., at Veterans Administration hospitals.

One consequence of this expansion and change of auspices (from medical to governmental) was that variation among the programs developed.[9] They differed in the number of patients treated (from a few dozen to almost a thousand in one clinic); the qualifications of the director (social worker, ex-addict, physician, administrator); type and qualifications of staff; the amount and type of counseling and medical services provided; methadone dose commonly prescribed (from less than 30 mg to over 100 mg); and policies about urine testing, take-home methadone, and many other aspects of treatment. By the end of the 1970s, methadone maintenance was far from being a uniform entity.[10] This change, as is discussed later, had both advantages and disadvantages.

By the 1980s, the great expansion of methadone maintenance treatment had ceased. No new treatment facilities were opened in New York City during a 10-year period.[11] There was some expansion or contraction of treatment programs in other cities or states, but it was primarily of local significance.

The 1980s were, then, a period of stability or retrenchment for methadone maintenance treatment in the United States. Although the programs that developed from the Dole-Nyswander model were generally underfunded,[8] during the 1980s even this level of financial support was reduced. As a consequence, programs were forced to curtail treatment and rehabilitative services, staff turnover was high, and the quality of care declined.[12,13] At the same time, many programs were beset with community opposition, lack of administrative support, and general public apathy or hostility.[14] Despite these considerations, methadone maintenance treatment endured.

Current Status of Methadone Maintenance Treatment

As of January 1, 1989 there were 667 methadone maintenance programs in the United States,[15] with a census of approximately 80,000 addicts. Most of these programs are located in large cities, with the highest concentration of heroin addicts and methadone maintenance clinics in East Coast cities. For example, there are 35,000 patients in New York State methadone programs, and most of these are residents of New York City.[16]

Mention has already been made of the variation in program characteristics, services provided, and other differences among methadone maintenance programs throughout the United States. In this regard, the role of the 50 state drug abuse agencies should be noted, as they exercise considerable control over the programs they administer: They establish and implement treatment policies for all programs under their authority.*

The status of methadone maintenance treatment throughout the nation was assessed in 1989 by the President of the Northeast Regional Methadone Treatment Coalition.[17]

> The existing drug treatment programs require an immediate infusion of fiscal and programmatic resources before any meaningful services expansion can be implemented. Standards of care and individual treatment capability vary widely from one state to another. The physical structure of drug treatment programs are in need of major renovation to reverse years of limited funding and general neglect. The present system does not have a stable cadre of career professionals. The rapidly changing characteristics of chronic drug users requires the long-term professional commitment of better trained personnel. Communities also need to be intensively educated about the value of drug treatment.

Current variations in program characteristics and services provided in methadone maintenance programs throughout the United States have both advantages and disadvantages. The advantages stem from the fact that we know little about what treatment characteristics are related to successful patient outcome. Therefore diversity among programs can provide a database from which appropriate models for methadone maintenance treatment can be established. In this regard, it now seems evident that a single uniform regimen of treatment for all addict patients is not a viable objective to pursue. The needs of different patient populations require, at the least, several models of methadone maintenance treatment and rehabilitation. For example, the need for vocational and rehabilitative counseling in a program where most of the patients are already employed at admission is different from that in a program where fewer than 10 percent of the patients are employed. Similarly, there are special needs for programs whose patients include a large proportion of mothers with young children, pregnant females, the illiterate, the aged, the handicapped, or the mentally ill. Furthermore, the racial and ethnic composition of the patient population often requires that programs accommodate special needs as well.

The disadvantage of having diverse treatment and rehabilitation services provided by methadone maintenance programs is that mere diversity is not conducive to the improvement of treatment, especially if the diversity is due to public opposition and financial austerity. Many programs have had to eliminate, reduce, or alter services because of lack of funds and other

---

*In 1987 there were 450,553 admissions of drug abuse clients in the United States, and 98,549 of them reported heroin as the principal drug of abuse.[16]

resources.[12,18] These changes have not been beneficial and hardly provide a framework for developing alternative model programs—quite the contrary. They only reinforce our knowledge of the deleterious effects of inadequate treatment.

The AIDS Era

The AIDS era has descended on drug abuse programs that treat intravenous heroin addicts with special force, as intravenous (IV) drug users are the second largest population (after male homosexuals) at risk for AIDS in the United States.[19] In New York City more than 50 percent of IV drug users in treatment are human immunodeficiency virus (HIV) positive.[20] In other cities, the positivity rate among IV drug users is lower but is rising.[21]

How the AIDS epidemic will affect methadone maintenance treatment in the long run remains to be seen. Thus far both HIV positivity and AIDS have arrived, but additional treatment resources have not. In the New York City metropolitan area the situation with respect to AIDS cases is already critical.[22,23]

Prior Research and Treatment Evaluation of Methadone Maintenance

A considerable body of scientific and medical knowledge has been published during the past quarter century about methadone maintenance treatment. Most of this research falls within two broad classifications: (1) pharmacological or clinical studies of the efficacy of specific drugs, dosages, or related treatment regimens, and (2) patient outcome studies that measure the overall effectiveness of methadone maintenance treatment. Investigators in both of these research areas have advanced our knowledge considerably, and these contributions have been reviewed in a series of research monographs sponsored by the National Institute on Drug Abuse (NIDA).[24,25]

Without reviewing the research literature in these two areas, it is nonetheless pertinent to comment on the scope and limitations of both pharmacological and outcome research studies. In the former classification, research tends to be experimentally designed to ascertain drug reaction or regimen effects in a highly controlled artificial setting (i.e., the laboratory or a specialized clinic). Although these and prior studies that established the basic mechanism of drug dependence (e.g., addiction, dependence, withdrawal, tolerance, detoxification) have provided a foundation for drug abuse treatment, they are largely restricted to the pharmacological and clinical aspects of drug abuse. These studies do not, for the most part, address etiology, epidemiology, treatment availability, quality of care, retention in treatment, and similar topics. The studies, then, are often unrelated to drug abuse treatment (although otherwise important).

Outcome studies of patients who have been in methadone maintenance treatment tend to be broad in scope and design.[25] Typically, patients are evaluated before and after methadone maintenance treatment to ascertain if positive change has occurred. These studies are designed to determine if an expected change has occurred among patients as a consequence of treatment. Thus data are obtained to determine if addict patients have reduced their drug abuse and criminality and have increased their employment and family stability after entering treatment. These outcome studies have sometimes been restricted to a single drug abuse treatment program, but multisite and multimodality studies have been undertaken that obtained follow-up data from numerous cohorts of patients.[26,27] These outcome studies have established that methadone maintenance (and other modalities of treatment) are effective in that some patients improve after treatment.[28–30]

The "Black Box" of Methadone Maintenance Treatment

During the 1980s a few researchers independently noted that there is a pervasive lack of knowledge about how treatment is actually carried out in methadone maintenance programs. Indeed, this somewhat perplexing void in our knowledge of drug abuse treatment has been dubbed the "black box" of treatment. It is worthwhile to recount these observations about the black box in order to assess the dimensions, significance, and reasons for this research void.

In a NIDA monograph that reviewed the status of drug abuse treatment evaluation, Lipton and Appel noted the following.[31]

> One concern expressed repeatedly has been that treatment is largely a "*black box*". The people, events, and interactions subsumed by labels such as "therapy," "counseling," "referral for services," and "remediation" remain largely undescribed in drug programs. As a result, variations in delivery and efficacy, which are crucial to treatment evaluation, are also unspecified. [Italics added]

To these researchers, then, the black box refers to lack of knowledge about the components and dynamics of treatment. It is especially significant that these authors asserted that even descriptive knowledge of treatment is absent. If so, it certainly follows, as the authors stated, that meaningful analysis of the delivery of treatment services is not feasible.

In another NIDA review volume on the status of drug abuse research and evaluation, Hall observed the following.[32]

Finally, many aspects of the treatment environment remain *untouched by research*. For example, issues of client staff ratio, the usefulness of aspects of the methadone regulations other than urine monitoring, and of program policy have not been researched to any extent. [italics added]

When stating that "many aspects of the treatment environment remain untouched by research," Hall described a void that is similar to the black box referred to by Lipton and Appel. The black box seems to be of considerable size, as Hall mentioned our lack of knowledge about such additional aspects of treatment as client/staff ratio, the usefulness of federal regulations and policy in general.

In an even broader context, Gottheil and co-workers, reviewing the status of both drug abuse and alcoholism treatment evaluation, found a pervasive lack of knowledge about treatment factors.[33]

There are also many treatment factors that may be related to outcome, *although few have been identified*. It is not enough to know that more treatment is better than less without knowing more about the effective components of treatment. . . . *There is an even greater need for* basic and systematic descriptions, classifications, and measurements of *treatment factors* than of patient characteristics. [Italics added].

These authors found that there is a general absence of research pertaining to treatment factors. In this regard, they stated that this lack of knowledge is not only of considerable magnitude but that it presumably involves inadequacies in basic methodological and design issues because there is a "need for basic and systematic descriptions, classifications, and measurements of treatment factors."

The idea that there is something amiss in our evaluation of drug abuse treatment appears to be developing, although the topic has not been systematically addressed in research studies. With regard to this developing awareness of the black box, two additional researchers summarized the state of drug abuse treatment research with the following comment.[34]

There was general agreement that outcome was affected by the patient's relationship *to something in the program* in addition to methadone, but whether it was a specific counselor, daily visits for methadone, special programs (educational, vocational, or psychotherapy), or legal interventions remains to be determined. [Italics added]

In this instance, Altman and Schnoll[35] also noted that "something in the program" was effective in treatment, and they went on to state that there was general agreement about this lack of knowledge. Therefore, some kind of consensus seems to be developing about the existence of a definite void in our research findings about treatment effectiveness.

With regard to possible reasons for this void about drug abuse treatment, another group of evaluators reported that this type of research is difficult to undertake.[35]

> The *complexity of treatment* is difficult to conceptualize and even harder to define and quantify. [Italics added]

In this instance, an experienced group of researchers (Hubbard, Rachal, Craddock, and Cavanaugh) implied not only that the void exists but that the state of our knowledge is such that we have not yet been able to conceptualize what treatment consists of. Thus, from this report it may be inferred that we are at a conceptual and methodological roadblock with respect to drug abuse treatment evaluation: We have yet to even define the relevant variables, let alone measure them.

Another researcher, in an introduction to a series of research papers on "Factors Affecting the Outcome of Methadone Treatment," concluded the review as follows.[36]

> The failures [of those patients who do not benefit from methadone treatment] need to be understood on the basis of *the complexity of the "black box,"* the characteristics of the patients and the therapist/counselors, and the mix. [Italics added]

In this instance, Meyer not only recognized the existence of the black box of treatment, but he regarded the efficacy of methadone treatment as also related to patient and staff characteristics.

After considering the general scope of the black box of treatment, it comes as no surprise that drug abuse researchers as well as policy decision-makers find it difficult to delineate what we know about the delivery of effective treatment or to formulate policy based on substantive findings. With regard to delineating what we know about treatment characteristics associated with successful patient outcome, Woody[37] observed that

> there are few studies comparing types of treatments offered within these programs [different modalities] and outcome. Thus, much of this paper consists of *impressions* found from treating patients and from reading the available literature. [Italics added]

Woody's paper is important because it recognized the need to address the topic of treatment characteristics. Furthermore, as a physician and director of a methadone maintenance program he is familiar with the operation of his clinic. Therefore it is all the more revealing when he stated that he relies on personal impressions in his research appraisal because of the "lack of relevant studies."

The plight of public officials and decision makers with regard to formulating policy about methadone maintenance treatment (or other modalities) is equally difficult. In this regard, D'Amanda stated the following.[9]

> *It is not easy* to find contributions from the large body of literature *suitable* for *policy decision-making*, nor is it easy to find references to policy(ies) which sustain(s) the myriad functions carried out in methadone programs.
>
> Evaluation of program efficacy was (and is) generally limited to statements about different client populations.

Therefore, the possibility of choosing one policy as better than another is not now available. [Italics added]

It is recognized, then, by a knowledgeable physician-administrator that the necessary knowledge base about treatment characteristics and outcome is absent. The black box is thus seen as an impediment to both treatment evaluation and policy determination.

Why a Black Box About Treatment Exists

It is important to determine why our knowledge of drug abuse treatment developed in such a way as to permit a black box to exist. Although a treatise of this topic is beyond the scope of this research report, it seems pertinent to at least comment on some of the disciplinary and empirical factors that come to mind.

There has been a general emphasis on the pharmacology of drug abuse and corresponding lack of interest in studying the dynamics of treatment programs.[6] This circumstance is partly a consequence of disciplinary considerations in that the "hard sciences" are not trained in program evaluation, and furthermore drug abuse treatment evaluation does not fall within the purview of any recognized profession or discipline. Adding to these academic considerations is the fact that on-site field studies of drug abuse treatment programs are difficult, costly, and problematical when compared with laboratory research.

The empirical and methodological impediments to research about drug abuse treatment, although certainly real and significant, seem less pervasive than the conceptual and disciplinary problems,[38] as it is the latter that more cogently explain the existence of the black box. Thus programs are not even regarded as a factor in most studies of drug abuse treatment. It follows therefore that treatment setting and characteristics have not been investigated. Hence a meaningful conceptualization of what constitutes drug abuse treatment may well be a precondition to the initiation of research to open the black box.

Four-Domain Schema for Treatment Evaluation

A new conceptualization of drug abuse and alcoholism treatment evaluation is presented here that recognizes the need to open the black box of treatment and systematically study its contents (Fig. 1.1). This research design formulation is slowly but simultaneously developing in the fields of drug abuse and alcoholism treatment evaluation. Thus in an article about alcoholism program evaluation Moos and Finney[39] began by stating that:

Until recently, a patient input–"black box" treatment–client outcome paradigm guided many evaluations of alcoholism treatment programs. The treatment pro-

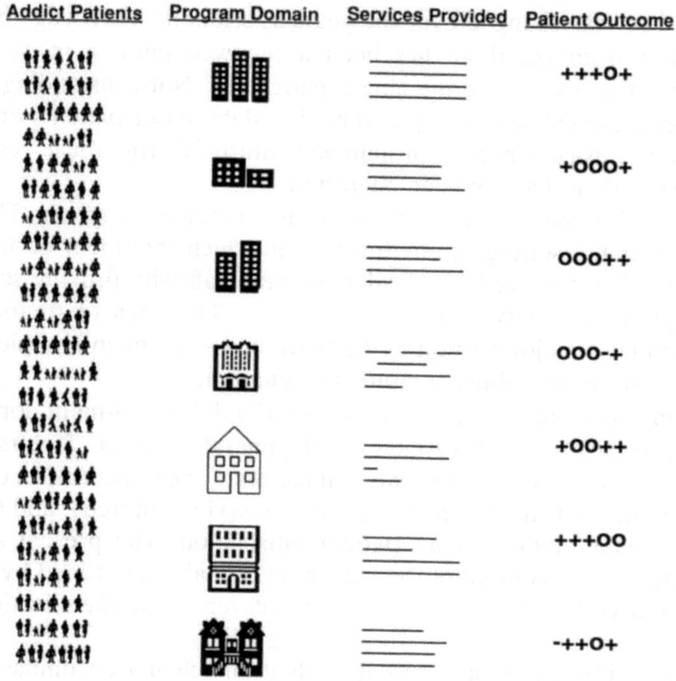

FIGURE 1.1. Four domains in the evaluation of treatment.

gram usually was assessed in terms of gross categories, such as treatment versus no or an alternative treatment. . . . Although it is popular (perhaps because of its simplicity), the summative approach [input-output] has at least one serious drawback: it provides no information as to why a program or treatment package is effective or ineffective.

From this beginning, they proceeded to delineate the scope and characteristics of the treatment domain. Their work is described more fully below. To conceptualize drug abuse treatment broadly, thereby opening the black box of treatment, it is efficacious to posit a schema that includes four domains of data collection and study: the patients, the programs, the services, and the outcomes. Each of these domains is delineated before discussing the overall efficacy of the fourfold evaluation schema.

First, with regard to patients, it has been recognized for some time that it is necessary to obtain detailed life history information and current health status data on addict patients. Thus, from the time of Terry and Pellens[40] (1928), to that of Pescor[41] at the US Public Health Service Hospital at Lexington (late 1930s), to the present, this area of research has not been neglected. As might be expected, however, consideration of which types of data to collect has changed over the years as scientific knowledge has advanced. For instance, there has been a renewed interest in obtaining psychiatric diagnoses of drug abuse patients.[42] Notwithstanding shifts in emphasis, the collection of preadmission data about patients entering treatment has usually been a prominent feature of drug abuse research. This domain, then, has not been neglected.

The second domain in the schema is the treatment program. This domain includes the setting or environment in which treatment occurs, the treatment policy followed, the leadership and staff who provide services, and the physical facility and other resources. This area of treatment—which includes a major portion of the black box—has been conspicuously neglected during drug abuse treatment evaluation.

Moos and colleagues[43] classified and described this treatment domain as consisting of five sets of variables: (1) general program factors, e.g., physical features, policy, organizational factors; (2) characteristics of staff; (3) work milieu; (4) treatment components (services offered); and (5) system performance indices, e.g., patient satisfaction. The present schema follows the general content of the treatment domain as outlined by Moos, Finney, and colleagues, but with some differences in classification and emphasis.

The third domain in the present evaluation schema encompasses the actual provision of treatment and rehabilitative services. In methadone maintenance programs this domain includes the number of methadone doses dispensed on-site and as take-home medications; dosages prescribed; hours of clinic operation; patient attendance; number, type, and duration of counseling sessions (e.g., individual or group); educational or vocational services; type and frequency of medical services provided on-site; referral services provided; psychiatric coverage provided; frequency of obtaining urine specimens and urinalysis procedure; and any other services provided. This services domain has also been neglected[44] but somewhat less so than the treatment domain.

The fourth domain of the schema is patient outcome following treatment or patient status during long-term stay. This area of study has not been neglected. Thus there has been a consistent realization that it is necessary to collect information about patient characteristics following treatment to determine if positive change has occurred.[45] For drug abuse treatment evaluation, common outcome criteria are a reduction of drug abuse (by type of drug), reduction of criminality, retention in treatment, improvement in employment, and reduction in welfare status.

The rationale for the fourfold schema is to emphasize the necessity of collecting data in all four of these domains whenever a comprehensive evaluation of drug abuse treatment is sought. One can, of course, study only one or even part of a single domain scientifically. Such specialized research efforts, however, are not designed as treatment evaluation studies. Collection of relevant data in the four domains is a prerequisite to comprehensive program evaluation.

Conceptualizing drug abuse program evaluation within a fourfold overall schema is only the first step in developing an appropriate research design. The variables and measurement procedures to be employed in each domain must be specified or derived before data collection begins and the overall plan of analysis formulated.

Conclusion

This study of methadone maintenance programs in New York City, Philadelphia, and Baltimore was planned to open the black box of methadone maintenance treatment. It was initially necessary to assess at first-hand how these programs operate on a daily basis to provide treatment to their addict patients. The plan of data collection explained in Chapter 2 includes a description of how comprehensive data about each of the programs was obtained through systematic observation, staff interviews, and record reviews at the three cities. The field procedures employed included face-to-face interviews with 633 male patients in these programs, 617 of whom completed valid Addiction Severity Index interviews.

The life history characteristics of 617 male addicts enrolled in these programs is discussed in Chapter 3. Their extensive drug abuse history, endemic criminality, and repeated failures in prior drug abuse treatment are recounted to establish baseline characteristics of these patients and thereby to posit realistic treatment goals.

How each of the six methadone programs operate on a daily basis as they provide treatment to their addict patients is described in Chapter 4. The detailed descriptions of these outpatient clinics are followed, in Chapter 5, by a comprehensive exposition of the entire treatment domain. In this presentation, the black box is opened, and the basic elements of methadone maintenance treatment are identified and delineated. This process includes (see Chapter 6) an enumeration and assessment of the medical and counseling services provided to the entire census of 1909 patients at the six programs.

The effectiveness of treatment is analyzed in the remainder of the volume. Research findings pertaining to the reduction of drug abuse and intravenous injections during methadone maintenance treatment are presented in Chapter 7, followed in Chapter 8 by consideration of the phenomenon of relapse among those who dropped out of treatment as well as the likelihood of cure. The issue of the prevalence of psychiatric symptomology among the 617 patients selected for detailed study is addressed in Chapter 9. In Chapter 10 a separate analysis is undertaken of the reduction in crime during methadone maintenance treatment. A statistical analysis of the effect of baseline patient characteristics, program elements, and treatment process variables upon successful patient outcome is undertaken in Chapter 11. Finally, the research findings of the entire study are summarized in Chapter 12.

References

1. Dole VP, Nyswander M (1965) A medical treatment for diacetylmorphine (heroin) addiction: a clinical trial with methadone hydrochloride. JAMA 193:80–84
2. Dole V (1989) Methadone maintenance. In Courtwright D, Joseph H, Des Jarlais D: Addicts Who Survived: An Oral History of Narcotic Use in America, 1923–1965. Knoxville: University of Tennessee Press, pp 331–343
3. Dole VP, Nyswander ME, Warner A (1968) Successful treatment of 750 criminal addicts. JAMA 206:2708–2711
4. Gearing FR (1972) Methadone maintenance: six years later. Contemp Drug Prob 1:191–206
5. Gearing FR (1970) Successes and failures in methadone maintenance treatment of heroin addiction in New York City. In: Proceedings of the Third National Conference on Methadone Treatment. Rockville: US Public Health Service, Pub. No. 2172, pp 2–16
6. Connell PH (1975) Review of methadone maintenance schemes. In Boström H, Larsson T, Ljungstedt N (eds): Skandia International Symposia: Drug Dependence-Treatment and Treatment Evaluation. Stockholm: Almqvist & Wiksell, pp 133–146
7. Newman RG, in collaboration with Cates MS (1977) The role of social and psychiatric services. In Methadone Treatment in Narcotic Addiction: Program Management, Findings, and Prospects for the Future. New York: Academic Press, pp 64–68
8. Lowinson JH (1981) Methadone maintenance in perspective. In Lowinson JH, Ruiz P (eds): Substance Abuse: Clinical Problems and Perspectives. Baltimore: Williams & Wilkins, pp 344–354
9. D'Amanda C (1983) Program policies and procedures associated with treatment outcome. In Cooper JR, Altman F, Brown BS, Czechowicz D (eds): NIDA Treatment Research Monograph Series: Research on the Treatment of Narcotic Addiction: State of the Art. (ADM) 83–1281. Rockville: US Department of Health and Human Services, pp 637–679
10. Bourne PG (1981) A 10-year perspective on the addiction problem. In Lowinson JH, Ruiz P (eds): Substance Abuse: Clinical Problems and Perspectives. Baltimore: Williams & Wilkins, pp 35–42
11. Kirn TF (1988) Methadone maintenance treatment remains controversial even after 23 years of experience. JAMA 260:2970–2975
12. Gerstein DR, Harwood HJ (eds) (1990) Treating Drug Problems, Vol. 1. Washington, DC: National Academy Press
13. United States General Accounting Office (1990) Methadone maintenance: some treatment programs are not effective; greater federal oversight needed. In: GAO Report to the Chairman, Select Committee on Narcotics Abuse and Control, House of Representatives (March). Washington, DC: US Government Printing Office
14. Klepak D (1978) Evaluation of treatment effectiveness: the New York State experience. Ann NY Acad Sci 311:248–252
15. FDA, personal communication, January 1989
16. Butynski W, Canova D, Jensen S (1989) State Resources and Services Related to Alcohol and Drug Abuse Problems—Fiscal Year 1988: An analysis of state

alcohol and drug abuse. Washington, DC: National Association of State Alcohol and Drug Abuse Directors
17. Parrino M (1989) Letter to Bennett WJ
18. Murphy S, Rosenbaum M (1988) Money for methadone. II. Unintended consequences of limited-duration methadone maintenance. J Psychoactive Drugs 20:397–402
19. Des Jarlais DC, Friedman SR (1989) AIDS and the IV drug user. Science 245:578
20. Des Jarlais DC, Friedman SR (1987) Target groups for preventing AIDS among intravenous drug users. J Appl Soc Psychol 17:251–268
21. Galea RP, Lewis BF, Baker LA (eds) (1988) AIDS and IV Drug Abusers: Current Perspectives. Owings Mills: National Health Publishing, Exhibit I-1, I-2, pp xxvii, xxx-xxxi
22. Novick DM, Joseph H, Croxson TS, et al (1990) Absence of antibody to human immunodeficiency virus in long-term, socially rehabilitated methadone maintenance patients. Arch Intern Med 150:97–99
23. Des Jarlais DC (1990) Stages in the response of the drug abuse treatment system to the AIDS epidemic in New York City. J Drug Issues 20:335–347
24. Cooper JR, Altman F, Brown B, Czechowicz D (eds) (1983) NIDA Treatment Research Monograph Series: Research on the Treatment of Narcotic Addiction: State of the Art. (ADM) 83–1281. Rockville: US Department of Health and Human Services
25. Tims FM, Ludford JP (eds) (1984) NIDA Research Monograph 51: RAUS: Drug Abuse Treatment Evaluation: Strategies, Progress, and Prospects. (ADM) 84–1329. Rockville: US Department of Health and Human Services
26. Hubbard RL, Marsden ME, Rachal JV, et al (1989) Drug Abuse Treatment: A National Study of Effectiveness. Chapel Hill: University of North Carolina Press
27. Simpson DD, Sells SB (eds) (1990) Opioid Addiction and Treatment: a 12-year follow-up. Malabar: Robert E. Krieger Publishing Company
28. Jaffe JH (1979) The swinging pendulum: the treatment of drug users in America. In Dupont RI, Goldstein A, O'Donnell J (eds): Handbook on Drug Abuse. Washington, DC: US Government Printing Office, pp 3–16
29. Cooper JR (1989) Methadone treatment and acquired immunodeficiency syndrome. JAMA 262:1664–1668
30. Pickens RW, Fletcher BW (1991) Overview of treatment issues. In: Improving Drug Abuse Treatment: NIDA Monograph. In press
31. Lipton DS, Appel P (1984) The state perspective. In Tims FM, Ludford JP (eds): NIDA Research Monograph Series 51: RAUS: Drug Abuse Treatment Evaluation: Strategies, Progress, and Prospects. (ADM) 84–1329. Rockville: US Department of Health and Human Services, pp 151–166
32. Hall SM (1983) Methadone treatment: a review of the research findings. In Cooper JR, Altman F, Brown B, Czechowicz D (eds): NIDA Treatment Research Monograph Series: Research on the Treatment of Narcotic Addiction: State of the Art. (ADM) 83–1281. Rockville: US Department of Health and Human Services, pp 575–632
33. Gottheil E, McLellan AT, Druley KA (eds) (1981) Reasonable and unreasonable methodological standards for the evaluation of alcoholism treatment. In: Matching Patient Needs and Treatment Methods in Alcoholism and Drug

Abuse. Springfield: Charles C Thomas, pp 371–389
34. Altman F, Schnoll SH (1983) Discussion summary. In Cooper JR, Altman F, Brown B, Czechowicz D (eds): NIDA Treatment Research Monograph Series: Research on the Treatment of Narcotic Addiction: State of the Art. (ADM) 83–1281. Rockville: US Department of Health and Human Services, pp 573–574
35. Hubbard RL, Rachal JV, Craddock SG, Cavanaugh ER (1984) Treatment outcome prospective study (TOPS): client characteristics and behaviors before, during, and after treatment. In: Tims FM, Ludford JP (eds): NIDA Research Monograph Series 51: RAUS Drug Abuse Treatment Evaluation: Strategies, Progress, and Prospects. (ADM) 84-1329. Rockville: US Department of Health and Human Services, pp 42–68
36. Meyer R (1983) Introduction to part III: factors affecting the outcome of methadone treatment. In Cooper JR, Altman F, Brown B, Czechowicz D (eds): NIDA Treatment Research Monograph Series: Research on the Treatment of Narcotic Addiction: State of the Art. (ADM) 83–1281. Rockville: US Department of Health and Human Services, pp 495–499
37. Woody GE (1983) Treatment characteristics associated with outcome. In Cooper JR, Altman F, Brown B, Czechowicz D (eds): NIDA Treatment Research Monograph Series: Research on the Treatment of Narcotic Addiction: State of the Art. (ADM) 83–1281. Rockville: US Department of Health and Human Services, pp 541–564
38. Tonry M (1990) Research on drugs and crime. In Tonry M, Wilson JQ (eds): Drugs and Crime, Vol. 13. Chicago: University of Chicago Press, pp 1–8
39. Moos RH, Finney JW (1987–1988) Alcoholism program evaluation: the treatment domain. Drugs Society 2:31–51
40. Terry CE, Pellens M (1970) The Opium Problem. Montclair, NJ: Patterson Smith
41. Pescor MJ (1943) A statistical analysis of the clinical records of hospitalized drug addicts. Public Health Rep Suppl 143. Washington, DC: US Government Printing Office, pp 1–30
42. Second Triennial Report to Congress from the Secretary (1987) Drug Abuse and Drug Abuse Research. DHHS (ADM) 87–1486. Rockville: US Department of Health and Human Services, pp. 59–75
43. Moos RH, Finney JW, Cronkite RC (eds) (1990) Alcoholism Treatment: Context, Process, and Outcome. New York: Oxford University Press
44. McLellan AT, Alterman AI, Woody GE (1991) A quantitative measure of substance abuse treatment programs: the treatment services review. J Nerv Ment Dis (in press)
45. Anglin MD, Hser YI (1990) Treatment of drug abuse. In Tonry M, Wilson JQ (eds): Drugs and Crime, pp 393–460

2 Research Plan and Data Collection Procedure at the Programs

The idea of a large-scale study to investigate the effectiveness of methadone maintenance treatment developed from a series of research review conferences sponsored by the National Institute on Drug Abuse (NIDA) during the mid-1980s. In these Research Analysis and Utilization System (RAUS) reviews,[1] the question arose as to "what extent should we invest in large-scale studies of process and effectiveness vs. smaller, program-based research?" Although a consensus was not reached by the assembled researchers as to how to answer this question, the need for multiprogram studies of treatment effectiveness was discussed. Therefore these RAUS discussions laid the groundwork for potential support of this study.

In 1984 the senior author and several colleagues were invited to the National Institute on Drug Abuse to discuss the feasibility of a large-scale study of methadone maintenance treatment. A principal concern of the NIDA staff was how to obtain the full-time commitment of a senior researcher to organize and direct such a project over a 5-year period. At this first meeting, the senior author soon became involved in delineating a suitable study and, somewhat unexpectedly, found himself "selected" to carry it forward.

At the beginning, then, there was an initial impetus and encouragement from staff at NIDA to undertake the study. This institutional support and encouragement waxed and waned over the ensuing years as bureaucratic priorities, funding levels, and staff organization changed; nonetheless, NIDA did provide continuous support throughout the years, which enabled the study to be completed.

Objective of the Study

The overall objective of the study was to investigate the effectiveness of methadone maintenance treatment in the United States. For reasons of practicality, it was decided to restrict the on-site data collection to three cities in three states on the East Coast. More specifically with regard to effectiveness, the study was to ascertain: (1) Does methadone maintenance as a general modality work? (2) If so, is this modality primarily effective for particular types of patients? (3) If so, are certain aspects of methadone treatment responsible for its effectiveness? In retrospect, this formulation overlooked the prospect that there might be different types of methadone programs (e.g., medical or rehabilitative in orientation, and that programs themselves might be a significant factor).

Development of the Research Design

The research design was developed primarily on the basis of prior field experiences of the senior author and the staff at the Institute for Survey Research at Temple University. With regard to the experience of the senior author, previous epidemiological research[2] and particularly completion of a statewide evaluation of 77 drug abuse programs in Pennsylvania were relevant to planning the present project.[3,4] With regard to the Institute for Survey Research (ISR), the experience of the director and staff in conducting local, state, and national surveys of drug abusers was relevant and invaluable. In this regard, Dr. Leonard LoSciuto, the Director of ISR, was a major participant in the design and execution of the project. Other colleagues who made significant contributions in the planning were Drs. David Nurco, A. Thomas McLellan and Zili Amsel. George Beschner, of NIDA, was a major source of support when planning and initiating the project.

In the original protocol, 12 methadone maintenance programs were to be selected for study in five states, and 2400 newly admitted addict patients were to be followed during a 3-year period. For budgetary reasons, the scope of the project was reduced from 5 years to 3 years. As a consequence, the number of programs that could be comprehensively evaluated was reduced to six; and consequently, the number of patients who could be interviewed and followed was reduced. How this revised selection of patients was accomplished is discussed below. It is pertinent to note here that, in retrospect, the required reduction in the scope of data collection was probably fortuitous inasmuch as lengthening the years of data collection would have jeopardized the completion of the project, which at this writing has already taken 7 years.

Data Collection Paradigm—Four Areas

The data collection plan as well as the entire research effort was predicated on the assumption that meaningful evaluation of drug abuse treatment programs required that comprehensive data be obtained from four areas: (1) patient characteristics (especially baseline patient characteristics prior to admission); (2) the entire range of treatment domain elements (neighborhood, facility, aggregate patient census, treatment, facility, policy, and staff); (3) treatment and rehabilitation services provided ("output" from each program); and (4) patient outcome.

Selection of Six Methadone Maintenance Programs in Three Cities

It was decided to focus the data collection on three cities on the East Coast because this area has the greatest concentration of heroin addicts in the United States.[5,6] Indeed, the New York City, Philadelphia, and Baltimore metropolitan areas contain almost one-half of the methadone maintenance patients in the United States. It was held, then, that a study of program effectiveness in these three cities would provide an overview of the situation on the East Coast. Consequently, two programs were selected in each of the three cities.

The protocol for selecting methadone maintenance programs was elaborate. It involved the following procedure: (1) obtaining a listing of all methadone programs in the relevant cities; (2) retaining in the sampling frame programs of sufficient size, stability, and treatment resources to meet the requirements of the study (thus programs had to have a patient census of 200 or more, be in operation 3 years or more, and have an average staff/patient ratio); (3) selecting a best and average program from each city based on staff/patient ratios and the availability of services as enumerated in a federal listing of program characteristics.

The rationale for excluding markedly deficient programs was twofold. First, such programs would be more likely to cease operation or be unable to provide the cooperation necessary for a comprehensive evaluation. Second, the objective of the study was to ascertain which programs were effective so improvements in methadone maintenance could be implemented; finding that grossly inadequate programs were not effective would not contribute to this end. It was estimated that some 20 to 30 percent of the programs were markedly inadequate by our selection criteria as of 1985 (J.C. Ball, personal assessment).

This plan of program selection was followed, with modifications. Some substitution of programs was necessary before the data collection began; these aspects of the study are discussed later. In retrospect, too much time and effort was spent on the original "theoretical" program selection procedure. In fact, the available listing of programs was out of date, and the concomitant listing of program characteristics (e.g., treatment services available) was grossly inaccurate, as many, if not most, treatment services listed as available were not available.

On-site Program Data Collection by the Evaluation of Methadone Maintenance Treatment Staff

A unique feature of the overall evaluation plan was that comprehensive treatment domain data would be collected about each of the programs; the data included a detailed enumeration of all treatment and rehabilitative services provided to the entire patient census at each program, or the total output of services for each program. Furthermore, these data would be collected on-site by the "evaluation of methadone maintenance treatment" (EMMT) staff. Thus two major decisions set the stage for the program data collection: The first was that detailed program and delivery of services data (i.e., treatment domain and output data) would be collected at each program. The second decision was that this data collection would be undertaken by the project staff.

A comprehensive package of data collection schedules was devised for obtaining treatment domain and output of services findings at the programs. The broad content areas to be covered by these data collection schedules included the following.

1. Neighborhood and physical facility of each program
2. Hours of operation, attendance, patient flow, and security arrangements
3. Treatment policy and administration
4. Composition, qualifications, and experience of entire staff
5. Fiscal condition: sources of income and annual expenditure
6. Types of counseling services provided
7. Methadone dispensing staff, procedure, and output
8. Medical services provided
9. Urinalysis procedure, output, and utilization
10. Patient and program records
11. Present condition and needs of program

These areas of data collection included the entire treatment domain. Particular attention was directed toward determining the treatment and rehabilitative services provided to patients. Within each area, detailed forms were devised and arranged to facilitate on-site data collection by the EMMT staff. Thus designated forms were prepared according to the data collection procedures to be employed. These procedures included confidential face-to-face staff interviews; additional follow-up questionnaires for counselors; systematic observation and measurement of physical facility, security, patient flow, and clinic operations; compilation of required data from patient and program records; compilation of pharmacy data and urinalysis results, review of treatment policy statements; and compilation of program operation data.

These treatment domain and output of services data were collected on-site by a four-person EMMT team, which consisted of the principal investigator, a clinical psychologist, a pharmacist, and a supervisory drug abuse counselor. All four staff members had considerable prior research or clinical experience in drug abuse treatment. The collected data were deemed confidential, and the results were not made available to either the treatment or the administrative staff of the respective programs.

The first on-site collection of treatment domain and output domain data in New York City, Philadelphia, and Baltimore was undertaken during a 4-month period in 1985. This first comprehensive evaluation of the six programs (E-1) was repeated a year later in 1986. This second program evaluation (E-2) utilized the same on-site data collection procedure, instruments, and EMMT staff.

The rationale for the second on-site program evaluation was both methodological and substantive. With regard to method, it was necessary to establish both the continued feasibility of the field procedures and the reliability of the instruments used. With regard to substantive findings, the second measurement of the treatment domain provided a means of determining the stability or change of each of the treatment domain factors.

Selection of Patient Samples

There were two major foci of data collection planned for the EMMT project. One was to collect comprehensive data about the six methadone maintenance programs—the treatment domain. The other was to obtain detailed information about a sample of patients at each of the programs. The two sources of data were complementary. Thus it was necessary to collect data about the content and dynamics of treatment if the effectiveness of treatment was to be ascertained. Second, it was necessary to collect data about patients if one was to measure the effect of treatment. The two foci of the study are depicted in Figure 2.1

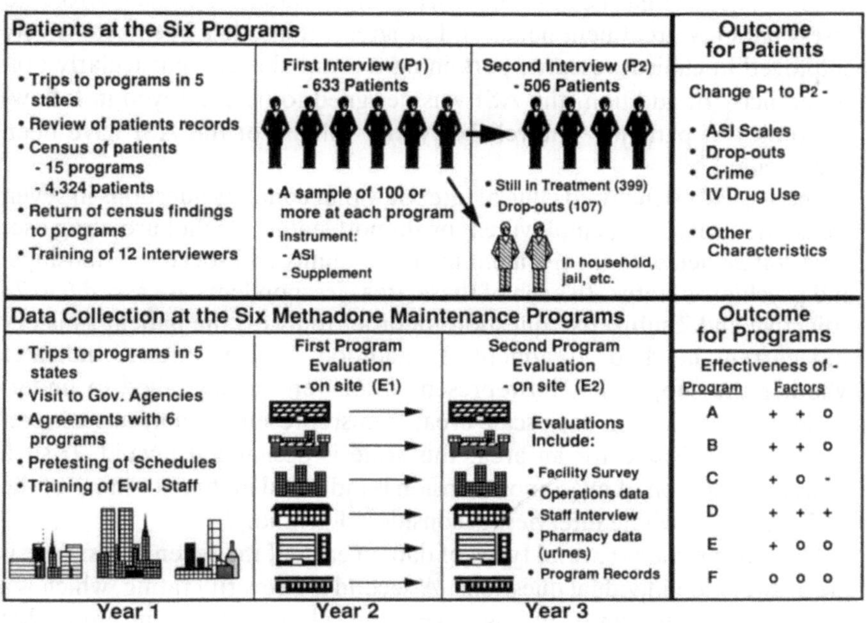

FIGURE 2.1. Design of data collection for 3 years.

With respect to collecting data about patients, the overall plan was to select some 100 patients for study at each of the six programs in 1985 and then to track these samples during the following year to determine if they had improved while in treatment. Those who left treatment would be followed up in the community. Two face-to-face interviews with the patients were planned: The first would take place at the programs during late 1985; the second would be at the same programs a year later or in the local community. In addition to the two interviews, detailed information about treatment provided to these patients was obtained from clinic records.

Patient Interview Schedule

The schedule used in the face-to-face interviews of 633 patients at the six programs consisted of 40 pages of questions. The two main parts of the schedule consisted of the Addiction Severity Index (Part I) and questions pertaining to each patient's prior treatment experiences, recent criminality, and services received while in his present methadone maintenance program (Part II). In addition to this schedule, follow-up locator information was obtained, an informed consent form completed, and a payment voucher signed in conjunction with each patient interview.

The Instrument: Part I (Addiction Severity Index)

The first part of the interview consisted of the Addiction Severity Index (ASI).[7] The ASI has been widely used in the United States and abroad to assess patients' treatment needs and progress. It also has been extensively employed in clinical research pertaining to drug abusers, particularly opiate addicts. In addition, the ASI was designed to be employed in follow-up studies of patients. The reliability and validity of the ASI have been documented.[8,9]

The ASI is a structured clinical interview that contains questions in seven areas: medical status, employment or support status, alcohol use, drug use, legal status including involvement in crime, family and social relationships, and psychiatric status. In each of these areas, respondents are asked 6 to 25 objective and 2 subjective questions in order to assess the patient's history and current need for treatment. In addition, the interviewer indicates whether the subject has misrepresented answers or has failed to understand the questions in each scale area. If misrepresentation or miscomprehension is indicated for an area, this scale is designated invalid. If such misrepresentation of miscomprehension is indicated in three or more of the ASI areas, the whole interview is considered invalid.[10,11]

The ASI provides several types of data in each of the seven areas. One is the answers to individual questions. A second is a severity rating, which is a rating by the interviewer of how severe the subject's problems are in that area and how effective treatment might be. (Severity scores range from 0 to

9, with a higher score indicating a more severe problem.) Third, composite scale scores are an important aspect of the ASI. In each of the seven areas an algorithm has been derived by which key objective items are weighted and combined to yield a score that is not influenced by interviewer ratings. Composite scores range from 0.0 to 1.0, with higher scores indicating that patients have more severe problems in this area.[12]

THE INSTRUMENT: PART II

Part II of the interview schedule consisted of 13 pages of questions to be asked each patient about his drug abuse treatment history, prior criminality, and services received in his current methadone maintenance program. In addition to detailed questions about these three areas, a few items to supplement specific ASI scale areas were included: such questions as age at onset of regular opiate use, and days of opiate use during the 30 days prior to admission.

The section of the interview schedule that asked each patient about his previous treatment experiences included questions on the number and type of previous drug abuse treatments, reason for leaving his last program, and his overall assessment of the effectiveness of methadone maintenance treatment.

The section on criminal behavior included a series of questions about the frequency of 14 types of offenses during each patient's last addiction period (i.e., when the respondent was "on the street" and addicted to opiates). This part was followed by a similar series of questions about criminality during the previous summer. The rationale and procedure for obtaining data pertaining to patients' last addiction period have been discussed elsewhere.[13] Obtaining data about criminality during the past summer was planned to compile information on a discrete and uniform time period. With regard to both time periods, questions were asked about the number of days per month that addicts engaged in each type of crime. The methodology of the crime-days approach has also been described elsewhere.[14,15]

A separate section of the interview schedule referred to the amount and the types of treatment and rehabilitative services received by each patient while in his current program. Questions were asked about the frequency with which each of the following services were provided: individual counseling; group counseling; physical examinations; medical care by a nurse, physician, or physician assistant; referrals for outside medical services; Narcotics Anonymous or Alcoholics Anonymous membership; family or couples therapy; psychotherapy; vocational assessment or referral; educational assessment or referral; General Equivalency Diploma or other classes; welfare assistance; legal assistance; home visits by staff; dental care; recreational activity; and any other services received. In addition to questions about the extent of treatment received during the past 30 days (or since admission), patients were asked to recount or assess various aspects of these services, e.g., the duration of counseling sessions and satisfaction with the methadone dose.

Patient Outcome Measures

The principal outcome measures employed in subsequent analyses refer to patients' drug abuse and criminal behavior at the time of their second interview. These measures were derived from prior research experience and review of the relevant scientific literature.[16,17] A series of these measures are discussed and analyzed in subsequent chapters. For example, patients' reduction in intravenous injections of drugs following admission to methadone maintenance treatment are analyzed by comparing monthly prevalence data for different time periods. The five outcome measures employed in the multivariate analysis of Chapter 11 are (1) heroin use during the past 30 days, (2) cocaine use during the past 30 days, (3) any serious drug abuse during the past 30 days, (4) intravenous drug use in the past 30 days, and (5) involvement in crime during the past 30 days. In addition to specific measures of drug use and crime, patients' outcomes with respect to the ASI and other criteria were ascertained.

Program Effectiveness

Although outcome measures of patient success during or after drug abuse treatment have been established for some time, the same is not true with regard to program success or effectiveness. Although program-based ratings for methadone maintenance programs were recommended by Dole in 1982, these studies were not carried out. Given these and other considerations, it became necessary to develop new ways of conceptualizing and measuring program effectiveness.

Until recently it was thought that program success could best be determined by measuring patient outcome in particular programs while controlling for preadmission patient variables. This approach has proved, however, to be a necessary but not sufficient means for determining program effectiveness, as such a plan of data collection and analysis omits consideration of the entire treatment and service delivery domains. Indeed, such a plan only perpetuates the black box of treatment because it does not provide any information about what it is about treatment that is effective or ineffective. Unraveling this question of what produces effectiveness in drug abuse treatment requires measurement and analysis of both treatment domain factors and treatment and rehabilitation delivery factors.

Therefore the outcome criteria of program success that were devised consisted of three types of measure: (1) aggregate patient data that demonstrate improvement, e.g., reduction in intravenous drug use and crime as a consequence of treatment at particular programs; (2) treatment domain factors that have a rational or empirical association with patient success rates, e.g., treatment policy, experienced director, and annual staff turnover rates; and (3) treatment and rehabilitation services actually provided. These factors include patient attendance rates (which is one measure of the total services received), the dosage of methadone prescribed, and the frequency of counseling services provided.

Data Collection at the Programs

Site Review of Prospective Programs in Five States

During the first year of the project, numerous site visits were made to methadone programs in five states that had agreed to participate in the study. These first site visits were exploratory in that we discussed our project with the program directors and other relevant staff to ascertain their interest in this cooperative project. As we became better acquainted with each program staff, we found it efficacious to observe the operation of the clinic, note the physical facility, its relationship with the neighborhood, the number of admissions per month, treatment policies, dispensing procedures, the location and content of patients' records, and other pertinent matters such as accessibility to public transportation and the availability of parking space.

This early establishment of rapport and the concomitant appraisal of each program's overall treatment operation and facility was found to be indispensable: Clearly it was unlikely that the directors and staff at methadone maintenance clinics would become active participants in our 3-year data collection effort unless an agreeable and enduring working relationship was established.

Although site visits to the methadone maintenance programs have been emphasized, it should be noted that other means of developing or maintaining rapport with the programs were also employed. Frequent phone calls, letters, exchange of reports, and similar communications with each of the programs were common. It should not be inferred, however, that this communication was perfunctory; it was, in fact, purposeful and serious. We were amassing relevant program information and providing the participating institutions with relevant information about our data collection plans.

Exchange of Patient Census Data With 15 Programs

During the first few months of the project it was decided that it would be efficacious to obtain a current patient census from each of the programs. This census data would enable us to analyze aggregate demographic and length of stay characteristics of the addict patients at each program.

Second, each program's compilation of these data and our subsequent feedback of these findings would establish a working data-exchange relationship.

Fifteen methadone maintenance programs provided us with their census data; these programs included those selected for intensive evaluation as well as others that requested inclusion in this phase of the project. In return, relevant graphics were rapidly returned to each of the programs, and later a comparative analysis of findings from the 15 programs was provided. A few programs were unable to provide the required data sets.

The census data collection procedure facilitated the future success of both the overall program and patient data collection efforts that followed as it established a working data-exchange network between each of the programs and the EMMT project. In addition, this large-scale data collection effort demonstrated that current demographic data pertaining to 4324 patients could be obtained once an ongoing data exchange network was established.

Coordination With Local Drug Abuse Agencies

During the first year of the project, contacts and visits were made to drug abuse agencies that supervised methadone maintenance treatment programs in the five states. At these meetings the EMMT staff explained the overall design of our project, discussed issues of confidentiality, sought their advice and support, and otherwise exchanged information and opinions about the current status of methadone maintenance treatment. In addition, we attended regional and local methadone conferences to broaden our knowledge of the different state and local government policies pertaining to methadone maintenance treatment.

Final Selection of Six Programs and Two Patient Cohorts

Sometime after the middle of year 1, we were informed that the budget for year 2 would be significantly reduced. Therefore it was decided to reduce the geographic scope of the study to six methadone programs in three states: two in each of three cities. This course of action seemed preferable to a reduction in the scope and depth of data collection planned at each program. Consequently, the comprehensive plan of both program and patient data collection remained intact, but at fewer sites.

A further change in the research design necessitated by the funding reduction pertained to the patient samples. The original protocol specified that a sample of 100 consecutive admissions would be interviewed on-site at each program by ISR staff during a 6-month period. This plan of selecting admission cohorts could no longer be employed because of both funding and time constraints. Therefore a briefer period for interviewing was scheduled, and the patient samples were redefined to include both in-treatment and admission cohorts at each of the six programs. The six programs in New York, Philadelphia, and Baltimore that would continue to be included in the study were notified accordingly. A seventh program was involved as a test and demonstration site.

Cooperative Agreement With the Programs

During the first year of the project, the principal investigator and other EMMT staff met with key staff at each of the six programs numerous times. On these occasions we discussed our overall data collection procedures with each program's director and then proceeded to plan how these procedures could be implemented at each site. This latter planning was crucial to obtain space for interviewing patients and staff as well as to coordinate research needs with each program's daily schedule of operation.

In these preliminary discussions with key staff at each of the programs we came to a general agreement as to how the data collection and other relevant aspects of the project would be carried forward. Five principal points of agreement or understanding were established. The first was that the objective of our comprehensive study of programs and patients was to ascertain "what works" (or does not work) in methadone maintenance treatment and that the National Institute on Drug Abuse was supporting this research because of its interest in improving drug abuse treatment.

Second, because as university-based researchers we would objectively report and publish our findings, the discussion of dissemination of findings led to the issue of confidentiality. It was agreed that the patient interview data, the staff interview data, and each program's treatment domain and outcome data would be kept confidential. The last of these considerations was of pervasive importance for it was recognized that detailed treatment domain, data, and especially output data, could not be linked to specific programs without potentially disastrous consequences.

A third point of agreement with the programs (which was implicit throughout our approach) was that this project would be a cooperative undertaking between the director and staff of each program and the EMMT staff. In this regard, we (the EMMT staff) would exchange data with the programs, seek their advice, provide them with advice if requested, and otherwise treat them as equal partners in an important research effort to ascertain "what works" in methadone maintenance treatment.

A fourth point of agreement or understanding was that the task of program and patient data collection would be undertaken by the EMMT staff and the field staff of ISR. This point of agreement was crucial to the data collection procedure because the programs lacked the personnel, time, and resources to undertake comprehensive data collection.

Lastly, it was agreed that the principal investigator and EMMT staff would be directly involved and responsible for the entire program and patient data collection effort from beginning to end. This agreement meant that the EMMT staff were always "on call" and had to be available when problems arose about any aspect of data collection. In fact, this agreement was repeatedly implemented by means of on-site queries, later requests for assistance, emergency calls from interviewers, and similar matters.

Collecting Treatment Domain and Output Data in 1985

Program Data Collection Procedure

The first designated measurement of treatment domain and output data collection at the seven methadone maintenance programs (evaluation 1, or E-1) was undertaken during a 2-month period in the fall of 1985. A week was allocated for on-site data collection at each program, but only 2 days were spent on-site by the full four-person data collection team. The remainder of the week was spent in travel preparation, coordination, and, after the site visit, compiling and organizing the voluminous data obtained. There also were call-backs and a few follow-up visits to the programs by EMMT staff members for interviews or other data collection.

The core of the program data collection effort revolved around two designated days during which the full four-person EMMT team were on-site at each program. These two designated days spent at each site involved completion of two different but related tasks. Day 1 was an orientation and planning day. Day 2 was designated the output data collection day.

Day 1 was commonly scheduled for Monday at each program. By prearrangement, the entire treatment staff of the program was assembled to meet with the EMMT team on this day. At this meeting, prior relationships were renewed, the progress of the overall project discussed, the confidentiality agreements reviewed, and plans made for data collection during day 2. Ordinarily, day 2 followed on Wednesday in order to have a day in between for final scheduling and coordination with respect to staff interviewing and other matters.

On day 2 the four-person EMMT team began data collection when the program opened for dispensing in the morning. The principal data collection tasks were (1) face-to-face confidential interviews with the entire treatment staff (including the director); (2) a detailed survey of every room and part of the facility; (3) individual pharmacy output data for the entire patient census; (4) urinalysis procedures and results for the program; (5) observation and description of patient flow and security in the clinic; (6) gathering of administrative information and data on other aspects of program operation from program records.

After the first day 2 data collection effort was completed at the demonstration program, it was found that we had collected over 90 percent of the required data. No one refused to be interviewed; all of the supplementary questionnaires were returned by the counselors; the complete pharmacy data sets were obtained; and, in general, the required data were collected. In a few instances, however, it was necessary to obtain missing information later by telephone or additional visits. In the latter regard, those absent on day 2 were interviewed at a later date.

After the feasibility of the day 2 data collection plans had been demonstrated at this first preliminary site, the same data collection procedures were followed at the remaining six programs in New York City, Philadelphia, and Baltimore, during subsequent weeks. In general, the research team became more proficient as we became more experienced. The main differentiating factor in data collection at the various programs was difficulty of travel to some sites, different staff size, and the extent of turnover of administrative and treatment staff.

Observations After the First Program Data Collection Effort

As we returned from the last of our 1985 treatment domain data collection efforts at the end of October, it was time to consider what had been learned during the past months of field work. Three general observations provide an overview of our conclusions: (1) the original plan for program data collection had been feasible as we had obtained the comprehensive program data sought; (2) our data collection practices had improved, and our team approach was efficacious, and (3) there were such notable differences in the programs, patients, and neighborhoods that it was questionable if not erroneous to regard methadone maintenance treatment as a uniform modality of treatment. Each of these conclusions is discussed next.

After the completion of the seven on-site program data collection efforts in 1985, we were satisfied that we had been able to collect the program data in the three cities as scheduled: The entire treatment staffs had been interviewed; supplementary questionnaires had been completed by counselors; the full array of methadone dispensing data for 1874 patients was obtained; urinalysis results for the entire patient population were compiled; each physical facility was surveyed; and other observational and record information had been amassed. A sense of relief came with the realization that this important yet problematic part of our project was over.

Furthermore, it was evident that we had the full cooperation of the respective program staffs and that access to record data and other sources of information was not a problem. Thus no staff member refused to be interviewed, the entire dispensing records of each program were made available, all requested records and facilities were open to us and, in general, we were given full support and cooperation throughout the clinics. There could be no doubt, then, that we had access to whatever data were available.

It was concluded that the original plan for program data collection had been sound, although modifications became necessary. These modifications included greater reliance on face-to-face interviews and first-hand observation, rather than official records and reports. In this regard, it was crucial to determine quickly on-site which of the requested data sets were readily available and which were not readily available or not available at all.

Second, in the process of obtaining these comprehensive findings about staff characteristics, treatment services, and program operations, we learned to cope with the realities and vagaries of data collection in the midst of day-to-day drug abuse treatment operations. Our practices improved because we learned to anticipate and cope with numerous problems of data collection at the programs: how to obtain an up-to-date accurate list of the treatment staff, what to do about absentees, how to best arrange confidential interviews with the staff, how to find space, when to ask for certain data sets, who is likely to be most helpful (or most difficult)—in sum, what works and what does not work in program data collection.

In this regard, the advantages of our on-site team approach became more and more evident as our field work progressed. These advantages included the following.

1. The presence of four persons—our team—emphasized to the program staff the significance of our data collection effort.
2. That the four-person team included specialists in various disciplines (pharmacist, clinical psychologist, drug abuse counselor, and sociologist-criminologist) greatly facilitated our data collection.
3. We provided direction, advice, and encouragement for each other. The team approach enabled us to assist one another with scheduling, photocopying, tabulations, and getting supplies and messages to one another.
4. The presence of our four-person team furthered contact between relevant staff and specific persons of our team, thereby facilitating interviewing. Thus the busy program staff were often looking for the specific EMMT staff member who would interview them as soon as both had free time. One or another of our team could often direct the program staff member to the appropriate location.
5. The team approach made it possible to complete the data collection during a single day. This accomplishment was important, as it tended to facilitate future positive relationships between the EMMT and program staffs.

At the conclusion of the program data collection in 1985 there was a realization that our extensive travel to the slums and other neighborhoods of these three cities to study the operation of the clinics had markedly changed our knowledge and perception of methadone maintenance treatment. We could no longer think of methadone maintenance as a uniform abstraction. Instead, it became a treatment modality that varied by state, city, and neighborhood. Both programs and patients differed, although the extent of these differences, or similarities, would be more accurately determined by subsequent analysis. We observed differences in the neighborhoods, directors, medical staff, counselors, hospital affiliation, physical facilities, services provided, and characteristics of the patients treated.

Patient Interviews in 1985 and 1986

Collection of Data in 1985

A major part of the EMMT Project was to interview patients in treatment at the six methadone maintenance programs. These face-to-face interviews were undertaken to assess patients' status in methadone maintenance treatment and to provide baseline data on patients' preadmission and life history characteristics. Prior to conducting the interviews at the programs, it was necessary to prepare an appropriate schedule for the face-to-face interviews, train special interviewers, select the patients, and otherwise plan and supervise various aspects of the patient data collection at the programs. These tasks are reviewed next (except the content of the interview schedule, which has already been described).

The patients selected for study at each of the six programs consisted of two cohorts. The first cohort was composed of 126 consecutive patients who were admitted to the programs during a 2-month period when the designated interviewers from ISR were on-site during late 1985. The second cohort consisted of 507 in-treatment patients who had already been at these programs for 6 months or longer at the time of their selection during late 1985. The original sample of 633 patients selected for study in 1985, then, consisted of 126 new admissions and 507 in-treatment patients. Each of the six programs was represented by approximately 100 of these patients.

The criteria for patient selection were minimal, except that females were not included. The reason for restricting the study to male patients was primarily budgetary; it was estimated that including both sexes in the study would require twice the available funding. The decision to limit sample selection to English-speaking patients was also budgetary. (It is relevant to note, however, that foreign-language versions of the ASI are extant.)

All male new admissions who qualified and agreed to participate were included in the study (the refusal rate for the 1985 or T_1 interviews was 6.9 percent). The admission cohort, then, was representative of male patients (with the qualification noted) admitted to these programs during late 1985.

The in-treatment sample of 507 males were selected by the EMMT staff from randomly generated lists of each program's patients who had been admitted on or before May 1,1985. Thus, in general, the in-treatment patients were a representative sample of each program's male census.

Interviewers from the Institute for Survey Research

Plans for conducting the patient interviews in both 1985 and 1986 were developed in cooperation with the ISR. Indeed, the staff of ISR not only conducted more than 1100 field interviews of the addict patients selected for study, but the senior staff had been involved in the preparation of the original research protocol.

Twelve interviewers from the field staff of ISR were assigned to conduct the patient interviews at the six programs. These 12 were specifically selected and trained for this task. Four of the interviewers were black and eight were white; there were four male and eight female interviewers. They were experienced interviewers (with a mean 9.5 years of experience), and two-thirds of them had prior experience interviewing drug abusers.

To ensure that proper procedures were followed when conducting the interview, a special 3-day training course was scheduled for the 12 interviewers in Philadelphia. The training session was conducted by the senior field staff of ISR in conjunction with two consultants (Drs. A.T. McLellan and John Cacciola) who had extensive experience in the use of the ASI. Also present during the training were the principal investigator and EMMT project coordinator.

Training of the 12 interviewers consisted of didactic as well as role-playing sessions. Among the topics covered were procedures for obtaining informed consent and location information for follow-up interviews, the purpose and use of the ASI, and procedures to follow with Part II questions of the schedule. This training was intensive. Thus every item to be asked in the interview was explained, and questions about procedure or interpretation were addressed by the instructor. This instruction was followed by supervised practice sessions in which interviewer scoring and other procedures were checked and, if necessary, corrected. After completion of the training session, the 12 interviewers returned to their respective cities and shortly thereafter began interviewing patients at the six programs. Two interviewers were assigned to each program.

Face-to-Face Interview Procedure (at T_1)

Patients who had been selected for study were referred by program staff to the ISR interviewers at each of the programs. The purpose of the study was explained and the confidentiality of the data emphasized; if pertinent, it was mentioned that a Certificate of Confidentiality had been obtained from NIDA that denied access by criminal justice or other officials to the data collected by the project. The interviewer asked the patient if he wanted to participate in this study. If the patient agreed to participate, he signed an informed consent statement and the interview began.

The confidential interview was usually conducted in a private office and lasted about 45 minutes. In this face-to-face situation, the interviewer asked each relevant question of the schedule and recorded each response. At the completion of the interview, the patient was paid for his participation ($10 or $15 depending on the program), and the completed schedule was sealed in an envelope and mailed to ISR.

Second Interviews of Patients (1986)

The second interview of the patient samples at each program was undertaken during late 1986, a year after the first interview. By this time, about one-third of the patients had dropped out of treatment. Approximately one-half (48 percent) of these dropouts were interviewed at their homes, in jail, "on the street," or at other locations. The 506 second interviews, then, consisted of two cohorts: the still-in-treatment cohort of 399 patients and the dropout cohort of 107 patients.

The same interview procedure and the same ISR interviewers (11 of the 12 interviewers) were employed in 1986 as in 1985. As previously, face-to-face confidential interviews were conducted with the patients in treatment. Because these were "repeat" interviews with, in most cases, the identical interviewer who first contacted the patient, rapport was easily established and the refusal rate was low (fewer than 2 percent of the patients and ex-patients refused the second interview). Still, continued cooperation of the clinic staff was necessary to arrange and facilitate these interviews.

The second interview with the former patients who had dropped out of methadone maintenance treatment was more difficult and time-consuming.[18] As indicated, it was decided to locate and interview approximately one-half of these patients, as funding restrictions precluded locating and interviewing the entire dropout sample. The sample selected and interviewed was partly designated and partly made up of those who could more readily be found. A comparison of the 107 dropouts who were reinterviewed with those dropouts who were not reinterviewed revealed that the two groups did not differ significantly with regard to demographic or addiction characteristics.

The standard follow-up version of the ASI was employed during the 1986 patient interviews, along with relevant Part II questions. This latter part of the interview contained questions about services received since the first interview, recent criminality, and employment status. A separate version of the Part II items was prepared for those who were interviewed in the community. An important addition to the 1986 schedule was a series of questions pertaining to each patient's current (or last) frequency of intravenous drug use and concomitant needle-sharing behavior.

Treatment Domain Data Collection in 1986

Second Program Data Collection, 1986 (E-2)

The overall program data collection plan that had been developed and implemented in 1985 was following for the 1986 effort. Fundamentally, the same data sets were obtained from the same six methadone maintenance programs. The same four-person EMMT team collected the data at the sites, and the same procedures were followed. A few further comments about methodology and experiences during the 1986 procedures are relevant.

The rationale for a repeat measurement of the treatment domain involved, as noted previously, two considerations. First, repeat measurement of treatment domain factors would ascertain how stable these factors were from year to year and permit determination of change. Thus repeat measurement of the treatment services provided by the methadone maintenance programs addressed the issue of consistency of treatment provided at each program: If there were marked changes in the treatment services provided, one could hardly relate patient improvement to the consistent delivery of specific treatment services. Consequently, it was necessary to ascertain which treatment services were consistently delivered before one could determine their effectiveness.

The second reason for undertaking repeat measurement of treatment services and related program characteristics was methodological. Repeat measurements were necessary to establish the reliability of the instruments and procedures employed.

Revision of Data Collection Instruments

The same data collection instruments utilized for the 1985 program data collection effort were employed for the 1986 effort; the same programs were also involved both years. There were, however, relevant revisions made in the data collection instruments based on the first field experience and subsequent knowledge of the results obtained. Most of these changes were minor revisions rather than major changes, as we were committed to replication rather than new directions in data collection.

With regard to field work, it was decided to adhere to the prior schedule of two on-site days at each program during a designated week. As before, the first day would focus on staff orientation and the second on staff interviews and other program data collection tasks.

In this regard, it was found that a repeat of an orientation day of a year ago was necessary as it facilitated the data collection that took place later in the week (usually 2 days later). Thus during orientation day we reviewed the current progress of our project with the treatment staff at each program and distributed our first research findings to them. In addition, we reiterated that the forthcoming staff interviews would be kept confidential, renewed prior relationships, compiled an up-to-date list of staff, and then made arrangements for scheduling interviews and other data collection efforts when we returned later in the week.

SECOND FACE-TO-FACE INTERVIEW WITH THE TREATMENT STAFF

As in 1985, each member of the treatment staff at each program was interviewed by one of the EMMT team. These face-to-face interviews were confidential, and informed consent was obtained from each person before the interview began. Usually this written consent was almost perfunctory, as it was the "second time around" for most of the treatment staff and the issue of confidentiality had already been addressed during orientation day. Still, in a few cases the interviewee read the informed consent statement fully prior to the interview and asked pertinent questions; this situation was most likely to occur with staff who had been absent on orientation day.

Final plans for day 2 data collection were made by the EMMT staff after day 1. Individual program staff were assigned to specific EMMT staff for interviewing. As in 1985, one team member interviewed all counselors, another interviewed the medical staff, and a third the admission staff, the fourth member collected the pharmacy data. This interviewing and data collection were allocated by relevant discipline for the most part; thus a counselor interviewed the program counselors, and a pharmacist collected dispensing data from the pharmacy. In this way, there was specialization of interviewing based on relevant prior experience. This procedure was adhered to in 1985 and 1986. Consequently, most of the treatment staff were interviewed by the same team member both years.

In addition to the planned on-site data collection procedures followed at the program in 1985 and 1986, the research team members also had occasion to tour the neighborhood, talk with staff and patients about topics of mutual interest, observe the operation of the clinic, and otherwise became more familiar with each of the seven methadone maintenance programs. This first-hand familiarity with the programs—director, treatment staff, administration, facility, hours of operation, dispensing routine, security, neighborhood—greatly increased as a consequence of our second intensive program data collection effort in 1986. Thus by the time of our second on-site effort, we not only felt more confident working at the programs but our knowledge of how treatment services were delivered had markedly improved.

Record Data Collection and Assessment in 1986

Record Review of Patients' Treatment Progress

A separate compilation of data from clinical records at each program was undertaken in 1986 to ascertain the amount and type of treatment provided to patients during the past year or since admission in 1985. This compilation of record data on the admission and in-treatment cohorts was termed "linkage" data, as these findings were intended to link the patient and program data sets. Thus the clinical records would document services provided to each of the 617 patients, and these findings would corroborate the patient interview data. Concomitantly, aggregate data on services provided by each program would corroborate the output findings. In addition to this linkage function, the record compilation was utilized to review and evaluate each program's records and thereby obtain additional treatment domain findings.

Preparation of special schedules for obtaining information from records at each program about patients' treatment history and services received took place during early 1986. Development of these schedules was undertaken in conjunction with feasibility studies at the programs to ascertain what record information was commonly available. On the basis of these assessments of the clinical records, two forms were devised to obtain data pertaining to services received by patients in the two cohorts; one form was for new admission patients (i.e., those admitted during late 1985), and the other was for patients from the in-treatment cohort. Each form contained a series of items pertaining to the specific treatment services provided to patients during the past month and year. These items referred to attendance, methadone dosage, dosage change, take-home doses, urinalysis results, number and type of counseling, and medical services received.

This record data collection (linkage) was undertaken at the programs during a 3-month period in 1986. Two members of the EMMT staff compiled the data from records at each site; the length of stay at each site was 2 days.

Record Assessment

The status of each program's records was also assessed; that is, we ascertained the extent to which the clinical records were obtainable (i.e., lost or not), up-to-date, or otherwise complete and accurate. The extent of missing data as well as other considerations were utilized for preparing a composite rating of the adequacy of each program's records. In addition to the assessment of records, information was obtained about the adequacy of record room space, filing and security procedures, clerical staff, and similar treatment domain matters.

Other Sources of Data

Although the comprehensive program data collection, patient interviews, and linkage record data compilation were the main data collection efforts of the EMMT project, additional sources of data were utilized to augment these findings or to support special studies. It is pertinent to mention these additional data sources, as most of them have furthered our knowledge of methadone maintenance treatment. Seven additional data sources or special studies are worthy of note: (1) an analysis of the content of individual counseling sessions based on counselors' reports; (2) an observational study of counselors' daily routine and allocation of time to various tasks; (3) a study of the 12 interviewers' experiences and assessment of the truthfulness of addict respondents; (4) structured conversations with addicts about select aspects of methadone maintenance treatment; (5) comparison of self-reports of criminality among addict patients with official records; (6) the effectiveness of a long-term (10 years or longer) medical maintenance regimen; and (7) a detailed history of one methadone maintenance program.

Conclusion

The research plan and data collection procedures have been emphasized in this chapter because obtaining detailed information about the four domains (patients, programs, services, and outcome) is the crucial and distinguishing feature of this project. Obtaining these data sets provided the foundation for subsequent analysis. Thus in later chapters the relation between variables in specific domains and among variables in all four domains are the topic of analysis. It is the underlying data collection procedures within the four domain schema, however, that provide the database for subsequent analysis.

Looking back over 3 years of data collection at methadone programs in New York City, Philadelphia, and Baltimore, a number of conclusions seem warranted. The principal conclusion that emerged from implementation of the research plan was that the intensive program data collection effort and the patient interviews and follow-up procedure were feasible. Thus the required data in all four domains were obtained.

Second, it should be stated that the program data collection was markedly more difficult and problematical than the patient data collection. This was because obtaining comprehensive treatment domain and services output domain data involved not only the development of new instruments and new field procedures but use of them in active methadone maintenance programs. Originally, the feasibility of these data collection procedures was problematical. Conversely, interviewing addict patients was comparatively more straightforward because a standard interview instrument was utilized (the Addiction Severity Index along with Part II sections), experienced professional interviewers were utilized, and field work routines developed by the ISR were followed.

Stating that one aspect of data collection at the programs was less difficult and problematical than another is not meant to imply that any aspect of data collection at these programs was easy or without numerous problems. In this regard, there is a certain misrepresentation implied in this chapter: The orderly discussion of data collection procedures leads one to the impression that the data collection experiences in the three cities were routine and uneventful, whereas the real day-to-day story of the site visits and data collection were anything but that. How to explain the realities of field work in these inner city neighborhoods and programs remains to be resolved.

Lastly, our experiences at the methadone maintenance programs over the years led to a number of observations about how comprehensive treatment domain data and service domain data could and could not be obtained. It was found that on-site data collection by an independent staff was the only feasible way to obtain the comprehensive program data required. The program staff by themselves were not suitable for this task because of the confidentiality required in interviews, the problem of in-house bias, and other considerations. Concomitantly, we considered it unrealistic for city, state, or federal agencies to mandate comprehensive in-house evaluations of drug treatment programs. Although in-house program audits and accountability reviews are necessary, they are different from an independent evaluation based on intensive on-site data collection.

References

1. Tims FM, Ludford JP (eds) (1984) NIDA Research Monograph 51: RAUS: Drug Abuse Treatment Evaluation: Strategies, Progress, and Prospects (ADM) 84–1329. Rockville: US Department of Health and Human Services
2. Ball JC, Chambers CD (eds) (1970) Epidemiology of Opiate Addiction in the U.S. Springfield: Charles C Thomas
3. Ball JC, Graff H (1974) Phase I evaluation of drug treatment programs in Pennsylvania. In Fisher S, Freedman AM (eds): Opiate Addiction. Washington DC: Winston & Sons, pp 175–183
4. Ball JC, Graff H (1975) Drug treatment programs in Pennsylvania: a statewide evaluation. Am J Public Health 65:592–598
5. Butynski W, Canova D (1988) An analysis of state alcohol and drug abuse profile data. In: State Resources and Services Related to Alcohol and Drug Abuse Problems: Fiscal Year 1987. Washington DC: National Association of State Alcohol and Drug Abuse Directors
6. Some 260,000 narcotic addicts were reported for New York State; New York State Division of Substance Abuse Services, 1986–87. Annual Report. Albany: Executive Park South
7. McLellan AT, Luborsky L, O'Brien CP, Woody CE (1980) An improved diagnostic evaluation instrument for substance abuse patients: the addiction severity index. J Nerv Ment Dis 168:26–33
8. Kosten TR, Rounsaville BJ, Kleber HD (1983) Concurrent validity of the addiction severity index. J Nerv Ment Dis 171:606–610
9. McLellan AT, Luborsky L, Cacciola J, et al (1985) New data from the addic-

tions severity index: reliability and validity in three centers. J Nerv Ment Dis 173:412–423
10. McLellan AT, Luborsky L, Cacciola J, et al (1985) Guide to the Addiction Severity Index: Background Administration and Field Testing Results. Washington, DC: U.S. Government Printing Office
11. Cacciola J, Griffith J, McLellan AT (eds) (1988) Addiction Severity Index: Instruction Manual, 4th Ed. Washington, DC: NIDA Research Project DA02559 and the Veterans Administration
12. McGahan PL, Griffith JA, Parente R, McLellan AT (1982) Composite Scores from the Addiction Severity Index. Washington, DC: NIDA Project DA02554 and the Veterans Administration
13. Nurco DN, Cisin IH, Balter MB (1981) Addict careers. II. The first ten years. Int J Addict 16:1327–1356
14. Ball JC, Rosen L, Flueck J, Nurco D (1981) The criminality of heroin addicts: when addicted and when off opiates. In Inciardi JA (ed): The Drug-Crime Connection, Vol 5. Beverly Hills: Sage Publications, pp 39–65
15. Ball JC, Shaffer JW, Nurco DN (1983) The day-to-day criminality of heroin addicts in Baltimore—a study in the continuity of offence rates. Drug Alcohol Depend 12:119–142
16. Cohen M, Howard A, Klein DF, Newfield K (1976) Evaluating outcome criteria used in methadone maintenance programs. Int J Addict 11:283–294
17. Wells EA, Hawkins JD, Catalano RF (1988) Choosing drug use measures for treatment outcome studies. I. The influence of measurement approach on treatment results. Int J Addict 23:851–873
18. Johnston LD, Nurco DN, Robins LN (eds) (1977) Conducting Follow-up Research on Drug Treatment Programs. Rockville: US Department of Health and Human Services

3 Pretreatment Characteristics of 617 Male Methadone Maintenance Patients

The 617 patients selected for longitudinal study were a representative sample of male patients at six methadone maintenance programs in three eastern cities. At the time of sample selection in late 1985, there were 2394 patients enrolled in these six programs of whom 1874 were in methadone maintenance treatment. Consecutive admissions and a sample of those already in treatment were selected from each treatment program. Some 100 male patients, then, were selected for intensive study from each of the six programs.

Characteristics of the Addict Patients

Age of Patients at First Interview

The 617 addict patients were primarily young to middle-age adults (Table 3.1), with 72 percent of the patients being between 25 and 39 years (61 percent were in their thirties). Only 3 percent were under age 25, but 25 percent were 40 or older. Their mean age at time of interview was 36.6 years. The older age of these methadone maintenance patients reflects the fact that most have had a considerable history of heroin addiction prior to their present treatment.

Minority Group Status

With respect to race and minority group status, 51.2 percent of the 617 patients were black, 40.7 percent were white, 6.3 percent were Hispanic, and the remainder were American Indian, Oriental, or other races (1.7 percent). In general, race and minority group composition of the patients at the six programs reflected each program's catchment area because most patients seek treatment that is convenient to their place of residence and ethnically congenial. Although some patients traveled from various parts of the metropolitan area to their treatment program, both the patients and

TABLE 3.1. Age of 617 Male Patients at First Interview

	White		Minority		Total patients	
Age	No.	%	No.	%	No.	%
19–24	16	6.4	1	0.3	17	2.8
25–29	35	13.9	31	8.5	66	10.7
30–34	92	36.7	120	32.8	212	34.4
35–39	69	27.5	97	26.5	166	26.9
40–49	34	13.5	88	24.0	122	19.8
50–59	4	1.6	26	7.1	30	4.9
60–76	1	0.4	3	0.8	4	0.6
Total	251	100.0	366	100.0	617	100.0
Mean age	34.6		37.9		36.6	

Note: underscore in past digit of total percent indicates that above column does not sum to zero due to rounding.

the programs in the three cities were concentrated in center city neighborhoods.

Education

When considering the life history of these 617 addicts in greater detail, it is pertinent to note that commencement of heroin addiction (which was a culmination of their earlier involvement in a drug subculture) generally occurred at the end of their teenage years when they were terminating school. For most, it is unlikely that these two events were causally related (i.e., leaving school did not directly lead to addiction). It seems more likely that the demands of heroin addiction are such that most addicts find formal education increasingly irrelevant to or incompatible with their daily life "on the street."

The years of formal education of the addict patients was considerably below that of the general population (Table 3.2). Thus only 58 percent had completed high school compared with 87 percent of the US population (age 30–34 years). The educational deficit of the addict cohort was most evident with respect to the completion of college education: Only 4 percent of the 617 males had finished 4 or more years of college compared with 27 percent of the US population (age 30–34 years). Although the percent of minority patients who completed high school was somewhat lower than that of the white patients (52 versus 68 percent), it appears that there is an overall leveling and inhibiting effect of addiction on higher education as both white and minority patients were markedly less likely to complete college than their US age cohorts.

TABLE 3.2. Years of School Completed by Methadone Maintenance Patients Compared with US Population

	Percent of patients or population with specified years of education[a]							
	Elementary school			High school		College		
Cohort or population (no.)	1–4	5–7	8	1–3	4	1–3	4+	% High school graduates
All pts. (n = 617)	0.4	3.3	3.7	34.5	35.7	18.8	3.6	58.1
White pts. (n = 251)	0.4	4.0	3.2	24.8	40.8	20.4	6.4	67.6
Minority pts. (n = 366)	0.3	2.7	4.1	41.3	32.2	17.8	1.6	51.6
US population, 25+ years	2.8	5.0	6.6	12.4	38.4	15.8	19.1	73.3
US population, 30–34 years	1.2	1.5	1.8	8.3	38.7	21.5	27.0	87.2
US population, black, 30–34 years	1.7	1.2	2.9	16.2	45.3	17.9	14.8	78.0

[a]US Bureau of the Census, (1985) Statistical Abstract of the United States: 1986 (106 ed). Washington, DC: US Government Printing Office, Table 218.

Onset of Daily Heroin Use

The early age at which opiate addiction commonly began was a crucial event in these patients' lives. With few exceptions, the onset of daily intravenous injections set the stage for a deviant course of life that has proved difficult to change. With respect to early onset, almost two-thirds had began daily use of opiates by age 19 (Table 3.3 and Fig. 3.1). The highest incidence years were ages 15, 16, 17, and 18, with more than 10 percent of the cohort beginning regular opiate use during each of these years. An appreciable number (10 percent) began their daily opiate use at

TABLE 3.3. Age at Onset of *Daily* Opiate Use for Male Addicts

	White		Nonwhite		Total[a]	
Age at onset	No.	%	No.	%	No.	%
9–14	25	10.0	39	10.7	64	10.4
15–19	150	59.8	186	51.0	336	54.5
20–24	50	19.9	93	25.5	143	23.2
25–29	19	7.6	33	9.0	52	8.4
30–45	7	2.8	14	3.8	21	3.4
Total	251[a]	100.0	365[a]	100.0	616[a]	100.0
Median age	18.3		18.9		18.5	

[a]There were 616 valid cases.

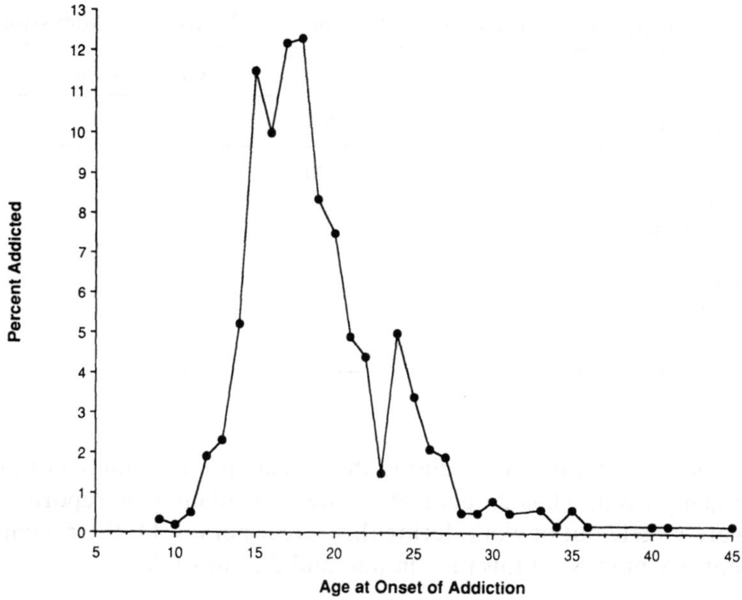

FIGURE 3.1. Age at onset of opiate addiction for 617 male patients

age 14 or earlier. There was an overall similarity between the white and minority cohorts with respect to age at onset of addiction.

Employment History

Most of the patients had a considerable work history by their fiirst (T_1) interview, although about one-third had serious employment problems. Thus 71 percent reported that they have a specific occupation, e.g., a trade or skilled work, and 94 percent reported that they had pursued some line of work for at least 1 year. The average length of the longest full-time job was 5.6 years. The usual occupation for these males was (1) major or minor professions 10.0%, (2) clerical work 9.4%, skilled manual labor 36.1%, semiskilled manual labor 20.6%, unskilled labor 23.3%, and never worked 0.6%.

The new admission patients present an overview of the employment status of patients in the study prior to methadone maintenance treatment (Table 3.4). During the 3 years prior to their current admission, 56 percent of the addicts were engaged in full-time work. An additional 14 percent worked part time, either on a regular basis or intermittently. Thus 70 percent reported that they worked during the past 3 years, but 14 percent of this employment was only part time. Still, more than one-half were engaged in full-time work prior to treatment.

TABLE 3.4 Principal Employment Status During Past 3 Years, New Admissions

	New admissions	
Employment status	No.	%
Full time	71	56.3
Regular part time	10	7.9
Irregular part time	7	5.6
Student	2	1.6
Unemployed	32	25.4
Jail or prison	4	3.2
Total	126	100.0

Of those who did not work during the 3 years prior to admission, most were unemployed. Thus 25 percent of the new admissions reported that they were mostly out of work during this 3-year period. Of the remainder, 4 patients spent most of this time in jail, and 2 were students.

Family Life

With respect to current marital status, 28 percent of the 617 males were married, 29 percent were separated or divorced, 2 percent were widowed, and the remaining 40 percent had never married. The high percentage of those who never married is noteworthy.

Further information about these addicts' family life is afforded by noting their usual living arrangement (Table 3.5). During the 3 years prior to admission, 46 percent were living with a wife or partner, 35 percent were living with their parents or other family members, and only 20 percent were living away from their families. The latter group of patients mostly

TABLE 3.5. Patients' Usual Living Arrangement During Past 3 Years

	White		Minority		Total	
Living with	No.	%	No.	%	No.	%
Wife and children	72	28.7	118	32.2	190	30.8
Wife or surrogate	37	14.7	54	14.8	91	14.7
Parents	55	21.9	28	7.7	83	13.5
Other family	45	17.9	87	23.8	132	21.4
Friends	6	2.4	7	1.9	13	2.1
Alone	33	13.1	67	18.3	100	16.2
Not stable	2	0.8	2	0.5	4	0.6
Jail or prison	1	0.4	3	0.8	4	0.6
Total	251	100.0	366	100.0	617	100.0

TABLE 3.6. Drug Abuse History of Methadone Maintenance Patients: Years of Regular Use[a]

	White		Minority		All males (n = 617)		
Drug	No.	%	No.	%	No.	%	Mean years of use for positives
Heroin	232	92.8	358	98.9	590	97.0	11.2
Other opiates	129	51.4	51	14.3	180	29.6	8.9
Barbiturates	94	37.8	47	13.1	141	23.2	4.5
Other sedatives	115	46.2	87	24.2	202	33.2	5.5
Cocaine	94	38.1	190	52.3	284	46.6	5.8
Amphetamines	72	28.9	71	19.7	143	23.5	3.1
Cannabis	196	78.7	229	63.1	425	69.4	10.5
Hallucinogens	70	28.9	19	5.4	89	14.9	2.9
Inhalants	25	10.0	7	2.0	32	5.3	2.8
Alcohol to intoxication	124	50.0	181	50.1	305	50.1	8.5

[a] Regular use was defined as use of a drug at least three times a week for 6 months or longer.

were living alone, although a few were living with friends, as transients, or were in jail. The information provided about current living arrangements indicates more family ties and dependency than the more formal classification of current marital status.

Drug Abuse History

The addict patients included in this study had a long history of regular drug abuse prior to treatment (Table 3.6). As might be expected, opiates were the principal drugs of abuse. Thus 97 percent reported regular heroin use prior to treatment, and this addiction was maintained on the average for 11.2 years. In addition, 30 percent of the addicts were regular abusers of other opiates; their mean extent of such abuse was 8.9 years. For all opiates, the combined occurrence of regular use (or addiction) was 13.5 mean years. (The ASI defines regular annual use as use of a drug three or more times per week for 6 months or longer.)

Although their lifetime abuse of other drugs was less enduring than their abuse of opiates, it was considerable. Thus, 46.6 percent of the patients had a history of cocaine abuse and their mean duration of regular cocaine abuse was 5.8 years. Comparable lifetime data for sedatives were that 33.2 percent abused these drugs for 5.5 mean years; for barbiturates, 23.2 percent of the addicts abused these drugs regularly for an average of 4.5 years. Amphetamines were abused by 23.5 percent of the addicts for 3.1 mean years, and some 14.9 percent of the addicts had been regular hallucinogen abusers for 2.9 years.

Both cannabis and alcohol were extensively abused prior to treatment.

Thus 69.4 percent of the patients were regular marijuana abusers, and they had 10.5 mean years of abuse. Similarly, 50.1 percent abused alcohol to intoxification, and their mean duration of such abuse was 8.5 years.

In sum, the drug abuse history of these patients reveals a primary addiction to heroin that had lasted for 11 years or more. For most, opiate addiction had been combined with long-term abuse of marijuana or alcohol, or both. In addition, almost one-half of the patients had abused cocaine for an average of almost 6 years. The other classes of drugs that had lifetime prevalence rates of more than 20 percent were sedatives, barbiturates, and amphetamines; only a minority of patients abused these drugs regularly, but such abuse was not inconsiderable, averaging 3 to 5 years.

Although nonopiate drugs were abused by most patients prior to treatment, it should not be inferred that these subjects were primarily polydrug abusers who readily substitute other drugs for opiates. The life history data indicated the contrary. The vast majority of these patients were confirmed opiate addicts who preferred these drugs to others and used nonopiate drugs only in an adjunctive or secondary fashion. This fact does not deny the significance of dual addictions or imply that concomitant drug abuse does not have serious consequences; it is to maintain that for most of these patients their primary drug abuse problem has been opiate drugs, heroin in particular. The fact that this principal drug of abuse is commonly taken intravenously further exacerbates the problems associated with heroin addiction.

Criminal History

Most of the 617 male addicts had a long criminal history prior to their current methadone maintenance treatment: 85 percent had been arrested one or more times. These 532 addicts accumulated 4723 adult arrests, with their mean number of arrests being 8.9.

The types of offense for which these addicts were arrested is shown in Table 10.1. Both the overall range of offenses committed by the cohort as a whole and the specialization of offenses by groups of individuals are notable. The tabulation of arrest types—shoplifting, burglary, robbery, assault, parole violation, forgery, weapons offenses, homicide, rape, drug offenses, and others—runs the general spectrum of criminal offenses. At the same time, there is evidence of a concentration of certain offense types (i.e., drug offenses) as well as specialization within types. This aspect of their criminality is discussed below.

The most frequent single reason for arrest was drug charges, which accounted for 30 percent of the 4723 arrests. Sixty-two percent of the addicts had been arrested for such offenses.

The principal nondrug offenses for which the addicts were arrested included shoplifting, burglary, and robbery: 32 percent for shoplifting, 38 percent for burglary, and 23 percent for robbery. Together these three offenses accounted for more than one-third of their total arrests. Arrests for assault, weapons offenses, and parole violation were also frequent: 25 percent of the male addicts were arrested for assault, 29 percent for weapons violations, and 30 percent for violating parole.

Arrests for forgery were less frequent than those already mentioned, as only 13 percent had such arrests. Forgery and other "paper crimes" are far less likely to result in arrest, however, so these figures grossly underrepresent offense rates.

Homicide and rape were among the least frequent types of arrest reported, although even these rates were far from inconsequential. More than 5 percent of these addicts had been arrested for homicide and almost 2 percent for rape.

Criminality

The magnitude of criminal behavior among these 617 addicts was markedly higher than their arrest rates indicate because most crimes addicts commit do not result in arrest. Indeed, the findings of this analysis as well as those from other comparable studies in the past reveal that fewer than 1 percent of the crimes committed by heroin addicts result in arrest. (This topic is addressed further in Chapter 10.)

To ascertain the extent and frequency of their criminal behavior, each patient was asked, in a face-to-face confidential interview, to enumerate the specific types of crime in which he engaged during his last addiction period; he was also asked to recount how frequently he committed each type of crime. These data were then standardized to an annual basis. The measurement obtained for each addict was the type and number of crimes committed per year during his last addiction period when he was "on the street."

The scope and frequency of their criminal behavior during their last addiction period is tabulated in Table 10.2. Overall, these 617 males committed 293,308 offenses per year when addicted to heroin, which constitutes a mean of 484 annual offenses per individual when addicted.

Three main aspects characterized the prior criminal behavior of these addict patients. First, as a cohort they engaged in a wide range of criminal behavior, from store theft and auto theft to loan sharking and pimping. Second, there was considerable specialization by individuals regarding the types of crime they committed. Third, most of these addicts were frequent offenders: Daily commission of crime was the rule, not the exception. Each of these aspects is discussed next.

The wide range of criminal behavior engaged in by these addicts when "on the street" was similar to that previously presented for arrests, except that they pursued far more "professional" or organized crimes than their arrests indicate. The prominence of numbers racket offenses (12.5 percent of 293,308 offenses), fencing stolen property (11.1 percent), confidence game swindles (6.1 percent), pimping (5.1 percent), and loan sharking (1.8 percent) are noteworthy. Together, these five offenses accounted for 36.6 percent of the crime committed during the last addiction period by these 617 males.

Still, with respect to the range of offenses committed, it is significant to note that criminal involvement in the drug business (e.g., sale of drugs) constituted some 30 to 33 percent of both arrests and criminal behavior (see Tables 10.1 and 10.2). The frequency of even these events, however, is vastly different, as there were several hundred times more drug business offenses than drug-related arrests on an annual basis. This situation occurred even though arrests for possession were included in the category of drug arrests, whereas drug business offenses (which included selling and touting) did not include possession or use of drugs.

The common crimes against property and persons were evident in both the criminal behavior enumeration and the arrest tabulation. Store theft, burglary, robbery, and assault were the principal such offenses committed during these patients' addiction periods, and these crimes are represented in the arrest tabulation (see Table 10.1). In each instance, however, these more "traditional" crimes constituted a smaller *percentage* of the total annual crimes committed than of the total lifetime arrests; this comparison supports the conclusion that arrests are more likely to occur for commonplace crimes than for more organized crimes (e.g., numbers or prostitution).

Second, considerable specialization in criminal behavior was evident during these addicts' active periods of heroin use. Most were engaged in only a few types of crime, but these crimes were pursued intensively. Most of the 617 males who engaged in a particular type of crime committed more than 100 crimes of this type per year. The mean number of offenses per year for the 14 major types of crime committed during the last addiction period ranked as follows (also see Table 10.2): pimping, 302 offenses; drug business, 279 offenses; numbers, 200 offenses; fencing and loan sharking, 167 mean annual offenses each; store theft, 166 offenses; con games, 166 offenses; other theft, 126 offenses; prescription forgery, 112 offenses; burglary, 91 offenses; general forgery, 91 offenses; robbery, 82 offenses; auto theft, 66 offenses; assault, 55 offenses per year. Significantly, for all 14 types of crime the annual offense rate for those who committed each type was more than 50 offenses per year. As noted, for 9 of the 14 types of crime the mean number of offenses was 100 per year or more.

The third and most striking aspect of these addicts' criminality is the sheer magnitude of their criminal behavior during their periods of active heroin use. The commission of 293,308 crimes per year for this cohort is a staggering figure: It constitutes a mean of 484 offenses per year per addict. If these findings on annual rates of offending are extrapolated to their prior 11.2-year heroin addiction history, the lifetime offenses committed by these 617 addicts is more than three million offenses, which constitutes a mean of 5263 offenses committed per addict prior to current treatment.

TABLE 3.7. Lifetime years of Incarceration Prior to Current Treatment

Years in prison	White No.	White %	Minority No.	Minority %	Total No.	Total %
None	120	47.8	92	25.1	212	34.4
<1	56	22.3	74	20.2	130	21.1
1–1.9	17	6.8	36	9.8	53	8.6
2–4.9	32	12.8	76	20.8	108	17.5
5–9.9	15	6.0	54	14.8	69	11.2
10–27	11	4.4	34	9.3	45	7.3
Total	251	100.0	366	100.0	617	100.0
Mean Years	1.5		3.2		2.5	

Incarceration History

As might be expected from their repeated and long-term involvement in criminal behavior, most of the addict patients had spent time in jail or prison: 65.7 percent of the 617 patients had been incarcerated, and a sizable proportion of them had considerable histories of imprisonment (Table 3.7). In this regard, more than one-third (36.0 percent) of the patients had been in prison for 2 years or more prior to their current period of treatment.

Prior Treatment for Drug Abuse

In addition to imprisonment, these patients usually had had numerous prior treatments for drug abuse. Indeed, 94.3 percent of the patients reported one or more prior treatments and most had three or more such treatments (Table 3.8).

TABLE 3.8. Number of Prior Treatments for Drug Abuse for 617 Patients

No. of prior treatments	White No.	White %	Minority No.	Minority %	All patients No.	All patients %
None	9	3.6	26	7.1	35	5.7
1	39	15.5	87	23.8	126	20.4
2	51	20.3	75	20.5	126	20.4
3–4	81	32.3	107	29.2	188	30.5
5–9	56	22.3	54	14.8	110	17.8
10–19	8	3.2	13	3.6	21	3.4
20–95	7	2.8	4	1.1	11	1.8
Total	251	100.0	366	100.0	617	100.0
Mean	4.3		3.4		3.8	

Of the total 2316 drug treatment experiences amassed by these 617 males, 43.4 percent were for detoxification, 43.1 percent for previous methadone maintenance treatment, and 13.5 percent for other modalities of treatment for drug abuse. With regard to prior methadone maintenance treatment, 72 percent of the 617 patients reported that they had had this type of treatment previously.

Commonality Among the Addict Patients

Addicts in the Three Cities

When comparing the patient samples from New York City, Philadelphia, and Baltimore, it was found that there was an overall similarity with respect to demographic variables, drug abuse history, and pretreatment criminality. Conversely, there were important differences with regard to their current treatment experiences at the six programs in the three cities. The latter variations in program services and patient outcome are discussed in subsequent chapters. In this chapter attention is focused on pretreatment characteristics of patients.

The ages of the patients from the three cities at the time of interview during late 1985 were similar; the mean age of the New York sample was 34.8 years, 36.9 years for Philadelphia, and 36.5 years for Baltimore; the New York patients were, then, slightly younger.

With respect to minority group composition, the Baltimore sample consisted of more whites than were found in the other two cities (52 percent for Baltimore versus 38 percent for New York and 31 percent for Philadelphia). The other notable difference was the larger representation of Hispanics among the New York addicts (18 percent versus 2 percent in Philadelphia and none in Baltimore).

Methadone patients in the three cities were similar in terms of their educational attainment. The frequency distributions of years of schooling were almost identical. Mean years of schooling for the three samples were 11.6, 11.6, and 11.5, respectively. The percent of each sample who had more than 12 years of education was 21.1 for New York, 23.3 for Philadelphia, and 23.9 for Baltimore. (In this and other comparisons, the younger age of the New York patients should be kept in mind.)

The three samples were also similar with regard to marital status: In New York 27.7 percent were married, in Philadelphia 27.6 percent, and in Baltimore 32.9 percent. More variation was evident with regard to the number of dependents for the three samples: a mean of 0.8 in New York, 1.0 in Philadelphia, and 1.6 in Baltimore.

There was also a similarity in the drug abuse histories reported by the patients in the three cities. The mean age at onset of heroin addiction was 18.5 years in New York, 19.9 in Philadelphia, and 18.4 in Baltimore. Lifetime years of heroin addiction was also similar: 9.8 in New York, 12.0 in

Philadelphia, and 11.4 in Baltimore. Lifetime prevalence and years of regular use of barbiturates, amphetamines, and cannabis were similar in all three cities. Indeed, the similarity of these data on prevalence and length of regular use is striking. For example, 70 percent of the New York sample were regular cannabis users compared with 76 percent of the Philadelphia sample and 70 percent of the Baltimore sample. Furthermore, their mean years of regular use were 10.9, 9.4, and 10.1, respectively.

It was only with respect to cocaine usage that notable differences were evident. The New York patients were more likely to have used cocaine regularly and to have done so for more years than the other samples. The lifetime prevalence of regular cocaine use was 73 percent in New York, 52 percent in Philadelphia, and 55 percent in Baltimore; the mean duration of cocaine use for those who abused this drug were 6.3, 2.8, and 4.7 years for the respective cities.

The lifetime prevalence of having overdosed on drugs for patients in the three cities was similar. In New York 35 percent of patients had had such episodes, and their mean number was 2.5. In Philadelphia 37 percent had overdosed, and their mean number was 2.7. In Baltimore 39 percent had overdosed, and their mean number was 3.6.

Criminality in Three Cities

There was a notable similarity in the criminal history of addicts from each of the three cities. The lifetime prevalences by type of arrest were similar, as were the frequencies of arrest. With respect to the New York addicts, 78 percent had been arrested, and their mean number of arrests was 9.0. For the Philadelphia addicts, 89 percent had been arrested, and their mean number of arrests was 10.9. Of the Baltimore addicts, 92 percent had been arrested, with 7.8 mean arrests.

The incarceration history of these three samples was almost identical. Among the New York patients, 61 percent had been incarcerated, and their mean time in prison was 3.6 years. For the Philadelphia patients, 65 percent had been incarcerated, and their mean years in prison was 3.7. Lastly, 70 percent of the Baltimore patients had been in prison, and their mean time of incarceration was 4.0 years.

Minority Group–White Similarities

In general, the race-ethnic differences in pretreatment characteristics were greater than the intercity differences, although the leveling effect of the addict career was still evident. As noted earlier, 41 percent of the 617 males were white, and 59 percent were minority group members. The latter group was mostly black, although there was a small Hispanic representation. For convenience of analysis and description, the white patients are compared with the entire group of minority patients.

The 366 addicts from minority groups were significantly older than the

251 white addicts; their mean ages were 37.9 and 34.6 years, respectively. This difference was attributable to the higher percentage of white patients in their twenties (20.3 percent versus 8.8 percent) and the higher percentage of the minority patients who were over 40 years of age (31.9 versus 15.5 percent). The percentage in their thirties was similar for both whites and minorities (64.2 versus 59.3 percent).

The white and minority cohorts did not differ with respect to marital status or the number of dependents claimed by the patients. The educational attainment of the minority group patients was only slightly lower than that of the white patients.

Despite the educational similarity, there was evidence of lower socioeconomic status among the minority group patients. There was more unemployment during the past 3 years (35 percent versus 17 percent for the whites) and more need for employment counseling at the time of interview (ASI employment composite scale scores were 0.706 versus 0.444 for the minority patients and whites, respectively). In addition, only 27 percent of the minority addicts had a valid driver's license and 19 percent had use of an automobile; these figures compared with 62 percent of the whites who had a license and 53 percent who had use of an automobile. (For a discussion of drug addiction in the black community, see Primm et al.[1])

The white and minority group patients differed considerably in terms of their drug abuse histories, although the overriding dominance of opiate addiction remained as a focal point of their drug abuse history. In the latter regard, 93 percent of the whites and 99 percent of the minority addicts were heroin users; their mean years of heroin addiction were 8.7 and 12.8 for the whites and minorities, respectively. This shorter history of lifetime heroin addiction among the whites was counterbalanced by their increased use of other opiate drugs: 57 percent of the white addicts had used other opiates regularly, and their mean years of such use was 7.6 years. Conversely, only 16 percent of the minority addicts had regularly used other opiates, although their mean years of use was similar, 7.3 years.

When regular use of all opiate drugs is considered together (heroin use combined with that of other opiates), the lifetime similarity of their addiction histories is striking. The mean years of opiate addiction for whites was 12.5 years versus 13.4 years for minority patients (the minority patients are slightly older).

With regard to lifetime differences in the abuse of nonopiate drugs, the minority group patients were less likely to have a history of regular abuse of barbiturates, other sedatives, hallucinogens, or inhalants. Conversely, they were somewhat more likely to regularly abuse cocaine—58 percent versus 43 percent for the whites. The lifetime abuse of amphetamines, cannabis, and alcohol to intoxication was similar for the two cohorts.

With respect to criminal history, the minority and white patients were similar in that 89 percent of the former and 82 percent of the latter had been arrested. The mean number of lifetime arrests for those who were arrested was 6.5 for the white addicts and 8.7 for the minority addicts.

The minority group patients were more likely to have been incarcerated, and they had spent more time in prison than the whites: 75 percent of the minority patients had been in prison, and their mean time incarcerated was 3.2 years, in contrast to 52 percent of the whites having been imprisoned for a mean duration of 1.5 years.

The white and minority group patients differed somewhat with respect to their treatment histories, although less so than with their criminal histories. The whites had somewhat more prior treatment for their drug addiction than the minority group patients. The mean number of prior treatments for the whites was 4.3 compared to 3.4 for the minority patients. Almost all members of both groups, however, had a history of drug abuse treatment. Only 4 percent of the whites and 7 percent of the minority patients reported no prior treatment for drug abuse.

Methadone Patients in the United States

The 617 patients selected for study from six methadone maintenance programs were representative of male patients in treatment at these programs during late 1985. To what extent the 1874 patients at these six programs were representative of the estimated 80,000 patients in methadone maintenance treatment in the United States cannot be accurately determined because the characteristics of the total methadone maintenance population is not known.[2] The available evidence, however, indicates that methadone maintenance patients in a given city tend to be generally representative of the "hard core" addicts in that city.[3,4]

The extent of the opiate problem in the United States and the characteristics of addict patients have been the topic of research for some time.[5–8] The contemporary challenge is not only to delineate these populations more accurately but to fiind ways to reduce the scope of this social problem and to mitigate its consequences through treatment and other means.

In general, the addict patients were remarkably similar in terms of their preadmission or life history characteristics. This similarity was evident when comparing life history characteristics among the city cohorts. Thus not only were the modal values usually similar (e.g., with regard to years of opiate use or crime-days per year when addicted), there was a marked similarity in the frequency distributions. A discussion of the similarities and differences in patient characteristics by city and race-ethnic cohorts indicated the extent of this commonality of addiction characteristics.

Conclusion

It is necessary to understand the life course of addiction among the patients admitted for treatment if one is to provide effective rehabilitation and have realistic expectations of success and failure. Therefore it is efficacious to recapitulate the main contemporary findings about the natural history of heroin addiction among the patients studied. Second, it is pertinent to determine the baseline preadmission characteristics of these patients before proceeding to investigate the effectiveness of methadone maintenance programs.

A review of the life history of the 617 male patients reveals that most became enmeshed at an early age in a drug-oriented peer group subculture that glorified drug abuse and the exciting way of life it denoted, that their daily use of opiates and other drugs continued during their adult years, and that their preoccupation with obtaining and using drugs was associated with an ever-present network of friends and associates who supported this way of life. These young, inner-city males became confirmed addicts who found it difficult to extricate themselves from the daily demands of drug use and criminal behavior.

The fact that 94 percent of these 617 patients have previously been enrolled in drug abuse treatment programs and 72 percent in methadone maintenance programs is provocative. It raises the question of whether these past failures were due to treatment inadequacies or patient deficiencies—or to some combination of the two, which seems most likely. Still, the extensive history of treatment attempts does establish that most of these patients were not naive about drug abuse treatment prior to this treatment and that in the past they had not been sufficiently motivated to stay in treatment until rehabilitation was effected.

Although there is a commonality of addiction characteristics in the three cities, it should not be inferred that all addicts are the same or that differences are unimportant. Addict patients do differ in age, length of addiction, extent of drug use, involvement in crime, and other significant characteristics, and these considerations are important for clinical practice and program planning. At the same time, it is important to recognize the broad parameters of opiate addiction in order to cope with this difficult population realistically. It was found that for most patients there was a long history of intravenous drug use and street crime that preceded their current treatment admission.

Treatment Implications

Attention has been focused on the life history or pretreatment characteristics of addict patients because this information is the baseline from which treatment begins. Determination of the effectiveness of treatment requires that comprehensive baseline data be obtained. Beyond this methodological point, several implications for treatment seem warranted about this population.

It was noted that opiate addiction is a chronic condition that often persists from adolescence into adulthood as a complex and persistent behavior problem. Given that most addicts who seek treatment have been involved in regular drug use for 10 years or more, it is evident that rehabilitation requires a long-term effort. Successful rehabilitation involves, in most cases, changing the addict's way of life—his values, attitudes, habits, behavior, friends, how he earns and spends his money, and much more. Because these changes cannot be effected overnight, it follows that long-term concerted effort on the part of the patient and the treatment staff are necessary. Most patients need continual support and encouragement for several years or longer. Furthermore, the likelihood of success is mitigated by the fact that many patients do not remain in treatment until they are rehabilitated, and those who drop out usually relapse to drug abuse.

Although the task of treating contemporary opiate addicts is clearly formidable, it is feasible if realistic expectations of success are maintained. Long-term treatment is indicated. When such treatment is provided, one can expect that patients' day-to-day existence and health will improve as they begin to stabilize their lives and give up hustling "on the street." To what extent long-term treatment leads to successful rehabilitation is the subject of subsequent chapters. Before turning to this topic, however, it is pertinent to delineate methadone maintenance treatment in some detail.

References

1. Primm BJ, Cook DR, Drew J (1981) The problem of addiction in the black community. In Lowinson H, Ruiz P (eds): Substance Abuse: Clinical Problems and Perspectives. Baltimore: Williams & Wilkins, pp 703, 705, 711
2. National Drug Control Strategy (1990) The White House (January). Washington, DC: Superintendent of Documents, p 34
3. Maddux JF, Desmond DP (1981) Careers of Opioid Users. New York: Praeger
4. Nurco DN, Wegner N, Baum H, Makotsky A (1979) A Case Study: Narcotic Addiction Over a Quarter of a Century in a Major American City 1950–1977. NIDA Services Research Report. Rockville: US Department of Health, Education, and Welfare
5. Terry CE, Pellens M (1970) The Opium Problem. Montclair, NJ: Patterson Smith
6. Ball JC, Chambers CD (eds) (1970) The Epidemiology of Opiate Addiction in the United States. Springfield: Charles C Thomas
7. Kozel NJ, Adams EH (1986) Epidemiology of drug abuse: an overview. Science 234:970–974
8. Arif A, Westermeyer J (1990) Methadone in the Management of Opioid Dependence: Programs and Policies Around the World. New York: Praeger

4
Candid Descriptions of the Six Programs

From the outset of the study, it was recognized that detailed descriptions of how numerous methadone maintenance programs operate were needed. Preliminary visits to dozens of sites revealed not only that program characteristics and treatment procedures varied widely among individual programs but that, for the most part, the black box of treatment included a descriptive void as well as research neglect. Furthermore, it was found that city, state, and federal regulations did not reflect what occurred at the programs. At best, these regulations provided rough guidelines to follow; at worst, they were inappropriate or out-of-date bureaucratic rules. In practice, the regulations were often merely heuristic statements about what should be done. Another reason why accurate descriptions seemed necessary was the almost total dearth of publications about how contemporary methadone treatment clinics function, although a few partial program descriptions are available.[1–3] The black box of treatment remained closed.

On-Site Data Collection During 3 Years

To open the black box with respect to methadone maintenance treatment, it was necessary to collect detailed information about how each of the programs operate. This was done through field work at the programs over a 3-year period, including systematic observation of each program, face-to-face interviews with the staff, record reviews, and other on-site data collection procedures as previously described.

Purpose of Program Data Collection

The overall purpose of undertaking on-site data collection about the programs in New York City, Philadelphia, and Baltimore was to describe in detail the operation of each program and to determine the type and amount of treatment provided. The collection of program data, then, involved the classification, description, and measurement of program characteristics as well as determination of the services provided. The day-to-day operation of each of the six programs selected for study is described in this chapter. In later chapters, attention is focused on measurement of the programs and the treatment services they provide to patients.

Description Based on Comprehensive and Supplementary On-Site Visits

The detailed descriptions of the six programs is based on two primary sources of information. The first was the scheduled comprehensive on-site data collection efforts, which included facility surveys, staff interviews, systematic observation (e.g., of patient flow), and compilation of record data. The second source of descriptive information was derived from more informal visits and contacts with the programs. In this regard, it is pertinent to note that dozens of supplementary visits were made to the six programs during the course of the study by one or more members of the research staff. These additional visits to the programs in the three cities served to further substantiate and supplement our knowledge of how each of the methadone programs operate. For example, conversations with the staff and patients often clarified questions about how treatment procedures were implemented or services were provided. Observation about dispensing procedures and urinalysis arrangements provided further information about the coordination of treatment services.

Treatment Policies and Procedures

As the data collection trips and other visits continued over the years, it became apparent that methadone maintenance programs varied not only in their overall characteristics; they differed fundamentally in their treatment orientation. It was found that the programs had diverse objectives and rationales for treatment. Some programs were committed to short-term treatment and subsequent detoxification of patients. Others believed in long-term maintenance and social rehabilitation. Still others emphasized medical or psychiatric aspects of treatment.

Detailed Descriptions

Each of the six programs is described in detail in the remainder of the chapter. The delineation of each treatment domain and its overall functioning includes consideration of designated topics: treatment setting or neighborhood, physical facility, aggregate patient population, treatment policy, role of director and key staff, admission procedure, methadone dispensing procedures, patient flow in the clinic, security at the site, medical services provided, urinalysis procedure, counseling services available, and special features of each program.

There are several points to be noted about the program descriptions. The first is that the objective of the descriptions is to accurately portray each program in operational terms—how it functions on a day-to-day basis. Second, the purpose of the descriptions is not to engage in invidious comparisons among the programs. Rather, the intent is to portray different types of programs in some detail in order to emphasize the diverse treatment policies and procedure encompassed within this modality of treatment. A third point about the portrayals is that the unique aspects of particular programs as well as the general aspects of methadone maintenance treatment are considered in each report. The general descriptions provide a heuristic framework for discussing how programs carry out major treatment functions. Thus in one description the provision of medical services may be delineated in detail whereas in another attention is focused on counseling services. Although in each case the descriptions are detailed accounts of what occurred at the programs, it should not be inferred that these descriptions are measurements of the services provided.

A fourth, more analytical point follows, i.e., that a detailed or candid description of how programs operate is different from the measurement and analysis of treatment domain and service delivery variables. The latter undertaking is the topic of subsequent chapters. A fifth point is that the individual programs are not named and the respective cities are not identified, thereby maintaining the confidentiality of the information collected.

A Word to the Program Directors and Staff

Because the program staffs opened their programs to intimate inspection and otherwise graciously assisted this project in innumerable ways over the years, it is only courteous to explain why unseemly or unfavorable aspects of these programs are included in the descriptions of the individual programs. There are two reasons.

The first reason for including descriptions of unseemly material (e.g., noting dirty bathrooms, overcrowded conditions, or lack of medical staff) is accuracy and verisimilitude. These unfavorable aspects of methadone maintenance programs exist, and there is an obligation to portray the programs accurately—not to embellish the favorable aspects or ignore the unfavorable.

The second reason for describing unflattering aspects of the programs, along with the more favorable aspects, is to inform the public of the difficult conditions and circumstances under which the programs operate. So long as the public, interested professionals, and officials are misinformed about the programmatic realities of methadone maintenance treatment (e.g., as erroneous talk continues about "Cadillac programs" and "comprehensive care") and therefore fail to comprehend the scope and nature of assistance required, it is unlikely that methadone maintenance treatment will be improved. This second reason is the driving force behind the realistic program descriptions.

Still, a word is in order to the program directors. After carefully considering comments about these descriptions from an earlier draft, the descriptions remain largely unaltered, as significant changes would interfere with the overall process of portraying the programs as we found them.

But, the overall tenor of these six reports does not sufficiently convey the staff dedication and ongoing accomplishments effected at the programs on a day-to-day basis in providing treatment to this difficult population of addict patients. Nonetheless, some indication of this staff commitment is evident in the six descriptions that follow.

The Six Programs

*Program 1: Metrocare**

Treatment Setting

Metrocare is located on a busy commercial side street in Metrocity. This methadone maintenance program is a free-standing clinic that is open 7 days a week to a heterogeneous patient population. The program was established more than 10 years ago by the director, who perceived a need for methadone maintenance treatment in this part of the city. Since then the program has grown and expanded until it now is one of the largest in the city.

The neighborhood in which the clinic operates is a commercial warehouse area adjacent to a major thoroughfare leading to metrocity. The clinic is located in the middle of a side street off this thoroughfare, but traffic is also heavy on this street. Along the street are warehouses and similar establishments. The street is active during the day, with trucks coming and going, pedestrians passing by, and patients arriving by car, truck, and on foot. Counselors from the clinic occasionally patrol the immediate neighborhood to prevent patients from loitering.

Facility

The Metrocare building is formidable in appearance. The one-story warehouse-type building makes a fortress-like impression: Barbed wire and razor wires cover the roof, and an oscillating video camera is located above the steel front door. The outside of the brick and concrete building is drab, massive and obviously maintained with a keen concern for security. In the latter regard, there is a fenced-in and padlocked parking space alongside the clinic for some ten staff cars.

---

*Metrocare is a fictitious name; the other five programs have also been given such names. In subsequent chapters, different orders or different designations of the six programs are provided to ensure confidentiality of the treatment domain and outcome data

There are no notable deficiencies in the building. The roof did not appear to leak, and there were no holes in the walls or other major problems. The building, however, gave the impression of being fenced in and run down.

The fortress-like impression continues as one enters the building. There are interlocking doors (i.e., one door cannot be opened without the other being closed) that lead into a large reception and waiting area. The center of this large room is dominated by a circular counter behind which two or more security clerks sit; they face the entrance and control the flow of patients into and out of the clinic. Three toilet rooms occupy one side of the reception area; they are utilized by patients when providing urine specimens. Benches along the other side of the reception room are used by patients waiting for admission or by visitors accompanying patients to the clinic. Adjoining the large reception area are three dispensing stations.

The interior of the building is clean but it still makes a sort of decrepit impression. Once one gets out of this central area, the rooms are small, and every bit of space is utilized. Counselors have private offices (just enough room for a desk and a side chair), and they have names on their office doors. In many of the offices, the wall dividers do not go all the way to the ceiling, so privacy is minimal.

As in most methadone maintenance programs, there are four functional areas in the clinic: (1) dispensing area, (2) counseling offices, (3) medical rooms; and (4) administrative area. The dispensing area is described later.

One-half of the counselors' offices are located toward the front of the building near the large central waiting room. This front counseling area includes the head counselor's office, a small waiting room with six seats and a children's playroom. This last room is attractively decorated and contains toys for young children; it is utilized while mothers obtain treatment at the clinic. The rear counseling offices are more isolated from the other parts of the clinic.

The space devoted to medical services consists of two offices and a small waiting room. The two offices—which also serve as examining rooms—are occupied by the physicians' assistants (PAs) and a part-time physician. The physician's room is small and crowded, but the room used by the PAs is larger. Both rooms have an examining table and computer terminal.

The main administrative area is located in the rear of the clinic, down a hallway from the main waiting room. This area consists of a large open office with two desks, a table, files, and a photocopying machine. Through this large office area is the director's and administrator's office. The two share one large office, which is also utilized as a computer station by various staff (there is a shortage of space in the building).

At the rear of the central office a door leads to a narrow file-filled hallway and then to a file room with a desk. On the other side of the director's office is a large conference room that is utilized for staff meetings and, when not so used, for clerical work or other clinic functions.

The physical quarters are crowded and inadequate for this large methadone maintenance program. The clinic is virtually bursting at the seams, with all available space utilized.

PATIENTS*

Metrocare treats addict patients who come to the clinic from throughout the city; most are private, paying patients who are not local residents. Almost 50 percent of the patients have been in treatment less than 1 year, but one-fifth have been in their current methadone maintenance for 5 years or longer. Most of the patients are white, although there also is a sizable black and Hispanic population. As is common elsewhere, about three-fourths of the patients are male.

TREATMENT POLICY

Metrocare functions as a methadone dispensing clinic that also provides ancillary medical and counseling services. The program emphasizes overall efficiency of operation, especially dispensing and medical services. Long-term methadone maintenance is the principal regimen, but detoxification is also available.

As with other methadone clinics, definite rules and regulations have been promulgated for patients. These rules address such matters as selling methadone, loss of take-home methadone, handing in counterfeit urine specimens, disorderly behavior in the clinic, attendance at scheduled time and days, loitering outside the clinic, return of empty take-home medication bottles, and providing urine specimens. Infractions of these rules are cause for staff admonition, reduction of methadone dosage, or dismissal from the program.

DIRECTOR AND PROGRAM STAFF

The director of Metrocare is a physician who established this methadone maintenance program more than 10 years ago. He is an active director who is continually involved in both administrative and treatment issues at the clinic.

The director functions as medical supervisor of the program. In this capacity he supervises the PAs, part-time physician, and other relevant staff on medical matters. Furthermore, as a physician he sees some patients for evaluation and treatment.

In addition to supervising medical care, the director also is responsible for the overall treatment policy and procedures of the clinic. In these re-

---

*Program staffs commonly refer to their census members as either patients or clients. For consistency the term patient is used throughout this text.

gards, he serves more as a policy setter and decision maker than as a day-to-day administrator.

The treatment staff at Metrocare, in addition to the director, consists of counselors, a supervisory counselor, dispensing nurses, a part-time physician, PAs, and an administrative staff. This last group of employees includes an administrator, administrative-secretary, office secretary, and part-time clerks. This last group includes desk clerks employed to provide administrative assistance and security in the reception area of the clinic.

Admission of New Patients

The basic requirement for admission is that a patient have at least a 1-year history of opiate addiction. If the patient is transferring from another treatment facility, documentation of his last status at that program is required. Efforts are made to exclude persons who might disrupt the clinic because of violence, drug sales, or other deviant behavior.

There is no waiting list for admission to Metrocare. The admission procedure operates as follows. First, the interested patient phones the clinic and is told when he can come in. When the patient arrives he is referred to whichever counselor is available. At the first visit, current drug use and treatment history information are recorded and a supervised urine specimen obtained. Personal identification is also checked closely to prevent misrepresentation or concurrent methadone maintenance treatment. Finally, the patient is interviewed by a member of the administrative staff or one of the senior counselors. If a medical problem is suspected, the patient is seen by the physician.

The next stage of admission takes place 1 to 2 days later when the patient sees a counselor to complete forms and provide a psychosocial history. The patient then is seen by the physician and is given a physical examination. His current drug abuse status is ascertained, and he is prescribed an initial dose of methadone, which he then receives from the dispensing nurse.

Methadone Dispensing

Oral methadone is dispensed to patients at three nursing stations. Each station consists of a small open-topped room in which a nurse sits behind a counter with a computer terminal. Patients enter one at a time and sit down behind a low counter facing the dispensing nurse. Two large metal coffee containers, holding Tang or water, stand on the counter. Each patient gives the nurse his (or her) identification card. She enters his name and number in the terminal to determine if there are any special instructions to be given, if not, she orders his medication which is mechanically dispensed into a small paper cup. After adding juice or water to this liquid methadone, the patient drinks the dose and leaves the clinic. In addition to methadone, these nurses dispense other medications: Antabuse, INH, rifampin, and psychotropic drugs in appropriate cases.

The three dispensing stations operate simultaneously and independently, as each room has a computer terminal and an automated methadone dispensing machine. Consequently, there is a minimum of waiting time for patients.

Role of Nurses

The principal role of nurses at Metrocare is to dispense oral methadone to patients who enter the three small dispensing offices that adjoin the central reception room. Each nurse is busy when on shift in her small dispensing station office where she sits by a computer terminal and enters data to effect dispensing and patient monitoring.

In addition to dispensing, nurses perform an important monitoring function for the clinic, as they serve as a control point for patient compliance. Patient fee payments, appointment schedules, test results (e.g., urine specimens positive for illicit substances), and similar information are noted by the nurse from the terminal screen at the time of medication dispensing. If there is a "hold" on a patient, he cannot receive his methadone medication until he has completed the assigned service (e.g., counseling appointment). She informs him of this fact and tells him what he must do before he can be given the methadone. An important part of this monitoring function is the collection of patient fees. Private patients pay $42 per week for treatment, and the nurses record and keep track of these payments through the online computer system. Inasmuch as nurses are primarily engaged in dispensing and related duties at this program, most medical care is provided by the physician and PAs.

Patient Flow in the Clinic

Two interlocking vestibules lead from the street entrance into the dispensing area. They are monitored by a video screen system that scans the sidewalk approaches to the building as well as the street and adjacent parking lot. The interlocking doors are controlled by an attendant, who sits behind a counter that is in the center of the large waiting room. Patients are "buzzed" into the clinic, and there is continuous observation of their behavior as they enter or leave.

After the clinic opens and the first patients are checked in by the attendants at the central counter, the patients form a single line in front of the three dispensing offices to receive their methadone. While in line awaiting their morning medication, the patients are active and talkative. They joke or complain to each other, speak to the counter attendants, greet those coming or going, and otherwise pass the short time they spend standing in line (usually 5 to 10 minutes).

On one side of this large central waiting area are three toilet rooms: two for men and one for women. These rooms are used to obtain urine specimens from designated patients before they receive medication. Although most urine specimens are not directly observed, the bottles are checked for warmth. In addition, an attendant or counselor is available if direct supervision is required.

The overall daily patient flow then occurs as follows. Patients are buzzed into a large waiting area by an attendant; this waiting room is the central patient contact and control area of the clinic. The attendants who sit or stand behind the main semicircular counter direct patient flow into and out of the clinic by buzzing patients through the vestibule doors, checking them in, handing them urine bottles or take-home medication labels, and otherwise monitoring patient flow. The desk workers usually know the patients by name. From this central waiting area the patients proceed to one of the medication offices.

These two front desk attendants are continually busy checking patients in and out, as well as checking on take-home labels, urine drop lists, and similar matters. This waiting room control station also serves as a communication center as the main outside telephone answering service occurs here. A bulletin board on the wall behind the central desk provides space for clinic notices and messages; patients also obtain forms here for Medicaid payments or wait in this area for appointments with counselors or other staff. This large waiting room in the front of the clinic is, then, the area in which the greatest patient flow and activity occurs. During the busiest dispensing hours there may be 25 patients in this room.

Medical Services

Medical services at this large methadone maintenance program are provided by the PAs and physician. In addition, the medical director of the program evaluates difficult patients and provides some medical supervision.

Medical coverage at this program is generally provided throughout the day. The PAs are available on a full-time basis, and the part-time physician is on site every weekday. As a consequence, there is overlapping medical coverage, which enables the PAs and the physician to coordinate their treatment by exchanging clinical information and advice.

The two PAs and the physician are actively engaged in providing direct medical coverage at Metrocare. The medical coverage provided is continuous, coordinated (as between the PAs and physicians), and integrated with the overall treatment program. With regard to this point, the medical staff is able to supervise and coordinate the daily delivery of numerous services. One PA listed 24 medical services he commonly provides to patients. These orders or instructions are transmitted on-line to the nurses and other program staff. These 24 medical services provided through online computer coordination are as follows.

1. Change dose
2. Monitor attendance
3. Referral to venereal disease clinic

4. Referral for chest radiograph
5. Check positive or negative result of PPD
6. Relay medical information, i.e., pick-up prescription from clinic physician (or PA), instruction to patient for taking medication
7. Notification of abnormal laboratory results
8. Order supervised urine specimen for toxicology
9. Allow special take-home bottle (methadone)
10. Build up methadone dose
11. Detoxify patient (decrease dosage)
12. Hold dosage
13. Evaluate (by nurse) for signs of intoxification, sedation (oversedation)
14. Refer patient to counselor because of behavioral issue (drug abuse, clinical behavior)
15. Produce written verification of follow-up with VD clinic, chest clinic (positive PPD), psychiatric consultation
16. Referral to physician specialist: liver dysfunction
17. Notification of appointment for physical examination at this clinic
18. Order regarding permanent pick-up schedule
19. Urgent reminder to nurse regarding allergy to medication (e.g., penicillin, PPD, tetanus)
20. Physician identifies assigned counselor for patient
21. Notification that patient must have Papanicolaou smear by nurse
22. Reminder to nurse that patient is a "seizure patient"
23. Reminder to nurse to dispense Antabuse with methadone
24. Caution that patient may not be drinking methadone

Urinalysis

Urine specimens are collected from patients once a week. The laboratory that does the analyses prepares a computer-generated random list for each day of the week. (The problem with having the laboratory generate this list is that it is often about a week or two behind in terms of the current census at the program.) When the patient comes in for his medication, the person at the front desk checks to see if his name is on the urine specimen list for that day. If his name is on the list, the patient goes into the bathroom alone to provide a specimen. The specimen is provided either before or after the methadone has been received. (The laboratory provides two labels for each person with different days on each label. Thus if the patient misses one day there is a backup day for obtaining the specimen.)

According to the administrator, the urine results are discussed in weekly meetings. Urine bottle labels of patients who failed to provide specimens on a given day are picked up by the patients' counselors. Each counselor is supposed to find out why the specimen was not provided by his patient. The next specimen is then to be supervised. If a pattern of missed specimens (or positive specimens) persists, the patient is likely to lose whatever take-home privileges he has. If the drug of abuse is heroin, his methadone dose is likely to be increased. If the patient is abusing some other drug, detoxification may be begun if psychotherapeutic intervention fails.

The three bathrooms located near the dispensing area are not overly clean and smell of urine; in part, this condition is due to the high frequency of use of these toilets. Urine specimens are supervised (i.e., observed) when a counselor requests it.

Urine specimens are tested for all of the major drugs of abuse as well as for methadone compliance. The turnaround time on a routine test is less than 48 hours. When the laboratory results are returned, they are distributed to the appropriate counselors who are responsible for charting them.

Counseling Services

The counseling staff is composed of both men and women whose mean age is in the midthirties. Most of the counselors are not college graduates; none has an advanced degree. These counselors do, however, have several years of experience in the addiction field but considerably less experience at this program.

The counselors perform the intake screenings and admission processing, an activity that demands a large portion of their working time. They also provide case management for a sizable caseload of patients. In this program, caseload management is more of an administratively oriented than a treatment-oriented task. Thus, although casework management commonly involves monitoring urine tests, filing reports, documenting services, and providing individual counseling, there is little emphasis on treatment planning, coordinated implementation, or periodic case reviews. The individual counseling sessions are used primarily for disciplinary issues or crisis intervention. Patients are discussed at the weekly staff meetings but usually only with regard to program rule infractions. There is no group therapy practiced, but there are several regular Alcoholics Anonymous and Narcotics Anonymous meetings held at this site.

The counselors at Metrocare include two who have responsibility for determining patient fees and otherwise addressing the task of obtaining funds for the clinic from patients or third parties. Another counselor is the vocational-education coordinator; she refers patients to outside employment or educational agencies. Lastly, with respect to specialized functions, one counselor is in charge of the 21-day detoxification regimen.

The counselors in this clinic work in overcrowded, congested conditions; the patients have free access to the rear of the clinic once they are past the reception area. Though each counselor is assigned to an individual office, there is inadequate privacy, as most of the offices have open-topped partitions. The offices are tiny and usually barren of decoration or personal effects. All of the offices are equipped with a desk and chair for the counselor and another chair for a patient, which is all that space allows. Though there are telephones and an interoffice communications system, much of the interaction among staff occurs simply by speaking directly to each other from room to room. The atmosphere thus limits the personal and confidential aspects of counseling.

Special Features of the Program

The operation of this large clinic is certainly facilitated by an on-line computer system that enables staff to monitor patient attendance, dispensing, and other treatment services provided. This unique system ties the dispensing, medical, and administrative staff together by providing a coordinated means of monitoring and implementing patient care. (The counseling staff is less integrated into the system as there are no terminals for this staff group.) The daily care of individual patients is coordinated throughout the clinic; each patient's attendance, dosage, urine results, counseling status, and medical needs can be readily ascertained through the on-line data system, and this computer system is actively used by the staff.

Conclusion

This free-standing private clinic is highly organized. Program policy, treatment services, and administrative procedures are determined by the director. Although the available resources are being efficiently utilized, this clinic struggles to provide adequate services in a climate of severe fiscal constraint. Both the physical plant and the staffing could be upgraded to provide an improved treatment setting.

The principal emphasis at this program is on the efficient dispensing of oral methadone to patients who, for the most part, are engaged in full-time employment. In fulfilling this dispensing function, the program is exceedingly effective. Indeed, it might well serve as a model in this regard.

Whereas this program has an outstanding dispensing system, it places less emphasis on rehabilitative services. As a consequence, the treatment and rehabilitative needs of many patients are less adequately addressed. This lack applies especially to underclass patients whose needs are pervasive as well as to addict mothers and their children. (This observation about the limited care that addict mothers and their children receive applies to all programs studied.)

Program 2: City Clinic

Treatment Setting

The City Clinic methadone program provides daily outpatient service to some 250 patients in a commercial area of Metrocity. The clinic is part of a larger agency, although it operates independently in that it has its own policy and procedures. The clinic has been in continuous operation for some 12 years, although its location, staff, and policy has changed considerably over the years.

There have been a number of changes at this clinic during the past 2 years. At the time of our first on-site staff interviews and program data collection in 1985, a new assistant director had just been appointed. Inasmuch as this full-time person managed most of the clinic operations, it was a period of transition. Shortly after, the clinic was moved to new quarters. The assistant director then became acting director as well as continuing in his prior role as clinic manager.

There have thus been major changes in both staff and facilities during the past year. The move from one building to another was accomplished without significant disruption of treatment services. The change in directorship, however, is likely to have a more pervasive influence on the treatment philosophy of the program over the course of the next few years if the new director changes the present treatment policy.

The clinic is located on a main street near center city. Most of the nearby buildings on the street are stores, other city agencies, and similar establishments. The side streets adjacent to the clinic are slum neighborhoods consisting of mixed residential and warehouse properties.

Inasmuch as this clinic is located on a busy center city street, there is little involvement with the local community. Indeed, in this zone of transition there is minimal community organization evident.

Physical Facility

The building is a renovated two-story structure with an entrance on Main Street. The front of the building is newly painted. Small lettering on the glass front door indicates hours of operation and sponsorship of the two clinics in the building. The only parking available is at metered locations on a main street.

Patients

More than 80 percent of the 250 patients at City Clinic were black; the remainder were mostly white with a small Hispanic representation. As in most methadone programs, most of the patients were male, some three-fourths in this instance.

Treatment Policy

The treatment goal of this clinic has been to encourage patients on methadone to detoxify and become drug-free. Methadone is seen, then, as a means of effecting a transition from heroin addiction on the street to a drug-free-lifestyle. Therefore, long-term methadone maintenance is not encouraged. Instead, methadone substitution is advocated as a transition stage during which patients are encouraged to give up illicit drugs, stop their criminal behavior and, as soon as feasible, start gradual detoxification from methadone.

Clinic Rules and Regulations

All methadone clinics have stated rules and regulations that provide a framework for clinic operations. These rules and regulations differ by city and state as well as by individual clinic because various city and state regulations are superimposed on the omnipresent federal Food and Drug Administration regulations, and these local administrative procedures are interpreted and supplemented by the staff at each clinic.

At City Clinic, a handbook has been prepared to inform patients of current clinic rules and procedures. These rules constitute the operational procedures for effecting social control and the provision of services at the clinic. The handbook consists of several pages of rules pertaining to clinic operations that patients are expected to read and follow. They are required to acknowledge by signature their understanding and willingness to comply with these rules as a condition of admission to treatment.

Some three dozen rules pertaining to patient behavior and clinic policy are enumerated in the handbook. These rules refer to: intake requirements; keeping appointments; not missing methadone medication; drinking their liquid methadone dose in front of the nurse; how medication changes are to be made; how to inform the staff when prescribed medication other than methadone has been taken; that there is a 4-week grace period after admission to effect clean urine specimens; that a urine sample must be provided once a week; that no take-home methadone is allowed for the first 90 days; that take-home containers are not replaced if lost or stolen; the requirement to obey counselor or medical staff; if hospitalized or incarcerated, the need to have these institutions call to obtain confirmation of the dose; that methadone medication will be refused if the patient is under the influence of drugs or alcohol; the need to report an address change immediately; the need to present medical assistance card or to pay directly for methadone; the need to report expected absences to clinic; no loitering around building; outsiders cannot be brought to the clinic; that drug dealing, numbers taking, or other illegal activities are not permitted in the clinic; that patients must swallow their methadone dose when it is dispensed; evidence of sale of methadone is cause for dismissal; no weapons in clinic; violent behavior is not acceptable, including fights and misbehavior in the nearby community; assaults by patients must be reported to the police; pregnant patients must be temporarily transferred to a family clinic; prior notice must be given to make arrangements for out-of-town medication; no children are allowed at the medication window; all empty take-home bottles must be returned intact; how disputes between patients and staff are to be resolved; procedures for appeal of decisions of clinic staff; punishment designated for unauthorized absences, dirty urine specimens, and other non-compliant behavior.

The policy and organization of this methadone program promotes low-dose methadone medication, strict compliance with clinic rules, and a standardized professional approach to treatment and rehabilitation. In the last regard, treatment tends to be viewed as categorical services provided to patients (e.g., that patients have a contractual obligation to fulfill their part of the bargain by adhering to rules and "getting themselves together"). In this approach there is a legalistic emphasis on adhering to numerous rules along with a corresponding desire to utilize these rules as a socializing force to instill acceptable values and promote a law-abiding and productive life style.

Director and Program Staff

The treatment staff at City Clinic consists of the director, counselors, dispensing staff, two part-time physicians, and two secretary-clerks. There are no nurse practitioners or physicians' assistants at this program. Uniformed guards provide security at the front entrance.

The acting director of this clinic is a social worker who has assumed his new role from the former physician director. The new director had several prior years of experience at this clinic as a social worker. As a consequence of his former role as counselor, the director still carries a considerable caseload. He is, then, definitely involved in the direct provision of treatment as he works half-time or more as a counselor.

At the time of our second program data collection, the new director had not yet been officially appointed as director, though the former director had left 5 months before. As a consequence of this situation, the acting director was filling two positions: his official position as assistant director and his current role as acting director.

Patients and Admission Procedure

During the prior year, some 150 patients were admitted to methadone maintenance treatment at this clinic. These admissions were coordinated by a secretary-clerk who served as the intake worker.

According to the intake worker, patients are eligible for methadone if they are older than 18, are addicted to opiates, have a verifiable 1-year addiction history, and are currently addicted. The intake worker does not maintain a waiting list. A prospective patient calls or comes in and requests methadone treatment. The prospective patient is asked to provide a urine specimen and is then given an appointment to see the intake worker, social worker, and physician. These appointments are scheduled for a future date when the urinalysis results will be available to these staff.

When the new admission meets with the intake worker, she obtains required information from him, including the clinic's initial intake form and other required data. At this time, the patient is given information about the urine test policy and other rules and regulations of the program. The patient is then enrolled in the program and assigned a clinic number.

The patient's next meeting is with a counselor. The counselor completes a psychosocial history and prepares a treatment plan. Finally, the patient sees a physician, who completes a physical examination and prescribes the dose of methadone to be dispensed at the clinic. After seeing the physician the patient is ready to start his methadone medication. The admission process takes, on an average, four working days.

Dispensing

Dispensing is carried out by a staff of three, but on the date of our visit only two were working; one of the two functioned as the dispensary supervisor. Duties of the dispensing staff included scheduling medical appointments in addition to dispensing methadone.

The dispensary is a single room with ample counter space and one desk. Methadone is dispensed through a window with a plexiglass barrier. Access to the urine observation area is through the pharmacy. The dispensing staff is not responsible for monitoring urine collection; which is done by the counseling staff. This arrangement required counselors and other nonmedical staff to frequently enter the dispensing area. There were, then, a number of intrusions into the dispensary by outside staff. Although a lock on the dispensary door forced people to knock to get in, there was no obvious discrimination as to who on the staff had authorization to enter.

The dispensing procedure is straightforward. Patients are identified visually by the staff member, who hands each patient the prescribed dose. In addition, patients' names are on a daily alphabetical computer printout that lists their dose and take-home medication order. This printout is clear and easily understandable. Each patient's medication is prepared from Methadone Diskettes dissolved in warm water and orange drink. The liquid dose is given to the patient, who can add more water from a pitcher. Patients are required to speak to the dispensing staff person before leaving to ensure ingestion of their dose. The dispensing staff then initials the record to document administration of the methadone dose.

Patient Flow and Security

Patients enter the clinic from Main Street by a glass door that leads into a small waiting room (vestibule). A uniformed guard sits in this room, but there are no other seats available, so patients stand about while waiting to be admitted to the dispensing area.

This outer waiting room is active during dispensing hours. Patients give the guard their names and await their turn for medication. During the early morning (7–8 a.m.) patients who have jobs are medicated first. Those without jobs who nonetheless arrive early wait until 8 a.m. for medication, whereas others without jobs or on later schedules receive their doses after this hour.

The guard calls patients by name to proceed through a door to the dispensing window, which is some 20 feet away down a main central hallway. The guard has a small window in the wall through which he can observe patients in the hallway.

At the dispensing window the patient is identified by the dispenser and then signs for his medication. He is given a small paper cup that contains the dissolved methadone dose mixed with orange juice concentrate. Each patient drinks it while facing the dispenser and then leaves this area and goes back out the main entrance.

The time usually spent in the dispensing area is brief—about 5 minutes. Patients spend more time at the clinic if they have an appointment with their counselors or have other business pertaining to treatment.

Sometimes the vestibule and area in front of the dispensary are crowded, which occurs when numerous patients arrive for medication simultaneously, as at midday. Some patients loiter about on the sidewalk outside the clinic before or after medication; this activity is mostly ordinary conversation to be expected among people who share outpatient treatment on a daily basis.

Security personnel at the clinic consists of a uniformed guard who sits in the vestibule. He is not part of the clinic staff but is hired from an outside company.

Medical Services

Medical coverage at the clinic is provided by two part-time physicians, both of whom are general practitioners. One is new to the program and had no prior experience treating drug abusers. The other has been at this clinic for more than 5 years.

The two part-time physicians provide all of the medical coverage at the clinic, as there are no other medical staff who provide treatment (excluding dispensing). It is relevant to note that a psychiatrist at a nearby clinic does see one patient a week on referral from the clinic.

Urinalysis

Patients are supposed to provide a urine specimen for drug testing once a week. Two staff members confided, however, that patients are now being asked to provide only one specimen every 2 weeks. This change apparently was made for budgetary reasons. In addition, the drop schedule is supposed to be randomly drawn by computer, but it too does not seem to be the case. Thus it is common knowledge in the clinic that Tuesday is urine day. For the 2 weeks during which we collected data, 72% and 88% of the samples, respectively, were collected on Tuesday.

Two urine collection rooms are located next to the dispensary. The rooms (one for men and one for women) are clean and well lit. There is a two-way mirror in each room through which a staff member can observe the process. The observation room is entered via the dispensary. (Urine specimens were not being collected on the relevant on-site data collection day, so it was not possible to assess how closely urine drops are monitored.)

When a patient's name is drawn for a urine sample, two consecutive dates are generated for that sample to be given. If the patient is unable to provide a urine sample on the first day, he still is medicated. On the subsequent day the patient cannot get medicated without having provided a sample. If a patient has two positive urine samples in a row, his methadone dose is decreased by 5 mg.

Urine specimens are tested for all of the major substances: opiates, methadone, barbiturates, amphetamines, benzodiazepines, propoxyphene, cocaine, PCP, and alcohol. The turnaround time on a routine test is 1 day. When the laboratory data are returned the results are sent to the counselors and are filed in the "urine book," after which they are sent to a central office downtown to be entered into the computer. (The urine book is somewhat out of date, and some patients who have left the program are still in it. According to one dispenser, the only positive urine specimens that are taken seriously are ones for opiates and cocaine.)

Role of Counselors

The counseling staff consists of about an equal number of men and women. Their mean age is in the midthirties. Most of these counselors have advanced degrees as well as several years of experience at this program.

The counselors provide primary case management for their caseloads, and they function with a great deal of autonomy in their delivery of services to patients. With respect to admissions, patients first see the intake worker, who then assigns the patient to a counselor, usually on the basis of availability of slots in his caseload. The counselor then prepares a psychosocial history and develops and initiates a treatment plan. Patients are scheduled for biweekly counseling sessions but often see their counselors more frequently for brief contacts (e.g., checking in about clinic business, exchanging greetings, to complain, to ask a question).

Counselors at the City Clinic have considerable individual autonomy as they perform their casework and individual counseling on the basis of their personal philosophy and prior training rather than according to articulated clinic policy. Consequently, patients at this clinic receive counseling oriented toward principles of psychiatry, social work, or humanistic counseling depending on the counselor to whom they are assigned. Although this diversity of counseling approaches could provide for individualized treatment that matches patient needs with counselors' capabilities, such an arrangement would require selective assignment to predesignated counselors as well as an overall clinic-wide procedure for the systematic delivery of designated counseling services (i.e., particular types of individual counseling) to designated patients (in this and other programs.) Because such a coordinated system is lacking, the diversity of counseling provided is more akin to that of numerous private practices operating under the same roof. At the same time, there often is informal matching of patients and counselors on various bases, but it is ad hoc.

The counselors' independent autonomy leads to occasional lack of coordination of clinic services. Some treatment services are duplicated, overlapping, or absent. For example, counselors can, and do, request medical consultations from the clinic physicians, but so can the patients. As a consequence, a physician may change or restrict the patient's medication without the counselor's knowledge. This situation can, and does, result in conflicting instructions to the dispensing staff.

A recent move to a new building is viewed by the counselors as an improvement. Thus there has been a significant improvement in the morale among the counselors since last year. The counselors' offices are now grouped in a closed off (separated by a door) section of the building that restricts patient access to them. This change has eliminated a former problem of congestion in the hallways as well as frequent interruptions of counseling sessions by patients who were waiting for other services. Each of the counselors' offices is equipped with a desk, telephone, and several chairs. The offices are pleasantly decorated by each counselor.

Management of the Program

A considerable part of the budgetary and administrative aspects of running the clinic is performed off-site at a central agency. The director is therefore only semiautonomous with respect to hiring and firing and otherwise running the clinic. At the same time, this outside support and direction has provided a highly trained counseling and dispensing staff.

With regard to the management of the treatment staff, the clinic is without a permanent director and otherwise in a period of transition. How long this transitory status will continue remains to be seen, as does the future policy and direction of the program. The principal forces likely to determine this future policy are the ideas of the new director and the direction provided by the sponsoring agency.

Conclusion

During the 3-year period of study, it was found that a principal treatment emphasis at City Clinic was the provision of methadone to patients in order to reduce their opiate dependence. The expectation was that short-term methadone maintenance would be followed by detoxification and social rehabilitation. This observation is not meant to downplay the significance of the counseling or medical services that were also provided, but to note the general primacy of the methadone dispensing function at the clinic.

Program 3: MedPsych

Treatment Setting

MedPsych is a large drug abuse treatment program in Metrocity. In addition to some 250 male and female methadone maintenance patients who constitute the bulk of the program's census, detoxification and drug-free services are also provided to other drug abuse patients. The program is publicly funded, although it is affiliated with a local civic organization that provides some ancillary referral services and other support.

The clinic was established some 15 years ago and has been in operation continuously since that time, although the organization, treatment policy, and staffing patterns have undergone numerous changes. It should be regarded as one of the more stable and successful programs in the city (i.e., "successful" in the sense of providing continuous service to a difficult population of patients and still enduring). In this regard, several programs in this city have closed during the prior decade.

The clinic is located on a busy main street in a commercial neighborhood with heavy vehicular and pedestrian traffic. Most of the nearby buildings on the block are stores or small commercial establishments.

Physical Facility

This treatment facility has recently been remodeled and refurbished throughout. As a consequence, it is an unusually clean, attractive, and modern facility. Furthermore, it is spacious and well designed for this treatment modality. There are adequate waiting rooms for patients and appropriate low counters between patients in the waiting room and supervising secretary-clerks (instead of walls with peepholes or metal grills), and the dispensing area is designed for its function. The entire two-story building is occupied solely by this treatment program.

There are four distinct functional areas to the building. The first area consists of two large waiting rooms and the dispensing station. The second area consists of counseling rooms; these offices are well appointed and equipped with telephones.

The third area consists of administrative and physicians' offices, including the director's office as well as another for his secretary, the fee collection clerk's office, and that of the medical records supervisor. Two doctors' offices as well as one for another secretary are located in this area.

Fourth, there is the second story area that consists of a large conference room, staff lounge room, a children's playroom, and two large observation-type rooms that overlook the dispensing area. At present, these observation or group therapy rooms are not being used. There are ample bathrooms for both staff and patients in the building.

A word about security is in order. A uniformed security guard checks patients into the front waiting room, and another sits in the dispensing area to regulate and monitor the identification cards used for dispensing. Therefore the admittance-dispensing area is not locked during methadone-dispensing hours, but the adjacent counseling, medical, and administrative offices are closed off or locked so patients cannot wander through the rest of the building. At the same time, the ambience of the clinic is such that there is congenial patient–staff interaction in many parts of the clinic.

Patients

The 250 methadone maintenance patients are about equally divided as to race (i.e., one-half black and one-half white), and three-fourths are men. About one-third of the patient census had been in treatment less than 1 year. During the prior year there were more than 200 methadone maintenance admissions.

Treatment Policy and Procedures

The medical director of this program is heavily invested in the operation of the clinic and provision of services to patients. As a psychiatrist who specializes in the treatment of drug abusers, he has developed and implemented the overall treatment philosophy of the program. Most addicts are seen as having immature personalities characterized by a desire for immediate gratification and a corresponding inability to pursue realistic goals in life. The genesis of these personality problems is seen to be in early deficiencies in family dynamics, which lead to faulty upbringing. Therefore appropriate treatment seeks to address these personality deficiencies. It is done through psychiatric diagnosis, supervised psychosocial counseling, and the provision of necessary medication.

The psychiatric orientation of the clinic is evident in both the diagnostic emphasis and the follow-up treatment procedures implemented at the clinic. A psychiatric evaluation is a requirement of admission, and each patient's progress in treatment and medication regimen is closely supervised by the medical director. Long-term detoxification through methadone maintenance (i.e., in 6 months) has been a goal of this program for many years, but recently longer-term maintenance has been permitted.

General Role of the Director

The role of director in a free-standing methadone maintenance program commonly encompasses both in-house and outside responsibilities of considerable scope. On the other hand, if the clinic is part of a larger treatment program, the responsibilities and duties of the director may be considerably reduced.

In the case of a separate unaffiliated methadone maintenance program, the director is responsible for the overall administration of the treatment program. This arena commonly involves preparation and management of the annual budget; hiring, evaluation, and dismissal of personnel; formulating and implementing treatment and other policy; devising and maintaining records of various kinds; and otherwise supervising the staff and, to a lesser degree, the patients. In the latter regard, the extent to which a director becomes directly involved in the provision of treatment depends on numerous considerations, such as his prior training and experience, the size of the program, the type of staff available, and the particular needs of the program.

It is pertinent to note the extensive outside activities program directors may be called on to perform. Of crucial importance is their ability to establish and maintain working relationships with official city and state agencies that audit, inspect, and hopefully support drug treatment programs. Furthermore, most directors are also involved in local affairs that relate to their patients' presence in the clinic's neighborhood. The problem of community opposition to the presence of methadone programs in their neighborhoods is commonplace. (Even other public agencies often prefer not to be associated through close proximity with drug treatment programs that treat heroin addicts.) Directors also deal with the police and other local agencies, particularly nearby hospitals that provide emergency and referral services. In these and other regards, directors are often involved in community and public relations work in order to support or defend their treatment program and its operation.

In addition to in-house administration and outside agency and community commitments, many directors are also involved in professional activities on a city, state, or national level. They may participate in and contribute to professional associations and research efforts.

In sum, then, the responsibilities and duties of methadone maintenance program directors are broad in scope. They vary considerably, however, from program to program depending on the affiliation and characteristics of particular treatment programs.

Director and Staff

The director is an administrator with prior experience in the mental health field. He started as director a few years ago, replacing a long-time incumbent.

The staff at this program can be separated into two categories, treatment staff and administrative staff. The treatment staff of some score of individuals consists of physicians, counselors, nurses, and intake workers. The administrative staff is one-half as numerous and consists of the director, medical records administrator, secretaries, and clerks.

The medical records unit is an important part of the administrative staff. Two record clerks work at the task of preparing and maintaining these records in a separate record room that is of adequate size and well appointed. The record room is at a central location, where it is readily accessible to both clinical and administrative staff.

Admission Procedure

Admissions to the clinic are handled by two intake workers. One works full time and the other works 2 days a week. To be admitted, a patient makes an appointment with the intake worker. At present, the intake worker reports that prospective methadone maintenance patients are seen within 3 to 4 days.

At the initial appointment the patient fills out forms (informed consent, psychosocial history, addiction verification) and gives blood and urine for laboratory studies. The next appointment is set for 2 days later, by which time the laboratory results should have returned. At this second appointment the patient sees a physician for a physical examination and another physician for a psychiatric evaluation. The physicians make the decision regarding the modality of treatment to which the patient will be assigned. (This program offers detoxification as well as drug-free treatment in addition to methadone maintenance.) If the patient is to receive methadone, the first dose is given after the second physician has been seen.

Methadone Dispensing

The dispensary is located in a large room adjacent to an even larger waiting room. A dispensing window and locked door provide access between the two rooms. The large waiting area is under the supervision of a uniformed guard. Patients waiting to be medicated are under observation by this guard at all times. The guard also is in view of the dispensing nurse through the dispensing counter window. The nurses who dispense methadone would be able to call on the guard if any problems arose during the dispensing process. Nurses prepare the individual methadone doses by dissolving diskettes in water and orange drink prior to dispensing. A plexiglass window separates the clients from the nurses but does not prevent communication through this barrier. When patients are admitted to the dispensary waiting room and make themselves known to the nurse, she identifies them by sight and by identification (ID) card; she then hands the cup to the patient, who consumes the mixture while facing the nurse.

In addition to dispensing methadone, nurses collect urine specimens. (In most programs this job is done by counselors or specific urine monitoring staff.) The urine monitoring here is well designed in that nurses observe urine "drops" through a one-way mirror. The urine collection room is adjacent to the dispensary, allowing nurses to monitor urine collections without leaving the medication station.

The dispensary itself is well laid out. All of the material needed to dispense methadone is conveniently arranged and within easy reach of the nurse. Within the dispensing area are two desks that provide ample working area to do paperwork, e.g., calculating methadone inventory and making clinical notations on medication sheets.

Patient Flow and Security

The main entrance to MedPsych is on a busy street running into center city. There are no locked doors through which patients must pass to enter the clinic to receive medication: A swinging door opens into a vestibule that leads to a large waiting room. A security guard is posted at the entrance to this front waiting room to check patients in and out. (He records time in and time out as well as giving each patient his ID card.) Patients waiting for dispensing to begin in the early morning or who have an appointment with a counselor use this large outer waiting room. While seated in this room, male and female patients chat among themselves or talk to the security guard.

During dispensing hours patients without counseling or other appointments proceed to the rear of the building to check in with a second security guard in the dispensing area. He has them sign an attendance card and informs them as to whether they are scheduled to "drop" a urine specimen. Some 40 patients a day (200 per week) provide a urine sample.

After drinking their dose, patients leave the clinic by going back through the main entrance where the security guard checks them out. The dispensing station itself, however, is locked.

Patient flow through the clinic is rapid. For most, the length of stay is 10 minutes (as observed from the guard's tally sheet). If they see a counselor, the time is longer. The atmosphere in the clinic is lively and pleasant. There is considerable talk among patients and between patients and staff.

Medical Services

Two part-time physicians provide medical treatment to the 250 patients at MedPsych. One is a psychiatrist who is also the medical director. The other is an internist who is primarily engaged in performing physical examinations of new admissions and annual examinations of long-stay patients. Inasmuch as the nurses in this program are primarily involved in dispensing methadone, the role of the two doctors is crucial with respect to the provision of psychiatric and medical coverage.

Each of these two doctors has an office behind the dispensing area. As noted, they are part-time employees (less than half-time each), although they are assisted by a full-time secretary. The impact of the medical director on this drug abuse treatment program is considerable, even though he is employed less than half-time. This impact is due to a number of factors. First, he has formulated a comprehensive, yet practical, social-psychiatric treatment rationale that serves the program. In this regard, it is pertinent to note that he has been treating patients at this program for more than 10 years. Second, he has extensive clinical and teaching experience in the field of drug abuse treatment. Third, he provides direct psychiatric treatment to a considerable number of patients at MedPsych. Fourth, he monitors the methadone maintenance patients on a weekly or monthly basis, performing this service in conjunction with the counseling staff.

Urinalysis

At MedPsych urine specimens are routinely collected only from methadone maintenance patients. Each patient is supposed to give one urine specimen per week, and all specimens collected are analyzed. Patients are selected randomly by a computer program, and a list of those who are to provide ("drop") a specimen is given to the nurses. When the patient comes in to pick up his dose of methadone he is told that he must first provide a urine specimen. He enters a bathroom next to the dispensary, and while "dropping" the specimen he is observed by a nurse via a window cut in the wall. If a patient fails to provide a specimen, he does not receive his medication. (Only with the approval of the counseling supervisor can he be medicated without having provided a specimen.)

The nurses observe this designated urination and generally stand near the observation window. (There was a problem with the toilet in the "urine drop" room. While we were there it became inoperable and no more urine specimens were collected during that day. This problem had occurred at least one other time during the past month, when the bathroom was shut down for at least a day and a half.)

The urine specimens are sent out to a laboratory that tests them for an array of substances: opiates, methadone, barbiturates, amphetamines, benzodiazepine metabolite, propoxyphene (Darvon), cocaine, phencyclidine (PCP). The results are returned to the program in about 4 days. Counselors are informed of the results, and medical records personnel enter the values into patient charts and the computer.

Counselors' Role in Methadone Maintenance Treatment

A general description of counselors' caseload responsibilities is one way of delineating what methadone maintenance counselors commonly do. Each incoming patient is assigned to a primary counselor, who acts as the patient's contact and advocate within the clinic. Indeed, for most patients, the counselors are the clinic, as a designated counselor coordinates most aspects (medical, psychological, vocational) of a patient's treatment and consults with, as well as refers patients to, other professionals within or outside the clinic. A major responsibility of caseload management, then, is the coordination and documentation of services provided to each patient. The counselor develops an initial treatment plan from the psychosocial history done at intake, indicates any referrals or consultations made, monitors the weekly urine reports, monitors attendance, and writes notes for all scheduled counseling sessions or outstanding clinical or behavior problems. At 3-month intervals, each patient's status is reviewed by his counselor in conjunction with the counseling supervisor. On these occasions, the patient's overall progress is assessed and a revised treatment plan prepared if necessary.

Beyond the structured requirements of their role, counselors in methadone maintenance programs are faced with several unique issues. First, the methadone maintenance modality has been, and remains, controversial as a treatment modality. Although conditionally accepted within the medical community, methadone maintenance is viewed as a sanctioned addiction by many engaged in drug-free (abstinence) treatment. Therefore the counseling staff in some clinics are subjected to this theoretical conflict.

Second, within the methadone modality, there are no clear-cut, uniform treatment standards with reference to such matters as length of treatment, conditions for continued treatment, dose levels, or success. In the last regard, the criteria that constitute "successful" outcome are often unclear to the counselors who are providing treatment. In one clinic, increased employment, reduced criminality, and regular attendance may indicate success, whereas in another clinic clean urine specimens and improved social adjustment may be the primary criteria. Each clinic develops its own philosophy of treatment, which appears to be strongly conditioned by the director's personal philosophy. When a counselor's philosophy is congruent with that of the clinic, there is an evident reduction of job stress. Conversely, in those clinics where the counselors come from diverse disciplines, there is likely to be less staff unity and an undercurrent of unrest.

Counseling

The counseling staff consists of both males and females in equal numbers. Most are college graduates who also have a masters degree. Their mean age is similar to that of the addict patient population they serve. They have an average of 3 years of experience at this program.

In this clinic, each patient's primary counselor conducts two individual counseling sessions a month with him, to provide advice and support as well as to maintain an ongoing assessment of the patient's needs and progress. Each of these face-to-face counseling sessions lasts about 60 minutes. Initially, the counseling sessions are principally devoted to in-house matters as the counselor instructs and assists the patient in his adjustment to clinic rules and procedures. At this time an initial treatment plan is developed, treatment goals are established, and the patient assumes contractual responsibility for his own behavior as he agrees to and signs his treatment plan.

As the relationship between counselor and patient develops, the individual sessions become increasingly therapeutic. Addressing social, behavioral, employment and legal problems consumes approximately 60 percent of the counseling time. Once the treatment regimen is established (usually 6–12 months), the counselor's role becomes more individualized with each patient. For patients who are seriously committed to rehabilitation, their counselor becomes their friend. For others, treatment progress may be slower, more erratic, or problematical. In these cases the counselor functions more as a disciplinarian and behavior monitor.

The counseling supervisor does not maintain a caseload but does oversee the treatment of all patients and performs specialized or crisis counseling in the clinic. At the time of our on-site data collection, two of the counselors were in training and did not yet have caseloads.

Group therapy is not practiced in this clinic. The only counselor reporting any group work was actually conducting couples' sessions. Considering that group therapy is a potentially dangerous or destructive treatment tool in the hands of inadequately or poorly trained leaders, the lack of group work in this clinic may simply reflect a lack of qualified group therapists.

The counselors in this clinic enjoy (and appreciate) the functional benefits of a well designed treatment facility. The private counseling offices are grouped in a self-contained section of the building, so they are able to move freely among colleagues' offices for case consultations and are also immediately available for support if a patient should become unruly. Each counselor is provided with a roomy private office that is carpeted and equipped with a desk, telephone, and chairs. Decor is left to the individual, and most of the offices reflect the character and personality of the individual counselor. Some are bright and airy, others are soft and cozy. Most are inviting. Above the administrative section, and well removed from their work site, is a well equipped staff lunchroom that serves as a conference room during working hours. The room is not decorated and is furnished with only functional furniture (large table and hard chairs). Thus "break" time occurs in the more comfortable atmosphere of the counseling offices.

There appears to be a greatly improved morale since the first treatment domain data collection a year ago in the clinic. (At that time, there was considerable disorganization resulting from building renovations and a major revision of administrative policies, procedures, and supervisory personnel.)

Management and Administration

The day-to-day management of the clinic takes place by what may be termed a triumvirate leadership. The director serves as the overall administrator and coordinator who manages fiscal affairs and deals with personnel and the union, legal matters, and outside agencies. The medical director provides for the delivery of medical services to patients and to some extent supervises the counselors. The counselor supervisor provides direct management of these rehabilitation services.

Special Features

The physical facility at MedPsych is outstanding. The building was recently remodeled to accommodate this drug abuse treatment program. Consequently, the waiting and dispensing areas were specially designed for methadone maintenance treatment. The staff reported that the renovation had a beneficial impact on both patients and staff. In particular, patients were more inclined to respect this new facility.

Conclusion

This program is medical in overall orientation because of the long-term influence and active supervision of treatment services provided by the medical director. Still, designation of a program as primarily medical-psychiatric (or primarily oriented to dispensing or to social rehabilitation) is a relative matter. This program is more medical in orientation than the others studied. It should not be assumed, however, that this designation implies that the program is an exemplary medical program or, indeed, that it is even entirely adequate in this regard. In this last regard, I refer to the fact that few of the methadone maintenance programs in the United States have full-time physicians on their staff and fewer still have full-time directors who are physicians.

Program 4: The Haven

Treatment Setting

The Haven provides outpatient methadone maintenance treatment to some 250 addict patients in the midst of a black residential neighborhood in Metrocity. The program is housed in a two-story brick building that faces a side street. The appearance of the building is that of a somewhat neglected warehouse. The building occupies about one-half the area of a sizable lot that is surrounded by private homes. The homes in this working class area are mostly well kept.

The Haven is one block away from a main thoroughfare that runs into the city. The quiet residential neighborhood in which the program is located is adjacent to a commercial roadway with stores, restaurants, and other businesses. It is through this busy avenue that the addict patients reach the program by car or bus. The Haven has provided treatment and counseling services to drug abusers for more than 15 years. It operates as a separate, distinct program with its own facility, director, staff, and treatment policy. It is a nonprofit corporation with its own board of directors. Methadone maintenance is the principal type of service provided, although a pre-trial counseling program and a temporary detoxification research project are part of The Haven as well.

The large lot on which The Haven's building stands is surrounded by private working-class homes. There is parking on the lot for staff at the rear of the building, and this area is fenced in and locked at night. The windows are boarded up (with plastic or metal covering), and the building is in poor repair; the area around the building is littered. There is no name or other prominent identification evident outside to identify the program.

Physical Facility

The two-story building contains some three dozen rooms: offices for counselors, a dispensing area, nurses' offices, waiting areas, group therapy rooms; a staff conference room, administrative offices, computer room, chart room, photocopier storage room, staff lounge, bathrooms, closets, a darkroom, and a former dispensing area that is not utilized. The first floor contains the dispensing area, nurses' offices (one of which doubles as a doctor's office), and administrative quarters. The upper floor contains counselors' offices and group treatment rooms.

Patients

The methadone maintenance patients at The Haven include a greater percentage of females than is commonly found; more than one-third are female. With respect to race, there are slightly more white patients than black patients.

Treatment and Rehabilitation Policy

The Haven was founded with the philosophy that drug abuse and drug addiction are a result of various psychosocial pressures acting on the individual. As such, the program believes that given sufficient time, counseling and supportive services, an individual who is motivated to do so can eventually obtain a drug-free state. The program emphasis is on coordinated counseling and medical treatment for each individual in the program. This emphasis is implemented by development of a treatment plan based on the needs of the individual.

The treatment offered by the program falls predominantly into two categories: counseling services and medical services. It is the philosophy of the program that counseling is the primary mechanism for treatment of the addicted individual; chemotherapy is a secondary but essential aspect of this treatment. Because of the program's emphasis on both counseling and medical services, a team approach is utilized for patient treatment.

The dominant treatment orientation at The Haven is to provide social rehabilitative counseling services to intravenous heroin addicts who are, for the most part, unwanted by most social agencies and treatment programs. This program is a haven for unwanted addicts from various sections of the city.

Director and Program Staff

The treatment staff of the program consists of a director, a supervisory counselor, other counselors, dispensing nurses, a nurse practitioner, and part-time physicians. The administrative staff includes an administrator, secretaries, and a receptionist-clerk.

Most of the counselors and nurses as well as all of the administrative staff are full-time employees. As a consequence, most of the day-to-day treatment and rehabilitation are provided by the counselors and nurses.

The director was a former vocational education counselor at The Haven. He is responsible for establishing and implementing policy, hiring staff, and otherwise managing the overall operation of the program. Among his other duties, he is actively involved in local community affairs, as there has been continual neighborhood opposition to having a drug abuse treatment facility in this residential area. In particular, the neighbors object to addict patients moving in and out of the neighborhood and loitering.

Admission Procedures

The intake coordinator at The Haven does not maintain a waiting list. When someone calls the program to inquire about treatment, she gathers information from him (or her) over the phone to determine if he is eligible. The main requirements are that a patient have at least a 12-month verifiable history of narcotic addiction, he has previously undergone at least one methadone detoxification treatment, he is currently using opiates intravenously, and opiate addiction is the primary diagnosis. Patients are rejected and referred elsewhere if they do not seem to be adequately invested in treatment, if they left their previous treatment program less than 30 days ago, or if they are in their third trimester of pregnancy. If the patient seems eligible, an appointment to see the intake coordinator is scheduled. This appointment usually takes place within 7 to 10 days of contact. The patient is told to call the following Friday evening to confirm the appointment. (The intake coordinator schedules about eight appointments each week; she estimates that 50 percent of the appointments are kept.)

At the intake appointment, the coordinator obtains demographic and psychosocial information from the prospective patient. Basic clinic rules are explained and some preliminary forms completed, after which a urine sample is obtained.

Several days later the intake coordinator presents four or five new cases at the intake meeting. Present at the meeting are the intake coordinator, the medical staff (represented by the head nurse), the clinical coordinator, and as many counselors as possible. In essence, majority rules at this meeting.

The patients are told to call at a specified time on Monday afternoon to learn the outcome of the admission conference. If the patient has been accepted, he comes in on Tuesday to see the nurse practitioner for a physical examination and then signs the treatment contract. At this point the patient sees the physician and receives his first dose of methadone.

Methadone Dispensing

Patients enter the program from the street. They are checked in through a locked main door and then make their way to the medication station at the back of the first floor. Here they line up for their methadone dose in front of the two dispensing windows.

At each side of the dispensary, a dutch door, locked at the bottom but open at the top during dispensing, separates the nurse from the patients. Medication is handed over the door by the nurse to the patient. He immediately drinks his dose while facing the nurse, after which he is required to speak thereby preventing oral retention of the methadone for later use or sale. Before leaving the medication station, the patient must initial a medication card verifying his consumption of that day's dose.

Patients are medicated individually by the nurse, who identifies them visually. The nurses are familiar with the patients and are able to recognize new admissions as unfamiliar faces. All patients have photographs attached to their medication records. Therefore new admissions can be visually identified by both the regular staff and substitute nursing staff.

Nurses dispense methadone from stock solution of Methadose. Each nurse is responsible for her own stock bottle as well as for maintaining inventory control of the methadone it contains. The head nurse is responsible for reconciling the methadone supply for the entire dispensary each day. Each prescribed dose of methadone is prepared from the medication cardex and measured out with a micropipette into a paper dispensing cup. Water is added before the medication is given to the patient. Take-home medication is not prepackaged but is prepared when the patient appears for his daily dose.

The dispensing station is somewhat cramped. The medication flip charts are positioned behind the nurse on a rather flimsy table. By the time of our second on-site data collection, it was noted that additional shelving had made more space available in the dispensary, which made the room more functional and orderly. In addition, a somewhat cleaner appearance of the dispensary was evident.

Medical Services

Two part-time physicians provide medical treatment and supervision at The Haven. Both are at the clinic in the evening hours, after 5 p.m. Medical coverage provided by these two doctors during the week involves both direct patient care and supervision of other staff. With regard to supervision, approximately one-half of the physicians' time at the program is spent in supervisory work with the counselors, dispensing nurses, or nurse practitioner or doing administrative paperwork (e.g., signing charts).

Most of the nurses employed at The Haven to dispense methadone on a daily basis work full time at the clinic. These full-time nurses are experienced in dealing with addict patients as each has worked at The Haven for 2 years or more.

Active Role of Nurses

The dispensing nurses are active and intimate providers of treatment to the patients they medicate. Their activity is manifest in the number of patients they medicate, as well as by the busy, if not hectic, atmosphere that permeates the clinic during dispensing hours. During most of the dispensing hours patients are lined up waiting to receive their methadone, but the line moves forward rapidly as patients commonly stay in the clinic only 10 to 12 minutes each day.

Nurses quickly get to know each patient on a first name basis because they see him (or her) every day as they prepare his medication, observe him drinking it, converse with him, and keep records of his attendance and dosage. In addition, the nurses often provide patients with direct medical care and serve as a referral source to other medical services.

In addition to dispensing methadone, the full-time nurses at The Haven provide considerable medical care to patients. In the course of a week, one nurse scheduled urine drops for the entire clinic, tested two patients for tuberculosis, provided medical counseling to three patients, referred four patients for blood work and three for chest radiography, and distributed 50 booklets on health education. She also took part in a group needlework session for five patients held outside the dispensing area. Another nurse provided the following services during the week: provided personal and medical counseling for 7 patients, tested 10 for tuberculosis (PPD) and 20 for syphilis (RPRs), used a breathalyzer on 40 patients, and referred 2 to physicians; she also took part with a counselor in group session with four patients pertaining to their drug abuse problems. The head nurse was more involved in administrative tasks but still provided the following direct services: undertook medical counseling with 10 patients, tested 2 for blood pressure, referred 10 patients to clinic physicians, and referred 1 accident case to a hospital. The nurses also reported that they had brief conversations or personal contacts with almost all patients who attended the clinic each day.

A nurse practitioner is also employed part time at The Haven to conduct required physical examinations and teach health education. In the health education class, a specific topic is addressed each week, e.g., headaches, AIDS, or pregnancy. Attendance at these classes is high, and there is particular interest among the female patients.

Urinalysis

Patients are scheduled to provide two urine samples each month. The schedule for urine drops is set by the clinical director, who picks a specific day for the men and a different day for the women. All patients are expected to drop a sample on these scheduled days. In addition, new admissions or those with current drug abuse problems may be asked to provide extra urine samples.

Counselors

The counseling staff at The Haven constitutes well over one-half of the total treatment and rehabilitation staff. Indeed, in terms of full-time treatment staff, almost three-fourths of the program staff are counselors. This counseling staff consists of both males and females, whites and blacks. Most are college graduates, but many have less than 1 year's experience at this program.

The central role of counselors at The Haven can be summarized by noting the functions and tasks the counselors commonly perform. Counselors have the principal responsibility for the following.

1. Arranging and supervising the admission of new patients
2. Assigning each admission to a specific counselor, who then serves as his principal contact within the clinic (he is then on this counselor's caseload)
3. Instructing their patients about treatment and rehabilitation objectives
4. Seeing to it that patients are familiar with and adhere to program rules and regulations
5. Development of a treatment and rehabilitation plan for each patient (with input from other staff)
6. Scheduling and conducting individual and group sessions with patients
7. Monitoring patients' treatment and rehabilitation progress: attendance, urinalysis results, behavior in clinic, employment, income, legal problems, and so on
8. Coordinating treatment and rehabilitation services provided to each patient within the clinic
9. Serving as program liaison person for family and other outside contacts and problems (e.g., employment, legal)
10. Maintaining up-to-date familiarity with the rehabilitation and treatment status of each patient on his caseload
11. Keeping up-to-date charts (i.e., records) on each patient in his caseload
12. Disciplining and rewarding patients.

Although the assigned treatment, rehabilitative, and administrative duties of the counselors are considerable (if not grandiose), their actual work role is focused on a few principal tasks. First and foremost, they provide counseling services to patients assigned to them—their caseload. Second, as noted, they perform more general duties for the program.

Counselors at The Haven also provide training for new staff. At the beginning, new counselors receive pertinent skills training that takes place in closely supervised group counseling sessions. While learning to conduct individual and group sessions, new counselors monitor patients' progress, document services provided, and otherwise work under supervision while developing their counseling skills.

The second major work role of counselors at The Haven (in addition to looking after patients on their caseload) consists of more general programmatic duties, including admission screening and casework, treatment coordinating tasks (e.g., with respect to distribution and use of urine results), patient status and disciplinary team meetings, crisis intervention (e.g., a patient has just been arrested or been in an accident), as well as in-service training and other professional activities.

The counselors' relationships with their patients involve aspects of various roles: teacher, parent, and confidant. The counselors teach the patient about clinic rules and desirable behavior, advise him about family affairs and employment, admonish him about misbehavior, and provide discipline and rewards. They also listen to patients and discuss issues pertaining to each person's current concerns and needs.

From a separate content-analysis of topics addressed in counseling sessions at one program, it was found that both in-clinic and at-home issues were commonly discussed in counseling sessions. Of these two topics, out-of-clinic behavior was more frequently the subject of counseling sessions. The nine most frequently discussed issues, in order of importance, were family problems (far and away the single most frequently discussed content area in the counseling sessions), general irresponsible behavior, vocational issues, social relationships, drug use, dirty urine specimens, education, clinic discipline, and treatment progress evaluation.

Each counselor has a private, adequately furnished office in a restricted area of the second floor. This arrangement for a more private area for offices is viewed as a major improvement by the counselors who were at the program last year. Overall, there is a greatly improved atmosphere at this clinic. Though far from a showplace, the building maintenance and decor have been considerably improved. Staff morale is high with an enthusiasm that seems contagious. These high spirits are probably due, in part, to the newness of many counselors and their excitement with what they are learning. Morale, however, has also improved among other staff in the program. In contrast to last year, there is a more hopeful and purposeful attitude at the program. The credit for this change belongs to the director, the clinical supervisor, and the administrator, who are a close-knit triumvirate, dedicated to the provision of integrated services to their patients.

Special Features

Ambience of Program

As in a school, office, or extended family, the daily ambience is difficult to define or measure. Still, the impression or "feel" of a program is crucial, as it sets the tone and stage for whatever treatment or rehabilitation that occurs. Thus a given ambience permeates each program. At The Haven, the dominant ethos was social rehabilitation.

Each program's social control policy and procedures tend to reflect the treatment rationale and administrative policies of that program and its director. No guards were employed to supervise patients. Partly as a consequence of this absence of security personnel, patients were more boisterous and less disciplined than at other programs.

Management

As noted, the coordination of the counseling and nursing services was high, as the director, clinical supervisor, and head nurse were in agreement about treatment goals and program procedures. At the same time, there was less physician involvement in the program, largely due to the fact that the two doctors were part-time employees who were at the program only on specified evenings.

Community Relations

Inasmuch as The Haven is located on a quiet side street in a stable residential neighborhood, there has been considerable community opposition to this methadone maintenance program. The opposition is due to the aggregation of patients and their cars in the immediate vicinity of the clinic; loitering has been a continual problem. Patient flow in and out of the neighborhood is neither adequately controlled nor supervised. It is not that the program has paid no attention to the loitering problem. The contrary is the case; the director has been continually involved in local community affairs with respect to the loitering problem. The fact is, however, that loitering is a difficult problem for programs to address with their limited staff and lack of outside support.

Community opposition to the program has been expressed in various ways. Bricks have been thrown through the windows; the neighborhood association has formally complained about the program; and there has been a zoning hearing at City Hall to curtail the operation of the clinic.

In response to community protests, the program has tried to win support by trash clean-up drives in the neighborhood, open house meetings, and the establishment of an antiloitering policy for patients. These efforts have met with only a modicum of success because the program lacks the necessary staff resources and outside support it would take to overcome the loitering problem.

Conclusion

Despite current funding inadequacies, continual community opposition, and the almost insuperable problems that have beset this program over the years (e.g., neighbors throwing rocks at the building, zoning battles, high staff turnover due to low salaries), the director and key staff have persevered in their commitment to provide methadone maintenance treatment to needy heroin addicts.

Program 5: The Group

Treatment Setting

The Group is one of the oldest methadone maintenance programs in the United States. It is located in the midst of a large black slum area, and it has a close association with community leaders in this active yet deteriorated section of the city. More than most methadone programs, The Group is a part of the underclass culture in Metrocity. It is a part of the local community.

The Group is one of several methadone maintenance clinics operated by a parent organization that is devoted to providing treatment and rehabilitation to hard-core heroin addicts in Metrocity. This association with and dependence on a large treatment organization has both advantages and disadvantages.

The advantages are that the central administration provides direction and stability. The overall methadone maintenance treatment regimen and procedures are centrally established. In addition, staff recruitment is centralized, and external support staff are available for training and to assist clinics when special needs arise, e.g., illness of staff, accidents, or termination of employment. Furthermore, the central administration has responsibility for funding and assists with neighborhood problems and other matters.

The disadvantages of a central off-site administration are primarily bureaucratic in nature. Off-site administrators tend to rely on rules and regulations and lose contact with the day-to-day needs and problems of the patients and clinic staff. The clinic director often lacks authority to solve immediate problems and must await action from the higher administration.

Physical Facility

The clinic is located in an old three-story building that is only partly occupied by the clinic staff and patients. The occupied portion consists of five general areas: (1) dispensing space; (2) medical rooms; (3) counseling areas; (4) security offices; and (5) administrative rooms. The dispensing area on the first and second floors is described under Patient Flow below.

The medical area is located on the second floor behind the dispensing room. The medical section consists of several rooms: a physician's office, one for the nurse practitioner (containing an examining table), two for the dispensing nurses (who assist the nurse practitioner when not dispensing), one vacant office, one large workroom (containing four desks, a scale, a refrigerator, and similar equipment), and a waiting room with six chairs.

The counselor's area consists of offices, group session rooms, and one or more special vocational education rooms. Most of the counselor's offices are on the third floor, but the vocational counselor has a second floor office. The numerous group rooms are located throughout the building.

The security staff has separate offices on the first floor. Inasmuch as the security officers are an integral part of the program (e.g., they accept urine specimens and attend staff meetings), they have private offices that are similar to those of the counselors.

The director and most of the administrative staff have offices on the third floor. These staff include a secretary, clerk-typist, community liaison worker, and a medical records clerk. All of these staff members have adjoining offices, except the records clerk, who has an office on the second floor close to the file room. For the most part, this large, cavernous building is in poor repair, deteriorated, and dirty. The overall appearance is that of an old, massive, rundown apartment building.

Patients

At the time of our on-site program data collection in 1985 there were some 250 methadone maintenance patients enrolled at The Group. These patients were predominantly (three-fourths) black with most of the remainder Hispanic; one-fourth of the patients were female.

Although one-third of the patients had been in treatment for less than 1 year, two-thirds had been in treatment for 1 year or more, and some 15 percent had been in continuous treatment at this program for 5 + years. As with many programs, then, there was a high rate of dropouts among new admissions but a sizable number of long-term patients.

Treatment Policy

The Group and its parent organization see themselves as involved in providing specialized treatment services to hardcore heroin addicts who are predominantly minority group members. Most of these patients have a long history of heroin addiction, numerous arrests, minimum schooling, and few marketable skills.

In addition to providing comprehensive medical and rehabilitative services to its patients, The Group's treatment policy is community oriented. Indeed, the treatment philosophy of the program sees drug addiction as a community problem that has engulfed their patients.

Program Staff and Director

The treatment staff consists of a director, counselors, dispensing nurses, a physician, and a physicians' assistant. The administrative staff includes, in addition to the director, a secretary, clerk-typist receptionist, records clerk, and community liaison worker. All of these staff members are full-time employees except the physician; who is employed part-time. This high level of full-time commitment facilitates staff communication and the coordination of patient services. The high degree of staff coordination is most evident in the interdisciplinary team sessions, which are scheduled periodically to review and evaluate each patient's progress.

The director in this clinic coordinates the treatment staff and serves as the on-site supervisor for the central program administration. These two functions keep the director occupied, as the staff is dispersed on the three floors of this large building and the central administration is miles away in a separate office building. The director's role in this active clinic of more than 200 patients appears to be one of crises management. The demands on this small administrative staff seem overwhelming: patients waiting for assistance, crisis management, incessant outside telephone calls, administrative problems, and similar matters.

A special comment is relevant about the role of security personnel at The Group. The full-time security officers are closely integrated into the provision of treatment and rehabilitation services. They serve not only as gatekeepers, they also accept urine specimens from patients, coordinate treatment services, meet as part of the interdisciplinary teams to assess patient's progress, and are otherwise actively engaged in running the clinic. In this last regard, they check attendance and supervise the lineup of patients for medication.

Admission Procedures

During 1985 some 190 patients were admitted to The Group. The admission process takes place as follows. The intake worker (a designated security officer) coordinates the admission process. Potential patients are referred to the program or come in themselves. In either case, they are placed in contact with the intake worker, who obtains a urine sample from them, establishes the mode of payment, and sets up a record chart. An appointment is then made with a counselor. (There is about a 2-week wait for such an appointment.) In this interview, the counselor obtains a drug history from the patient and ensures that the necessary release and consent forms are signed. After meeting the counselor, the patient sees the mental health consultant, who completes a psychosocial history and other forms. The mental health consultant then makes the decision as to whether the patient is appropriate for methadone maintenance. At this juncture the patient has a preadmission physical examination. Finally, he receives an identification number and can then be medicated. This last part of the admission process takes about 2 to 3 days.

Dispensing

The dispensary at the rear of the second floor is small and unkempt in appearance. The dispensing station is inaccessible to patients, as nurses work behind a protective "cage" of wire fencing. Only one patient can be medicated at a time, as a single nurse prepares the methadone doses. This arrangement, however, does not seem to create undue holdups in the medication process.

The patient's dose is ascertained by the dispensing nurse from a computer printout of patients' doses. There are identification photographs in the dispensing book from which to identify the patient, but the presence of two staff in the medication area (the nurse and the security officer) provide sufficient ensurance of patient identification. Methadone Diskettes are dissolved in water and given to the patient while he faces the dispensing nurse. After drinking the dose, the patient signs a record to document that he was medicated. Take-home medication is also prepared at the dispensing station when patients appear.

Patient Flow

Patients enter the clinic from a side street through a set of steel doors. Once inside, they pass through an outer lobby to a large hallway area. Just inside the hallway a security guard sits behind a desk and checks them in.

Patients sign themselves in on a contact sheet as they reach the guard (the contact sheet is a daily list of patient attendance). The guard then gives each patient an identification card and directs him to proceed up two flights of stairs to the second floor. There is an observation mirror on the staircase by means of which the guard can watch patients ascend the second flight of stairs and pass down the hallway.

Once upstairs, patients go to the back of the building some 200 feet down a long hallway to the dispensing area. Other hallways leading to vacant or abandoned rooms intersect this long central hall.

At the entrance to the large dispensing room, patients wait their turn while a guard checks off their names (he usually knows them). When called, each patient approaches the dispensing counter and presents his (or her) identification card to the nurse. She checks each card and records the dosage given. Liquid methadone is given to the patient in a small paper cup to which he adds Tang or water from a jug on the counter. After drinking the dose, the patient leaves the clinic.

Patients wishing to see a physician inform the nurse and are referred to an adjoining area on the second floor after being medicated. Patients with scheduled appointments must complete their medical care before receiving medication. After being medicated clients are encouraged by the security personnel to quickly leave the area.

Medical Services

Medical services at the clinic are provided by a nurse practitioner and a part-time physician. Both are kept busy treating patients during clinic hours. The medical waiting room is full, and this part of the clinic is busy with a constant flow of patients seeking treatment.

The medical treatment provided falls into three general classifications: (1) intake and annual physicals; (2) medication adjustment; and (3) general medical care. The first type of treatment—admission or annual physical examinations—is a mandated service that takes about one-fourth of the available medical hours. The second type of treatment—methadone dosage adjustment—is a continual activity of the physician as she responds to patients' complaints. The provision of general medical care is the third type of service and occupies about one-half of the time of the two medical staff members. Examples of the general medical care provided are obtaining Papanicolaou smears, drawing blood samples, treating colds and other infections, dealing with problems of pregnancy, and making outside referrals for laboratory tests.

Urinalysis

Patients are scheduled to provide one urine sample per week on a randomly selected day. The day of the week is selected by the head security officer, and all attending patients provide a urine sample on this day. When patients enter the program on that day, they go to the urine drop area. Here a security guard sits at a desk in front of two bathrooms and monitors the flow of patients in and out of each bathroom. He does not enter the bathrooms but collects the samples and records who provided each specimen. If a patient cannot provide a urine specimen on the day he is supposed to, he is not medicated. The two bathrooms are of average cleanliness for urine collection facilities.

The specimens are tested for the major substances of abuse. The turnaround time on a routine test is 2 to 3 days. Urine results that are positive for illicit susbstances are dealt with by the respective counselors.

Counselors

This counseling staff is composed of approximately equal numbers of men and women, and their mean age is in the midthirties. Most have only limited experience with addict patients.

The counselors provide case management, which in this program includes the initial psychosocial history, 3-month treatment plans, weekly progress summaries, biweekly counseling sessions (weekly for the dual-diagnosis patients who are alcoholics), and interdisciplinary 3-month case reviews. Thus the patients are seen regularly by their counselors.

Although well educated, these counselors, as noted, are limited in their experience with addict patients. The counseling supervisor is new to the addiction field and appears to be engaged primarily in bringing structure and organization to the counseling process at this program. Unfortunately, the element that many of these counselors appear to lack is familiarity with the behavior and culture of addiction. Thus the frequency of the counseling is good, but the content of the sessions may not be appropriate to the needs of the patients. In addition, what many of these counselors are recording as individual sessions are rather brief "contact" meetings.

It is reasonable to surmise that the counselors' lack of experience with this difficult population and the clinic's focus on quantity rather than quality in the counseling process have created an atmosphere of frustration for the counselors. The frustration occurs because of the counselors' inability to determine the remediable needs of the patients and their lack of experience in assisting the patients toward any real life style change. This problem could be a factor in the generally poor morale (and resulting high turnover) among the counselors at this clinic. The counselors are primarily performing the documentation and referral responsibilities of case management, but they are delivering little counseling pertaining to patients' problems, available resources, and plans for rehabilitation. Moreover, the caseload of these counselors is far too high to allow for anything more than functional case management. It is unrealistic to expect any kind of effective individual counseling with such limited time available to see each patient and with the large caseloads involved.

Each counselor has a private office on one of two floors. The offices are dingy (as is the entire building), inadequately furnished (minimal furniture), and there has been little or no effort by the counselors to provide decoration. Though most of the offices have telephones, some do not work.

This program employs a designated vocational counselor to assist patients to obtain and maintain employment. She believes that a highly desirable rehabilitation goal is to assist patients in getting "real" jobs on the outside (i.e., competitive work rather than welfare-like jobs). She is not often successful in this endeavor because most of these addict patients lack realistic motivation. In this regard, she notes that a "not yet ready syndrome" is common in which patients agree to the idea of scheduled regular work but state that they are not ready for it yet. Furthermore, it is not only a matter of obtaining jobs but of keeping them. Thus, several patients have been placed in jobs recently, but often they cannot fulfill job requirements. For example, the counselor recently told a driver who was fired from his job because he repeatedly arrived late on his runs to get a city map so he would know how to find his way to locations. Within this underclass population of addicts, vocational counseling is difficult, as it often involves trying to surmount prior deficiencies in early socialization and elementary education.

Special Features

The program is strong in terms of the provision of general medical services to patients and it seems to be distinctive in that everyone pitches in and commonly performs more than one work role. A clerk takes over security at the dispensing station; security guards collect urine specimens, and the nurses assist with examinations.

Interdisciplinary Teams

A distinctive feature of treatment at this program is the extensive use of interdisciplinary teams to evaluate a patient's progress. These teams meet regularly and normally consist of someone from the medical staff, a counselor, and a security officer.

Community Liaison

The Group is heavily involved in local community affairs, especially as they relate to drug abuse and related problems. This commitment to community involvement is evident in the day-to-day operation of the clinic as, for example, when the staff attends and supports local activities or encourages patients to attend local recreational or civic events. The person primarily responsible for developing and supporting joint meetings and activities with neighborhood leaders and residents is the full-time community worker, who has a high-level position at the program.

Conclusion

The Group is dedicated to the social rehabilitation of hardcore heroin addicts who reside in metrocity slum areas. In this long-term endeavor, the program sees itself as not only treating and assisting individual addicts within the clinic but in being involved with the local community as well as the city in promoting overall social redevelopment and rehabilitation.

Program 6: The Family

Treatment Setting

The Family is one of the oldest methadone maintenance programs in Metrocity. It is an independent nonprofit corporation devoted to treating "hard-core" heroin addicts. Most patients have a long history of intravenous heroin use, multiple arrests, extensive incarceration, and repeated relapses to opiate addiction. The only treatment offered by this program is methadone maintenance rehabilitation. Some 250 patients attend this program regularly to receive oral methadone and rehabilitative services.

The Family is located on a busy main street leading out of center city. The neighborhood is commercial with most of the buildings on the block consisting of stores, offices, restaurants, and similar retail establishments.

Physical Facility

A single three-story building houses the entire program. The building is an old, rather attractive stone structure that is in good repair. A large outside sign identifies the program by name. The only parking space available is at metered stands or on adjoining streets.

There are five functional areas to the building: (1) dispensing area; (2) counselors' offices; (3) medical offices; (4) administrative offices; and (5) group rooms. The dispensing area is located on the first floor by the main entrance. This area has the greatest patient flow, as methadone is dispensed here 7 days a week.

The second major functional area is devoted to counselors' offices, which are located on the second floor. Each of the counselors has a well appointed private office; with his or her name on the door; each office has a telephone. There is a toilet on this floor, but the counselors' lounge is on the third floor.

The main administrative staff is located on the third floor. This area includes the director's office, that of the program administrator, and a secretary. There is also a large conference room on this floor and a record room that includes a photocopying machine. In addition to this third floor space, there is an office on the first floor next to the waiting room in which patient fees are collected. The remaining space includes a storage room for urine specimens and two rooms for group sessions.

Patients

During the 3-year period of program data collection, the census at The Family remained fairly stable at about 250 methadone maintenance patients. As with most programs, some three-fourths of the patients were male. With respect to race, there was almost an even split between black and white, with a slight edge among the whites. One-third of these patients had been in treatment less than 1 year.

Treatment Policy

The Family is avowedly a methadone maintenance program that is designed expressly to treat long-term opiate addicts. It is held that methadone maintenance allows addicts to function without a compulsion for street heroin and that successful treatment and rehabilitation involve three components: methadone as a long-term maintenance drug, regular counseling as a social and psychological support and medical services to promote good health.

The treatment rationale of The Family is based on the efficacy of daily methadone medication accompanied by active counseling services. Long-term treatment is planned to facilitate rehabilitation. The entire treatment staff is coordinated to supervise and assist patients in rehabilitation. In this sense, there is almost a therapeutic community orientation, or commitment, evident.

Director and Staff

The director has extensive experience and knowledge about drug abuse treatment and rehabilitation. He is the dominant force at The Family, as he has been responsible for the continuation and further development of this methadone maintenance program over the years.

The director is actively engaged in both the administration of the program and the delivery of treatment services. With staff assistance, he formulates and changes treatment policy and clinic rules. He is continually involved in staff supervision and program management. Moreover, he sees patients who have special problems, reviews new admissions and discharges, and otherwise takes an active part in providing treatment and rehabilitation.

One of his principal functions is to provide direction and support to the treatment staff and thereby to effect coordination and continuity of the treatment and rehabilitative services. This is done through meetings, policy statements, and personal contacts. In this last regard, his daily involvement in the operation of the clinic and his concomitant belief in the efficacy of rehabilitation through methadone maintenance engenders staff commitment to quality care and high morale.

The staff at this program can be separated into two categories, treatment staff and administrative staff. The treatment staff is comprised of full-time counselors and dispensing nurses; a part-time physician and a part-time physicians' assistant provide medical coverage with some assistance from the head nurse. The role of the nurses in this program is primarily that of dispensing methadone. Administration is provided by the director, administrator, a receptionist, secretaries, and clerks.

Admission Procedure

There is no waiting list for admission to The Family. The intake counselor has been able to give anyone who calls for admission an appointment within a week. The process starts when an addict calls the program; the intake worker screens the call and makes an initial judgment as to whether the addict will qualify for admission. To qualify, the addict must have at least a 2-year verifiable history of narcotic addiction, have failed in at least one effort at detoxification from narcotics, and failed at least one short-term methadone maintenance treatment. The intake worker estimates that of the 150 calls he receives per month about 40 pass this initial telephone screen.

Those who pass the telephone screening are asked to come in for a brief (20 minute) face-to-face interview. These interviews take place on Tuesday afternoons. Of 40 who come for the preadmission interview, some 20 to 25 are found to be appropriate for the full intake procedure. Patients not found to be suitable for intensive methadone maintenance treatment are referred to another program.

The 20 to 25 patients who pass the initial screening are asked to come in again a day or so later. At this second intake interview a drug abuse history is obtained, along with a psychosocial history, and then they see a nurse for a medical interview. At this time, they also complete administrative forms and provide a urine sample. Based on these findings, about 16 of these addicts are sent on to the next phase—admission for methadone medication and rehabilitation.

Methadone Dispensing

There are two dispensing stations in use. The bottom one-half of the entrance door at each station serves as a counter for methadone dispensing. This portion of the door is locked, but there is no other physical barrier between the nurse and the patient. The dispensing nurse prepares each patient's methadone dose and has him sign his medication sheet to document receipt. Thereupon the patient receives his methadone in a small paper cup to which he usually adds water from a pitcher on the dispensing counter. While facing the nurse, the patient drinks the medication and then leaves the clinic.

The dispensary area consists of a large open waiting room with an adjoining dispensary. The dispensary has ample space for the activity it supports. There is hot and cold running water, ample counter and desk space, and a suitable place (a separate locked closet) for the safe in which methadone is stored. Two nurses can dispense simultaneously from the two medication windows.

Oral methadone is dispensed by four nurses, two on a shift. Each is responsible for maintaining an inventory of her own bottle of Methadose; the head nurse is responsible for final reconciliation of the Methadose inventory for the entire dispensary. The nurses are readily accessible to the patients and screen their medical complaints and questions in an informal way. A friendly "family" atmosphere is evident in the dispensing operation, and it is apparent that the nurses' role extends beyond that of a mere drug dispenser to include some triage and supportive contact, even though this secondary role may not be part of their job description. Nurses and counseling staff work closely together. Nurses have the authority to refuse medication for a patient. In most cases they have the final say on this matter. Program policy in this regard is clearly spelled out and, like other policies, appears to be applied consistently.

If take-home medication is to be provided, it is prepared by the nurses from the stock bottles when the patient is at the dispensing window. (It is not prepackaged.) Take-home bottles are appropriately labeled and have a childproof cap and tamper-resistant seal.

Patient Flow

Patients enter the main door to The Family from the street by going up a few steps to a double set of locked glass doors. The lock is electrically released by the waiting room supervisor, who faces the door and checks in all patients and staff; from his central location, he supervises all patient flow into the program. He also is the telephone receptionist and factotum with respect to outside contacts and business: visitors, deliveries, urine collections, and so forth. There is a sign-in book for visitors at this front desk, and above the desk is a list of the staff by name and function.

By the time the clinic starts its morning dispensing of methadone, patients are lined up awaiting the opening of the dispensing window. When the window opens, each patient identifies himself to the dispensing nurse at the window and hands her his urine slip, used take-home bottles, and similar items. She, in turn, dispenses a designated dose. Identification of patients is not an issue, as the nurses know each patient by sight (most receive medication several times a week).

Medical Services

A part-time physician and a part-time physicians' assistant provide medical coverage at this program. They see patients late in the afternoon on scheduled days. The treatment provided by the physician is "mostly about methadone." He reviews patients' dosages and writes orders for other medication. Little primary medical care is provided. The physicians' assistant is primarily involved in conducting physical examinations and doing blood work on patients.

Urinalysis

All patients are expected to provide ("drop") three urine specimens each week; that is, each patient knows that he is supposed to drop a specimen on Monday, Wednesday, and Friday. An attempt is made to obtain an equal number of specimens from patients who are on reduced or irregular pickup schedules. Urine specimens from men are collected in a large, clean, well lit urine room that is next to the dispensing station. A male staff member whose only job is to collect these specimens is continually on duty. Women provide their specimens in a bathroom upstairs.

If a patient is unable to give a specimen, he has to give one the next day. Failure to drop a urine is considered a program violation and has an effect on such privileges as the length of time until the next reduction in a methadone pickup schedule. Two failures to drop during a 30-day period leads to a decrease in take-home privileges.

Urine specimens are tested for the current major substances of abuse. (Although each patient drops three specimens a week, only one is analyzed.) The turnaround time on a routine test is 4 days. When the results are returned, a list of patients with positive tests is generated and circulated; in this way, counselors are notified of the results that refer to their patients. The urine result slips are then filed.

Counseling

The counseling staff is mostly female, and the mean age of this staff is almost 40, which is 5 years older than the mean age of their patients. Almost one-half of the counselors have college degrees, and two hold masters degrees. Most of the counselors have more than 3 years' experience at this program, and there is unusual employment stability of this staff. In fact, the only turnover during the past year was caused by the death of one counselor.

Although the entire counseling staff maintains caseloads, three caseloads are considerably smaller than the others because these three counselors also have ancillary duties of considerable responsibility. The clinical supervisor remains an integral part of the counseling team even though she also maintains a major administrative role in clinic operations. Her role is to supervise all caseloads while paying attention to patients with special needs and filling in for counselors as needed. The counseling supervisor also maintains a small specialized caseload and provides ongoing supervision and training to the clinical staff. She does vocational assessments and planning on all incoming patients and provides vocational counseling for the patients when needed. In addition, one counselor is designated the Addictions Coordinator, and he has a reduced caseload as he is responsible for all admissions.

In addition to providing individual counseling and case management to the designated patients in their caseload, most counselors serve as co-leaders of group sessions. In addition, all of the counselors participate in various clinic committees according to their individual expertise or interest. These clinic committees address special issues relevant to their patients, such as alcoholism, cocaine abuse, family problems, and AIDS. In these regards, the counselors gather relevant information for the committees, undergo training, and develop strategies for clinic implementation. The strategies usually include educational and therapeutic sessions for the patients as well as the distribution of educational material throughout the clinic.

The counselors have various responsibilities: patient contact and advocacy, treatment planning and coordinating, conducting individual and group sessions, and documenting the services provided to each patient. When fulfilling these duties the counselors in this clinic appear to place great emphasis on the depth and quality of the services provided rather than on the mere administrative (or paperwork) part of the process.

This clinic enjoys a considerable reputation within the addiction treatment community as well as among the addict population. Although the staff is aware of general criticism about methadone maintenance as a treatment modality, they are proud of this program.

Special Features

Security

There are no security guards at The Family. Program security is maintained by the staff, especially the front desk supervisor and the counselors. The fact that the building is locked at all times and that the front desk supervisor admits all patients is significant. Moreover, admittance to this program is selective, so many patients become "family members" who have a commitment to the program and to their own rehabilitation.

Recreational Activities

The Family has offered various recreational activities over the past year: a picnic, exercise classes, holiday parties, bake sales, and a baseball team outing.

Conclusion

The Family places primary emphasis on effecting the social rehabilitation of its members. Methadone treatment is seen as a mutual commitment between staff and patients to restructure the lives of heroin addicts. Although methadone is seen as a crucial element in changing addicts' street life styles (because it alleviates and then stops the intense craving for opiates) successful treatment is seen as predicated on the establishment, or reestablishment, of a stable way of life, including gainful employment and assumption of responsibility toward the program, one's family, and other legitimate institutions.

Discussion

The six programs have been described in some detail in order to realistically portray the day-to-day operation of these methadone maintenance facilities in New York City, Philadelphia, and Baltimore. In delineating what occurs in outpatient methadone maintenance programs it is efficacious to note the commonality among programs as well as their more apparent differences.

The common factors that characterize methadone maintenance treatment include the fact that the clinics are continually open throughout the year 6 or 7 days per week; that patients attend the clinic on a daily basis or have a definite schedule of attendance per week; that on-site daily face-to-face dispensing of oral methadone occurs; that the continual provision of counseling services to designated patients is routine; that patients are required to provide urine specimens to the clinic upon demand; that medical coverage is provided at the clinics; that the goal of treatment is the reduction or elimination of illicit drug use and concomitant rehabilitation. These common features generally characterize methadone maintenance treatment in the United States.

Differences among the six programs have also been noted in order to provide an accurate and meaningful portrayal of what occurs at various sites as outpatient treatment is provided. Noting the differences among the programs is a way of presenting realistic descriptions of the unique ambience that characterizes each treatment site. In this regard, it is necessary to describe numerous programs if a general knowledge of methadone maintenance treatment is to be effected, just as a meaningful general description of an addict patient population cannot be based on information obtained from a single patient. In this context, differences among the programs are often a source of valuable information, as these observed differences are due to a variety of factors, particular city or state regulations, the treatment orientation of the director, the funds and resources available, the patient population enrolled, the training and experience of the staff, the existing physical facility and neighborhood, the history of the program, the relation with a sponsoring agency, and so forth. How a particular director or administrator copes with these various parameters of treatment is important for that program. This description does not, however, demonstrate that there is one best way to run a methadone maintenance program.

By noting that programs differ in their treatment rationale and regimen—that some emphasize efficient dispensing, others psychiatric or medical treatment, and still others social rehabilitation—does not imply that one or another of these approaches is superior to others (it is a matter for outcome evaluation to determine this point). Furthermore, the available evidence indicates that program orientation is only one of numerous variables of the treatment domain that affect patient outcome (see Chapter 11).

From the six descriptions, it would be incorrect to infer that there is evidence of greater or lesser effectiveness of the programs studied, as the descriptions are not measurements of the programs or the services they provide. Furthermore, one's intuitive surmise of a program's effectiveness is apt to be based on preconceived models of what methadone maintenance treatment should be. Indeed, these six descriptions were prepared before the patient outcome findings were available, and our opinions at that time about what these results would show were, in retrospect, merely guesses. It is held, then, that it is hazardous to attempt to predict program performance from program descriptions, although experts sometimes state that they can do so.

To recapitulate, the purpose of the program descriptions was to open the black box of methadone maintenance treatment and inspect its contents. In subsequent chapters the contents are classified, measured, and then analyzed with respect to their association with patients' success. It is only in this way that effectiveness can be determined.

References

1. Glasscote RM, Sussex JN, Jaffe JH, et al (1972) The Treatment of Drug Abuse: Programs, Problems, Prospects. Washington, DC: American Psychiatric Association
2. Drug Abuse Council (1973) Methadone Maintenance: The Experience of Four Programs. Washington, DC: The Drug Abuse Council
3. Arif A, Westermeyer J (1990) Methadone in the Management of Opioid Dependence: Programs and Policies Around the World. New York: Praeger

5
Treatment Domain

The treatment domain of methadone maintenance consists of the programs that provide medical and rehabilitative services to addict patients and the environment in which they operate. This domain includes the community setting of the program, the staff who provide treatment, and the services they provide. The treatment domain, then, encompasses both what a program is and what a program does.

The concept of a treatment domain is a holistic approach to understanding and studying drug abuse programs. The entire program is viewed as an environment in which treatment takes place, and analysis of this environment requires careful delineation and classification of its structure, content, dynamics, and output. Comprehensive data collection of the methadone maintenance treatment domain dictates that whatever is part of this treatment be included as a topic of study. The treatment domain approach, then, is the antithesis of the black box.

When conceptualizing the domain of methadone programs, it is necessary to go beyond instrumental and ad hoc views of drug abuse treatment and rehabilitation. Effective outpatient methadone maintenance programs must provide continuous treatment to former intravenous drug users so that patients remain in the programs and become invested in rehabilitation. The programs are not, then, mere dispensing stations or supermarkets wherein one transacts business.

Noting that methadone maintenance programs provide continuous treatment to addict patients implies certain similarities to public school attendance. In both instances there are compulsory daily attendance requirements and a designated staff at each site to educate or treat a designated population on a regular basis. In both instances the institutions are involved in a long-term process of effecting improvement through continual face-to-face interaction between staff and clients, and this occurs at specific local programs, each of which serves a designated cohort of clients.

Elements of the Treatment Domain

The day-to-day operations of methadone programs in New York City, Philadelphia, and Baltimore were described in Chapter 4. Attention was focused on what occurs in these busy outpatient clinics with respect to dispensing oral methadone, patient flow through the clinics, common staff roles, treatment and rehabilitation services provided, and other aspects of program management. The intent in presenting these six descriptions was to provide a vivid, accurate portrayal of what life is like for both patients and staff at these clinics. In this regard, common features of methadone maintenance treatment were emphasized, and the variations among the individual programs were noted.

Although accurate descriptions of what occurs is a first step in studying the programs, it is also necessary to identify, classify, and measure the fundamental elements of this treatment process in order to facilitate systematic analysis of the relation between program operation and successful outcome. In this regard, the treatment domain of methadone maintenance programs has been subdivided into seven basic elements. These seven elements characterize the setting (or environment) in which treatment occurs as well as the content of the treatment. The general structure and dynamics of the treatment domain are discussed in this chapter. Chapter 6 focuses on the treatment and rehabilitative services provided to patients in methadone maintenance programs.

The seven elements of the treatment domain have been classified as follows: (1) the community setting in which treatment takes place; (2) the physical facility utilized; (3) aggregate patient characteristics; (4) the director and treatment staff; (5) the services provided to patients; (6) the administration and available resources; and (7) the treatment rationale and policy. Each of these elements is discussed with respect to research findings from the six programs.

Community Setting

Most methadone maintenance programs in East Coast cities are separate service delivery entities housed in free-standing buildings (or separate quarters) located in inner city metropolitan areas. The individual programs (or clinics) are commonly isolated in the midst of a metropolitan slum or commercial neighborhood in that they are not part of a large hospital, city agency building, or other public service complex. Rather, each program stands alone in its city neighborhood and therefore finds itself a part of the local community. How each program copes with its unique community and how each community reacts to the daily presence of hundreds of addict patients is an important aspect of the treatment domain.

The neighborhood setting of methadone maintenance programs constitutes a fundamental aspect of the treatment environment because staff and patients must travel to this neighborhood, live in it during the day, and in various ways become a part of the community. Therefore individual programs usually find themselves necessarily involved in community affairs. This involvement includes addressing local complaints about loitering, drug sales, theft, and similar matters. These complaints often prompt zoning disputes and other efforts to curtail or remove these programs from the community. As a consequence, programs often find themselves at odds with the local community. (There are exceptions, as when a program is part of a hospital complex.)

In our visits to dozens of methadone maintenance programs in eastern cities, we found that maintaining working relationships with the local community was a major concern of the director and staff at most sites. At the six programs we studied in detail, all had, to a greater or lesser extent, problems with the local community; two programs had persistent and serious problems in this regard.

The extent to which the six program directors and other staff became involved in community affairs depended on each program's history as well as the seriousness of their current problems. The more persistent and serious the problems with the community, the more time and energy the program staff devoted to these concerns. For the most part, each director coped with community relations problems as best he could, given the limited time and resources available. How well he fared with complaints and local opposition depended on the character of the community, the history of their relationship to the program, and the amount of support he obtained from local civic leaders and government officials. In this last regard, most programs received little or no support from local agencies as they coped with community relations problems on a daily basis.

Physical Facilities—Building and Space Allocation

All six methadone maintenance programs occupied a separate building; three of them were free-standing, and the others had one or more adjoining buildings. For the most part, then, the programs were autonomous as to building occupancy. That is, they were free-standing or attached buildings of moderate size that were used for methadone maintenance treatment.

It is pertinent to delineate the treatment and administration space in use in these six programs in order to assess the adequacy of the physical facilities. Some two-thirds of the rooms in these six programs were devoted to the direct provision of services to patients: 125 of the 188 rooms were used to provide medical, counseling, and dispensing services. The remaining 63 rooms were used for administrative support.

The allocation of treatment space followed functional staffing patterns in these programs. More than one-half of the treatment rooms were offices for counselors. The other two major groups providing treatment services were the medical and dispensing staff. The medical staff occupied 15 rooms; the dispensing area is discussed below. The remainder of the treatment space consisted of special treatment rooms, waiting rooms and bathrooms. The special treatment space included rooms for group sessions, training and observation rooms, a children's playroom, and a darkroom for photography. The patients' bathrooms were used mainly for "dropping" urine specimens. Waiting rooms usually functioned as holding areas for patients who were waiting for medication or counseling.

Most of the programs had one or two rooms that served as a dispensing center or pharmacy. In all but the largest program, there were one or two dispensing stations per program; in the largest program, there were three automated dispensing stations.

Some one-third of the space in the buildings was used for administration purposes. These 63 rooms consist of offices, record storage areas, computer rooms, staff lounge areas, conference space, and bathrooms. Although there was some variation among the programs with regard to the number and type of administrative rooms, the general lack of space in most programs precluded allocation of separate rooms for many functions.

Aggregate Patient Characteristics

The two principal dynamic elements of the treatment domain are the patients and the program staff. The interaction of these two groups determines the dynamics of drug abuse treatment at each site. The impact of the patient population on the program environment is continuous and pervasive. It is continuous because patients attend the clinic on a daily basis so long as they remain in treatment and therefore constitute an enduring presence over the years. Furthermore, the patient population has a pervasive affect on programs because their pressing daily needs and demands dictate, to a considerable extent, how programs operate. In this regard, it is significant to note that patients at each program constitute an enduring subculture that itself becomes part of the treatment domain, e.g., when patients organize an advisory or advocacy group at a program.

Two observations about the patient population at methadone maintenance programs are pertinent with respect to how this patient census influences the treatment setting. First, the preadmission characteristics of the patients determine their treatment needs and, to a considerable extent, their in-treatment behavior. Young, aggressive, antisocial addicts are different from older, less hostile, psychologically depressed addicts. In this sense, the dominant types of patients in the census sets the stage for what occurs at each program. If the patients have serious and pervasive problems, successful outpatient treatment may be problematical. Conversely, if the problems are less serious or transitory, success may be more likely. Whatever the outcome, the types of patient selected for treatment (e.g., "hardcore" adult addicts, adolescents, mothers) determines to a considerable extent the program environment.

The demographic and drug abuse characteristics of the 617 patients at the six programs have already been discussed (see Chapter 3). It is relevant to note here that although there was a general similarity in addiction-related characteristics among patients in the three cities (e.g., age at onset of opiate use, length of addiction, extent and type of criminality) there were notable differences among patients at the various programs with respect to demographic factors. Patients at two programs were predominantly from minority groups (85 and 91 percent); at another program only 30 percent of patients were from minority groups; and at three others they were almost evenly divided as to white and minority group status. Similarly, pretreatment employment was common at one program but uncommon at another. The point to be emphasized is that the patient population is an integral aspect of the treatment domain, and the population differs from program to program. Whether demographic, addiction, or other patient characteristics are related to successful outcome is a topic for subsequent analysis, but these aggregate characteristics are clearly a crucial aspect of each program's treatment domain.

A second way in which aggregate patient characteristics influence the programs is with regard to length of stay in treatment. The overall progress of patients in treatment at a given time is of paramount concern to both staff and patients. One measure of patients' progress in outpatient methadone maintenance treatment is their length of stay: Newly admitted and unmotivated patients tend to leave; those who remain in treatment tend to become rehabilitated over the years. Consequently, determination of a program's current patient census by length of stay provides an initial assessment of the treatment domain because patients' progress in treatment and rehabilitation is commonly associated with time in treatment.

The length of time the 617 male patients in this study had spent in their current methadone maintenance programs is depicted in Figure 5.1 These data refer to each patient's length of treatment at time of the first interview in 1985.

Almost one-third of the 617 patients had been in treatment less than 1 year (30.2 percent). Another one-third had been in treatment 1 to 3 years, and the last one-third had been in treatment for 3 years or more. The patient census, then, is composed of three basic groups: new admissions, stabilizing patients, and long-term patients. Where the dividing lines are drawn depends on the research question being addressed and are therefore somewhat arbitrary; the point is that there are fundamentally different types of patients in methadone maintenance programs based on their length of stay in treatment. Length of stay is a measure of both the amount of treatment received and the extent of rehabilitation achieved. To be sure, length of stay is only one measure of "success," but it is an important factor to assess.

The importance of length of stay with regard to the treatment domain is that this mix of patients—by years of treatment completed—constitutes a

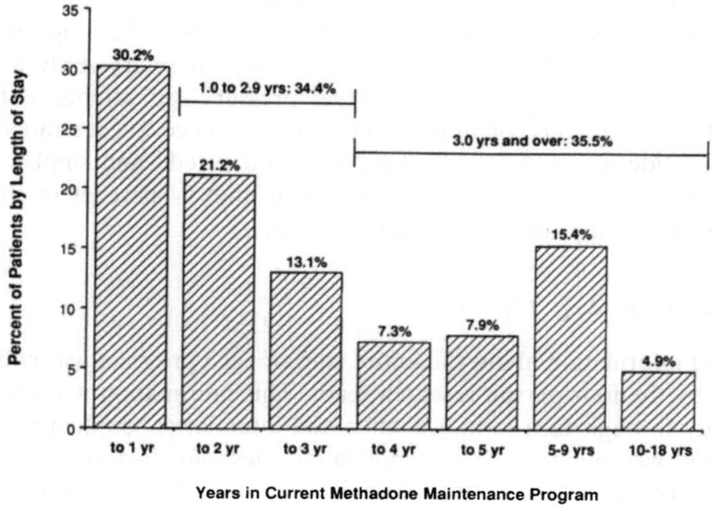

FIGURE 5.1. Length of stay in treatment for 617 methadone maintenance patients.

crucial part of each program's environment. A program that has a high proportion of new admissions, few long-term patients, and a high rate of dropouts, engenders definite expectations. Conversely, a program that has fewer new admissions, a lower dropout rate, and more long-term patients may denote more successful treatment. In this sense, then, the aggregate patient characteristics are a crucial aspect of the treatment setting.

With regard to the six programs under study, there were notable differences in the patient censuses based on length of stay. The percent of patients in treatment over 5 years varied as follows: 16.0, 16.8, 18.5, 23.6, 25.2, and 33.5. Thus there were twice as many long-term stay patients in one program than another. With regard to new admissions, the percentages also varied (27.1, 31.3, 31.9, 33.5, 36.2, and 48.0) but not as much. Again, the point is that these aggregate patient characteristics influence and are a part of the treatment domain. Subsequent analysis will investigate the relation of length of stay to patient outcome and other variables.

Staff at the Six Programs

The staff of methadone maintenance programs commonly consists of a director and small administrative staff, medical personnel, and counselors. The medical personnel include dispensing nurses (or pharmacists), physicians' assistants (or nurse practitioners), and physicians. Most of them are employed full time, except the physicians, who are usually employed on a part-time basis.

The two major functions of the staff are to run the program and provide available services to the entire patient population. These two functions are intertwined because providing services involves running the programs.

Admission to outpatient treatment is usually voluntary; only a small proportion of patients are under "legal pressure" to attend. Patients' motivation to attend is commonly expressed as a "need to get straightened out," to "tide me over," to "get detoxed and cured" and similar statements. In this regard, it is pertinent to note that 94 percent of the 617 patients have had prior drug abuse treatment.

Staff—Who Are They?

Detailed information about the entire staff of each program was collected on-site by the four-person research team. This information was obtained primarily through face-to-face confidential interviews; supplementary information was obtained from confidential questionnaires and record reviews. Inasmuch as the entire treatment staff of each program was interviewed twice by the research team, comprehensive and reliable data about personal characteristics, program duties, and the delivery of services were obtained.

As of late 1986, there were 135[a] persons employed at the six programs. This overall staff consisted of 100 treatment personnel and 40 administrative staff (Table 5.1). These figures, however, include both part-time and

TABLE 5.1. Total Staff for the Six Programs

	Number by FTE[a]	
Type of staff	No.	FTE
Counselors	59	55.2
Medical staff		
MD's—Physician	9	2.9
PA's—Physicians' Assistant	4	3.2
NP's—Nurse Practitioners	1	0.3
Dispensing Nurses	24	17.9
Dispensing Pharmacists	3	2.5
Administrative		
Personnel	40	35.5
Security	(S)	12.7
Totals:	135[a]	130.2

[a]There were 135 persons employed at the six programs in 1986; of these, 105 were full-time employees and 30 were part-time employees. Four of the full-time staff and one of the part-time employees had dual roles in the program (e.g., half-time counseling and half-time administration). These 5 employees are shown in both of their roles in the above columns, hence the number of staff positions sums to 140. Security staff are indicated in the FTE columns but not in the number of persons columns because many of the security staff were part-time contractual employees. (An FTE is a full-time equivalent and represents 35 to 40 hours per week of employment, depending on the program).

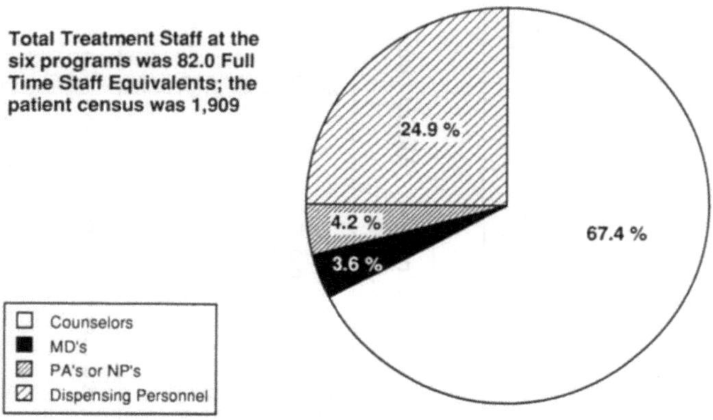

FIGURE 5.2. Type of treatment staff at six methadone maintenance programs.

full-time staff. With regard to full-time equivalents (FTEs) the staff consisted of 130.2 FTEs. Of these, 82.0 FTEs were treatment staff, 35.5 were administrative staff, and 12.7 were security guards. Thus 63 percent of the staff at the six programs were primarily involved in treatment and 37 percent in administration or security. As the role of the director commonly involved both administrative and treatment functions, his involvement in patient care varied and was calculated on a pro rata basis.

Two-thirds of the treatment staff at the six programs consisted of drug abuse counselors, the remainder being medical staff (Figure 5.2); 67.4 percent of the 82 FTE staff were counselors, 24.9 percent were dispensing personnel, and 7.7 percent provided medical care. This last group of staff was almost evenly divided between physicians' assistants (PAs), or nurse practitioners (NPs), and physicians; 4.2 percent of the treatment staff were PAs or NPs and 3.6 percent were MDs. Each of these staff types—physicians, NPs or PAs, dispensing personnel, and counselors—had definite treatment functions as well as related qualifications or experience.

Counselors

There were 57 counselors employed at the six methadone maintenance programs and two additional admissions counselors. As noted, they constituted some two-thirds of the entire treatment staff. These counselors were almost evenly divided with respect to sex; 50.9 percent were male and 49.1 percent were female. With respect to race-ethnic designation, 40.4 percent were white, 40.4 percent were black, and 19.3 percent were Hispanic or belong to some other minority group. Somewhat surprisingly, the counselors were not older than the patients they treated; the mean age of the 57 counselors was 35.2 years, and that of the patients was 36.6 years.

With regard to educational attainment, 33.9 percent of the 57 counselors

TABLE 5.2. Characteristics of 57 Counselors at Six Programs

Program	General information				Education		Experience			
	No.	Male (%)	Minorities (%)	Age (mean yr)	School (mean yr)	Advanced degree (%)	Ex-addicts (%)	Years as counselor	Years this program	Annual turnover (%)
U	≥10	50	50	36.0	17.2	80	30.0	6.0	3.0	50
V	≥10	30	50	39.2	14.2	10	30.0	9.5	6.5	10
W	9	44	44	31.3	16.9	22	0.0	2.4	0.9	70
X	6	67	33	35.2	18.0	83	16.7	9.5	5.0	43
Y	7	57	71	36.6	17.7	43	28.6	2.0	1.3	25
Z	≥10	60	73	33.9	13.4	0	66.7	4.2	1.5	29
Total	57	51	60	35.2	15.8	34	33.3	5.5	2.9	33.3

*In order to ensure confidentiality of the program data, the sequence and designation of the six programs has been varied in relevant tables.

held advanced degrees, 30.4 percent were college graduates, and 23.2 percent had no formal education beyond high school. As depicted in Table 5.2, there were marked differences among the programs with respect to the educational background of their counselors—from none with advanced degrees to 83 percent who had advanced degrees.

Of the 57 counselors at the six programs, 19 were ex-addicts. Thus one-third of the counselors had a personal history of drug abuse involvement. As might be expected, the ex-addict counselors were less educated than the other counselors (three held an advanced degree and ten had no formal education beyond high school) and were more likely to be from minority groups. At the same time, the former addicts were more experienced in treating addict patients, as they had been drug abuse counselors for a longer time. Although five of the six programs employed ex-addict counselors, two programs were rather different from the other four; one program did not employ any ex-addict counselors, whereas the other two-thirds of the counselors were ex-addicts (Table 5.2).

The 57 counselors had 5.5 mean years of experience in drug abuse or alcoholism counseling. With respect to experience at these programs, the counselors had an average of 2.9 years of experience. The differences among the programs in terms of years of experience of the counselors at their current positions were considerable: At three of the programs the mean period of experience at the current program was less than 2 years; at the other three the mean period of on-site experience for the counselors was 3 to 6 years.

The mean annual salary of the 57 counselors during the 1986–1987 year was $18,265. The mean for the six programs varied from $14,500 to $22,700. Partly as a consequence of these low salaries, the annual turnover rate of counselors between 1985 and 1986 was considerable: 33.3 percent had left. The turnover rate by program ranged from 10 to 70 percent (Table 5.2).

Medical Staff

The medical staff at the six methadone maintenance programs in 1986 consisted of 41 persons: 9 physicians, 4 physicians' assistants, 1 nurse practitioner, and 27 dispensing personnel. This latter group was composed of 24 dispensing nurses and 3 pharmacists. For the most part, direct medical care was provided by the physicians, physicians' assistants, and the nurse practitioner. The dispensing staff were primarily involved in the daily dispensing of methadone.

With respect to medical coverage, each of the six programs was served by at least one physician; there were two physicians at three of the programs. In addition, there was medical coverage by physicians' assistants at three programs (2 PAs at one program) and a nurse practitioner at a fourth. This enumeration, however, obscures the fact that most of these

14 medical personnel were only part-time staff; only three were full-time employees, and the remainder were employed half-time or less.

The nine physicians who provided medical coverage at the six programs were predominantly men (eight of nine) but diverse as to race-ethnic status. In the latter regard, four of the physicians were white, three were black, one was Hispanic, and one was Oriental.

With regard to experience at their current program, six of the nine physicians had been at the program for 6 years or more; the other three physicians were new to their respective programs, each with less than 1 year of experience. Taken together, these nine physicians had a mean of 7.5 years of continuous experience at their current position.

It is meaningful to delineate three basic roles physicians fulfill in methadone maintenance programs: (1) They may serve as direct providers of medical care; in this role they see and treat patients for their drug abuse or for medical or psychiatric problems. (2) They may serve as supervisors or consultants to other staff members who provide direct medical care and other services; this role is often referred to as case consultation and direction. (3) Physicians may serve as program directors and administrators who formulate and implement treatment policy. It is pertinent to note that individual physicians may fulfill more than one of these roles and, furthermore, that programs may emphasize or downplay particular roles.

In the six programs studied, eight of the nine physicians were primarily engaged in providing direct patient care. In addition, three served as active medical directors who were involved in formulating treatment policy. (The roles of medical director and program director are separate in most programs.)

Four physicians' assistants and one nurse practitioner provided direct medical care at four of the six programs. Two of these four physicians' assistants were employed full time at one program, and another was employed full time at a second program. These two programs, then, had full-time medical coverage by physicians' assistants. Two other programs had some coverage by either a physicians' assistant or a nurse practitioner, but the extent of this coverage was minimal, one-quarter time or less.

The 24 dispensing nurses and three pharmacists at the six programs were mostly employed full time. Each program had at least three persons engaged in dispensing oral methadone. The three pharmacists were accredited graduates, but most of the nurses (20 of 24) were licensed practical nurses rather than registered nurses. Some of the dispensing nurses—depending on the program—also provided routine medical care to patients when time permitted.

The treatment staff available at each of the six programs varied considerably, as did the mix of staff. Although both of these topics are analyzed later with regard to staffing per 250 patients, a few observations are pertinent here. The general similarity of the dispensing staff at the six programs was notable; the range in FTEs for five of the six programs is only 2.5 to 3.6 FTEs. This similarity undoubtedly reflects the uniformity of the dispensing function at all of the programs: to dispense oral methadone on-site, to prepare additional take-home doses, and to keep prescribed records. There is somewhat more variation in the number of counselors employed at the six programs (from 5.2 to 10.0 FTEs at five of the six programs): this variation reflects differences in such factors as staffing patterns and the difficulty of recruiting new staff. The greatest variation among the staffing patterns at the programs, however, occurred with respect to the medical staff. One program had nine times more medical coverage by physicians than another. How these differences in medical staff among the programs are related to variations in the medical services provided patients is discussed in Chapter 6, but it is relevant here to note the variation when delineating the overall staff at the six programs.

Administrative Staff

The administrative staff consisted of some one-third of the total staff at the six programs; the remaining two-thirds were the treatment staff. The administrative staff at the six programs consisted of program directors, administrators, clerks, secretaries, and security guards. Each of these staff members had particular responsibilities and duties to perform.

The director was a dominant administrative force in all six programs. He commonly was responsible for preparing a budget, hiring staff, running the clinic, and otherwise addressing whatever problems arose. This involvement in administrative duties was superimposed on treatment responsibilities because both of these functions fall within the director's purview.

All of the program directors were involved in administrative duties and responsibilities. The extent of this involvement depended on such considerations as whether there was another staff person who was an experienced administrator, the number of staff available for administration, and the demands of administrative duties or problems outside the program (e.g., with the community, the funding agency). Although all six of the directors were involved in administering their programs, their involvement in patient care varied considerably. Some were actively involved on a regular basis, whereas others seldom saw a patient. Five of the six directors were employed full time; one worked less than 20 percent at this position.

The demographic characteristics and professional qualifications of the six directors varied considerably. Five of the six directors were men; four were white and two were black; the mean age for the six was 43.2 years. Four of the directors held advanced or professional degrees (MD, MSW, or DSW), and two were not college graduates. With respect to experience as director at his program, the figure varied from 4 months to 13 years; two of the directors had been at their programs for 10 years or more, and three had 4 years or less of such experience. It is noteworthy that most of the directors' prior experience in drug abuse treatment was obtained at their present programs.

The secretaries, clerks, and other office staff employed at the programs were primarily engaged in answering telephones, taking messages, assisting patients with appointments, typing notes, entering data, filing records, photocopying forms, and fulfilling similar administrative duties. Although some programs had more such administrative support than others, generally the staff was inadequate for the extensive workload. Again, with one or two exceptions, the office space available for the administrative staff was also inadequate.

All six of the programs were confronted with the common security problems associated with methadone maintenance treatment: (1) theft of drugs and other valuables from the clinic; (2) sale of drugs on the premises or diversion of methadone for sale outside; (3) loitering outside the building, and (4) violent behavior by patients when in the clinic. Most of these security problems were dealt with directly by the program staff. Two programs hired uniformed guards to provide security on a contractual basis; one program had its own security officers; one hired "desk clerks" to monitor patient flow; and two assigned one or more administrative staff to this task. Commonly, security within the building did not pose a serious problem, as suitable controls were worked out during previous years of operation. At the same time, loitering of patients outside of the program was a persistent concern at most sites.

Administration and Organization

Because methadone maintenance programs are usually located in center city or commercial neighborhoods and each clinic stands alone in a separate building in the neighborhood, the administrative roles of the director and support staff are especially important. The staff are not only confronted with the unrelenting demands of running an active outpatient service for addict patients 365 days a year, they must accomplish this task as an isolated organization in an unfriendly environment. Although some local programs are part of a larger drug abuse treatment organization, most are not. Even when a local outpatient facility is part of a larger organization, it still is usually geographically isolated and depends on its own staff and resources to meet the daily demands of providing methadone and other services to its patients.

Noting that methadone maintenance programs tend to be isolated in the midst of center city or commercial neighborhoods is not meant to imply that their location is inappropriate. The point is that isolation in the midst of slum or commercial neighborhoods has various administrative consequences, one of which is the need to develop a self-contained treatment system.

The principal outside resource required by methadone maintenance programs is funding. Most programs on the East Coast are publicly funded, although private programs are far from uncommon. Five of the six programs studied were publicly supported; the sixth was about one-half publicly supported and one-half supported by patients' fees.

For the six programs, the mean annual funding per patient was $1459. This figure varied from a low of $865 per patient per year to a high of $2452 per patient per year. Four of the six programs, however, had mean annual per patient funding that ranged from $1400 to $2000 in 1986. All six supplemented this public funding by charging patient fees. Many patients were charged a minimal fee of $2 or $3 a week. For those who were employed or otherwise able to pay, the charge for treatment varied from $25 to $50 per week depending on the program and patients' financial situation.

Treatment Policy

In many ways the treatment policy established and implemented at methadone maintenance programs is a beacon that serves to provide direction for the treatment process. This beacon often flutters, however, and different programs have different beacons. Consequently, treatment policy at methadone maintenance programs tends to be amorphous and diverse. It is amorphous in that it often is not clearly stated nor consistently articulated with operational practices. It is diverse in that individual programs tend to adhere to several treatment rationales or orientations.

The treatment policy extant at the six methadone maintenance programs varied considerably, and it often was in a state of flux. This diversity of treatment policies is due to a number of factors that have been superimposed on the original rationale and regimen for methadone maintenance therapy developed by Dole and his colleagues during the 1960s. Contemporary factors that influence treatment policy are federal, state, and city regulations, the resources available, the desires of local funding agencies, the orientation of the director and senior staff, and such other considerations as the history and reputation of the program.

It was found that the treatment orientation of the six programs could be subsumed under two broad classifications: medical-psychiatric or social rehabilitation. Although all of the programs had some medical and some rehabilitation orientation, each tended to have one or the other of these two orientations as a guiding policy.

It was found that three programs had a primary medical orientation and three had a primary social rehabilitation orientation. Beyond this dichotomy, there were other treatment policy differences. One of the medically oriented programs stressed both long-term maintenance and efficiency of operations; the two other medically oriented programs stressed short-term treatment and, in one case, psychiatric diagnosis and coverage for patients. Conversely, the three programs oriented to social rehabilitation focused their treatment on changing the everyday behavior of patients. One of the social rehabilitation programs also stressed the role of the local community in its treatment rationale.

Measurement of the Treatment Domain

After completion of the second comprehensive program data collection effort in 1986, 89 summary treatment domain variables were selected from the voluminous data collected at the six programs during the prior 2 years (see Appendix A). These 89 variables provided a means of describing and measuring in detail the elements of the treatment domain. The 54 variables that refer to the six elements already discussed are described next. The remaining 35 service delivery or output variables are discussed in Chapter 6.

Neighborhood (Variables 1–4)

Most of the data about the neighborhood and physical facility of each program were obtained through direct observation and measurement by the research staff. Information about the community was obtained through tours of the neighborhood, conversation with local residents, and attendance at community meetings. Additional information was obtained from the director, staff, and patients about such matters as loitering outside the building, security arrangements at the program, community relations problems, parking availability, and ownership and maintenance of the building.

The evaluation staff also undertook a facility survey at each site, in which each room was measured, its occupants noted, and its contents catalogued; moreover, the adequacy of space, privacy, security, repair, equipment, and maintenance was recorded. As noted, the 89 summary variables provide only an overview of the data collected in each area.

Four variables summarize the neighborhood findings: (1) the type of neighborhood in which the program is located (middle class residential, working class residential, average commercial area, run-down commercial area, or slum area); (2) staff involvement with the local community; (3) extent to which the program experienced community relations problems during the 3-year field work period; and (4) parking space available for staff and patients at each program.

Measurement of the Physical Facility (Variables 5–9)

Five variables were selected to provide a summary delineation of the physical facility at each site: (5) the overall adequacy of the building (adequacy of space and structure); (6) state of repair of the building (exterior and interior); (7) cleanliness of the rooms and interior; (8) composite score of facility adequacy (average of variables 5–7); (9) adequacy of security provided with regard to patient flow in the building.

The first three variables (5, 6, 7) were derived from the facility survey; variable 8 was a summary measure of the facility based on the prior three variables. Variable 9 (security provided) was derived from an appraisal of how adequately each program was able to monitor or control patient flow and misbehavior in the clinic; this variable measured daily patient flow through the clinic with respect to scheduling arrangement, orderliness, presence or absence of complaints, and loitering.

Aggregate Patient Characteristics (Variables 10–14)

Five variables were selected to measure the patient census at each program: (10) the number of patients in treatment at a given time (i.e., the active census); (11) the percent of patients in treatment less than 1 year; (12) the percent of patients in treatment 5 years or longer; (13) the percent of patients who are nonwhite; and (14) the number of patients on the waiting list. The waiting list variable was found to be less evidently related to the treatment domain than the other four patient census variables. This occurred because most of the programs studied did not, in fact, have viable waiting lists. Nonetheless, this variable was included, as it might be significant in other programs.

Treatment Staff (Variables 15–37)

For convenience of exposition and subsequent analysis, the treatment staff were separated into three groups: director, counselors, and medical staff. Information about each of these staff groups was summarized in 23 key variables.

Six variables were selected to depict the director's role in each program and assess his performance: (15) his years of experience at this program; (16) his years of experience as director; (17) his years of education, (18) his employment commitment (i.e., percent of time employed at the program); (19) his involvement with patient care; and (20) his treatment effectiveness. The last variable was a composite measure derived from three items: his involvement with patient care (variable 19), his favorable impact on the overall treatment program (a rating based on interviews with the director and staff as well as on-site program observation), and his outside relevant professional activities.

There were nine variables that delineated the characteristics or functioning of counselors at each program: (21) number of counselors employed at each program; (22) number of full-time counselors (by FTE); (23) mean years of counseling experience at this program; (24) mean years of education of counselors; (25) percent of counselors with advanced degrees; (26) mean salary of full-time counselors; (27) percent of counselors who are ex-addicts; (28) percent of counselors who are minority group members; (29) annual turnover rate of counselors.

The medical staff at each program was delineated by eight key variables: (30) number of physicians employed at the program (by FTE); (31) number of physicians' assistants employed; (32) number of nurse practitioners;

(33) number of dispensing nurses; (34) number of pharmacists employed; (35) total medical staff employed (as in all the above, by FTE); (36) mean years of physicians' experience at the program; and (37) mean years of the physicians' assistants' or nurse practitioners' experience.

Program Administration and Treatment Policy (Variables 38–47)

Ten variables were derived to summarize the findings obtained with respect to program administration and treatment policy: (38) identification of program; (39) years of operation of program; (40) annual per patient cost for the treatment provided; (41) adequacy of funding; (42) status of patient records; (43) overall adequacy of administration; (44) management and coordination of treatment services; (45) extent of medical orientation; (46) extent of social rehabilitation orientation; and (47) extent of maintenance orientation. The first seven variables refer primarily to administration and the last three to treatment policy.

Record data sets were utilized for compiling these measures when feasible. Thus variables 38, 39, 40, and 42 are derived from available records. In addition, there was a need to devise other comparative measures of crucial aspects of administration that could not be directly compiled from existing data. Three such measures were derived: (41) was a comparative rating of the funding at the six programs, (43) was a composite rating of the adequacy of each program's administrative operations, and (44) was an assessment of how effectively treatment services were coordinated and managed.

Additional Areas of Measurement (Variables 48–54)

In addition to devising 47 variables that delineate the general scope of the treatment domain (the variables pertaining to the delivery of treatment services are reviewed in Chapter 6), data from other areas of special interest were also obtained. Three of these additional sets of variables about the treatment domain refer to staffing patterns, demographic concordance of staff and patients at each program, and the staff's rating of their program's effectiveness.

The first additional area of measurement refers to staffing patterns at each program when standardized to a census of 250 patients. Four variables were derived to measure staff allocation in this regard: (48) the number of counselors (by FTE) per 250 patients; (49) the number of medical staff (by FTE) per 250 patients; (50) the number of physicians (by FTE) per 250 patients; and (51) the total number of treatment staff (by FTE) per 250 patients.

These four variables depict the overall staffing pattern of the six programs standardized to 250 patients. Most of the treatment staff at each of the programs consisted of drug abuse counselors. There were, on average,

7.2 full-time counselors (by FTE) per 250 patients at the six programs. The counseling staff ranged from 5.2 to 12.5 full-time counselors per 250 patients; there were, then, one-half as many counselors at some programs as at others.

The medical staff consisted of the physicians, physicians' assistants, and a nurse practitioner as well as the dispensing staff. This latter group consisted of nurses and pharmacists who dispensed methadone, and this dispensing staff varied from 4.0 FTEs at one program to 1.9 FTEs at another. The mean number of dispensing staff at the six programs was 2.7 FTEs.

The staffing pattern for physicians and physicians' assistants (and nurse practitioners) at the six programs reflected both the limited medical coverage generally available and the considerable variation in this coverage from program to program. With respect to the limited medical coverage available, there was, on average, less than 1 FTE staff to provide medical services per 250 patients. With respect to variation among the programs, some had less than one-half the medical coverage of others. Significantly, the variation in the amount of coverage provided by physicians at the six programs varied by a factor of 9.

Staff-Patient Minority Group Concordance

Once data have been collected with respect to the designated elements of the treatment domain, it becomes feasible to measure and analyze relations among variables within programs. One such measurement derived was the extent to which staff and patients at particular programs were similar, or dissimilar, with respect to minority group status. The question is significant because concordance between staff and patients with respect to sex, race, age, social economic status, and certain other factors may influence the effectiveness of counseling and other services.

Approximately one-half of both the counselors and patients at the six programs in 1986 were minority group members (53.6 percent for counselors and 51.6 percent for patients), although the extent of this concordance at particular programs was markedly different. Thus at two of the programs the minority group representation of the patients and their counselors was similar: The difference was only 5 percent or less. Conversely, at two programs there was a notable lack of minority group concordance between staff and patients. At one, 85 percent of the patients were minority group members, whereas only 29 percent of the counseling staff were minority group members. At another program the situation was reversed: 71 percent of the counseling staff, but only 30 percent of the patients were minority group members. The extent of such minority group concordance (or discordance) between counselors and patients at each program is measured by variable 52. By itself this variable provides significant information about the treatment domain. In addition, it provides a means of relating this finding to both other treatment as well as outcome measures.

A third area of additional data about the treatment domain was obtained with respect to staff rating of the effectiveness of methadone maintenance treatment at their respective programs. Each staff member at each program was asked in the 1986 confidential face-to-face interview to assess the program's effectiveness. Specifically, each counselor and each medical staff member was asked to rate the program as below average, average, above average, or superior in terms of treatment effectiveness. The individual ratings were summed by type of staff for each program to provide an overall assessment.

Because the counselors were the largest staff group in the programs and most counselors were full-time employees, their rating of each program was utilized as a key program measurement. Two related variables were derived for this measure. Variable 53 was the mean counselors' rating of effectiveness at each program: (1) a superior rating, (2) far above average, (3) above average, (4) average, and (5) below average. The six mean ratings for the individual programs were 1.4 (superior for the counselors at one program) 2.6 (far above average for counselors at two programs), 2.9 at another, 3.0 (above average) at a fifth, and 3.4 at a sixth (the lowest rating).

Inasmuch as there was a tendency of the counselors to rate their own program as above average (similar to the psychological tendency of individuals to rate themselves favorably compared to others), another variable was devised to afford a more differentiating measure. Variable 54 was a measure of the percent of counselors at each program who rated their own program as "far above average" or "the very best." The percent of counselors at each program who rated their program in this highly favorable manner was 100.0, 42.3, 40.0, 22.2, 20.0, and 15.4. Thus all of the counselors at one program rated their methadone maintenance treatment as superior, whereas at three programs only a minority of counselors (22 to 15 percent) considered their program as superior in effectiveness.

Conclusion

The reason for employing the treatment domain schema in the study of methadone maintenance programs is to open the black box of treatment. To accomplish this objective it is necessary to identify, describe, and measure the component parts or elements of treatment. It is also necessary to recognize that individual programs are an entity, and that the characteristics of entire programs need to be considered and studied. The schema of the treatment domain, then, is intended to provide a framework for answering the question of what occurs at methadone maintenance programs. It also provides a foundation for measurement that facilitates further analysis of how treatment is related to successful patient outcome.

Seven basic elements of the treatment domain were identified and described: (1) the neighborhood setting; (2) the physical facility; (3) the aggregate patient population (i.e., the census); (4) the staff; (5) the output of services provided; (6) the administration of the program, and (7) the treatment policy. Relevant measures for each of these elements were described. The fifth element, services provided, is the subject of Chapter 6.

Studying methadone maintenance treatment from the perspective of the treatment domain schema has broadened, yet clarified, understanding of the setting, structure, and process of treatment. A number of substantive and methodological conclusions have come about in large part through use of this schema. Five of these conclusions seem especially relevant.

One of the significant findings of the present study is the crucial role played by individual programs. It would be an exaggeration to hold that *programs* have only now been discovered as a subject for study, as it has been recognized for some time that good and bad programs exist. It has not been sufficiently recognized, however, that individual programs, rather than an entire modality, may well be the crucial unit of analysis when determining treatment effectiveness.

Second, when conducting field work at methadone programs in New York City, Philadelphia, and Baltimore, it became more and more apparent that the community setting and patient population were an integral part of the treatment process. These two aspects of the treatment domain set the stage for a fuller understanding of how programs function.

A third conclusion about the treatment domain was that the on-site director of a methadone maintenance program played a crucial role in that he often was responsible for whether a program was effectively run. Concomitantly, it was found that the management and coordination of treatment services were important to program success. It was not sufficient to have services available; services had to be properly provided and coordinated. Thus counseling, medical, dispensing, and administrative services must be scheduled and highly coordinated if they are to be effective.

Lastly, from the treatment domain perspective, two methodological conclusions followed from the course of the study. First, it was evident from the beginning that collecting data according to the treatment domain schema necessitated on-site field work of considerable scope and duration. Second, it was recognized that it would be necessary to obtain repeat measurements of program elements in order to ascertain how consistently treatment services were provided. Therefore a comprehensive measurement of the treatment domain was undertaken twice, in 1985 and 1986. The treatment domain measurements obtained at the six programs in 1985 and in 1986 are compared in Chapter 6.

6 Treatment and Rehabilitation Provided to Patients at the Six Programs in 1985 & 1986

The scope, setting, structure, and organization of the treatment domain were delineated in Chapter 5. Here attention is focused on the actual delivery of treatment and rehabilitative services to patients. Although both of these chapters refer to the treatment domain, the topics of determining the specific services provided to methadone maintenance patients and the frequency of delivery are of sufficient importance to warrant separate and detailed consideration.

Measurement of Services Provided

Before discussing the findings regarding the services provided to methadone maintenance patients, it is pertinent to address two related issues: How can the provision of services to thousands of patients be accurately measured? How can the effectiveness of treatment services be determined?

An answer to the question of how the delivery of treatment and rehabilitative service can most efficaciously be measured is that it depends on the scope, depth, and reliability of the database required. If only superficial or limited information is sought from numerous programs, these data may be obtained from survey questionnaires or secondary sources. If, however, comprehensive and accurate data about the full range and frequency of service delivery to patients at designated programs are required, intensive on-site data collection by a specially trained staff is required. Each of these approaches—large-scale extensive questionnaire surveys or intensive on-site data collection efforts—has advantages and limitations. In the present study, on-site data collection by the research staff was deemed to be essential because of the detailed treatment domain data required.

Because the overall data collection procedures employed to measure the treatment domain have already been discussed (see Chapter 2), it is pertinent to comment here only on those aspects of the procedures that refer to the delivery of services. Four points summarize the procedure employed to measure the provision of services at the six programs. First, data collection at the programs was undertaken by the research staff, and these findings about the provision of services were deemed confidential. Specifically, findings about the services provided (or not provided) by each staff member were not revealed to program directors or administrators, and the total output data from each program were also confidential. Second, measurement was focused on the actual delivery of specific services during a designated week or month to all patients at each program; the objective, then, was to measure each program's output of services. Third, the measurement of output at each program was accomplished by structured interviews of the entire staff as well as by direct compilation from clinic records. These data were supplemented by such other confirmatory sources as patients' reports and systematic observation. Fourth, the entire on-site measurement of the output of treatment and rehabilitative services at each of the programs was repeated in 1986. Thus measurement of the services provided to 1874 methadone maintenance patients at the six programs in 1985 was followed by measurement of the services provided to 1909 patients who were at these same six programs 1 year later. The primary purpose of this second output measurement was to ascertain the stability or consistency of service delivery in methadone maintenance programs.

Comprehensive analysis of the effectiveness of methadone maintenance programs can only be undertaken after the various services that are regularly provided to patients in these programs has been ascertained and then measured. Once the delivery of services has been measured, the findings can be related to baseline patient characteristics, other treatment domain variables, and outcome measures.

Methadone programs provide four main services to their patients: (1) oral methadone medication; (2) urinalysis; (3) counseling; and (4) medical coverage. With respect to medication, all patients are scheduled to receive a daily dose of methadone each day of the year, and so most patients are required to attend their program five or more times per week. Most of the methadone dispensed to patients at the clinics is consumed on-site under staff supervision; the remainder of the daily methadone doses are dispensed at the clinic as take-home dosages. In addition to this dispensing function, programs provide counseling, medical, and other services to patients. Most of these counseling and other services are provided during regular weekday hours, but dispensing takes place 6 or 7 days a week at the clinics.

Daily Hours of Operation

Methadone maintenance clinics are busy, sometimes hectic places that provide medication and other services to addict patients on a daily basis. Most clinics are open during the week and during the weekend as well. Thus, the clinics are actively providing services 6 or 7 days a week.

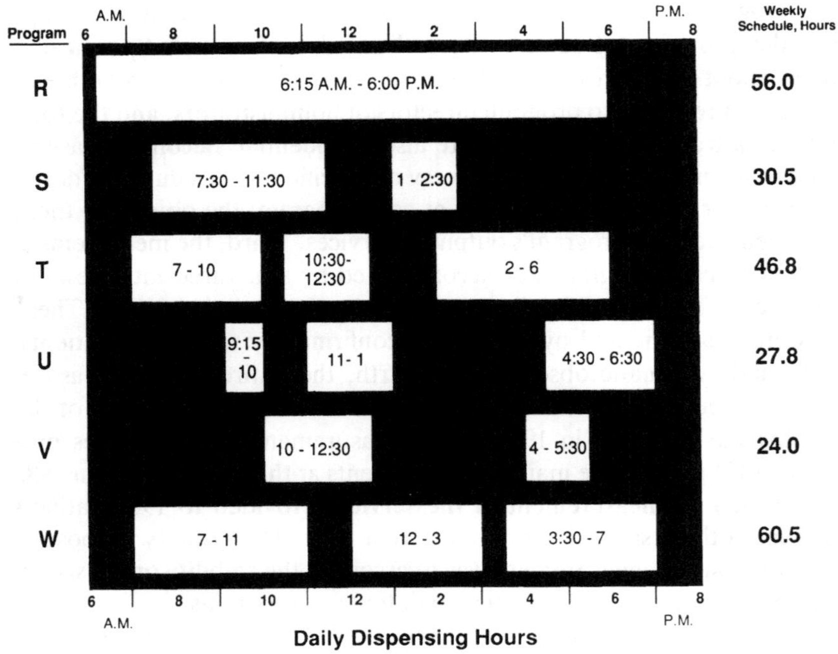

FIGURE 6.1. Daily dispensing hours at the six programs

It is worthwhile to delineate the hours of operation of the six methadone clinics to set the stage for considering how these programs function. In particular, consideration of how dispensing and other services are scheduled provides an initial description of what services are delivered to patients on a daily and weekly basis.

Dispensing Hours and Schedules

During the regular work week, all six of the clinics dispensed methadone in both the morning and afternoon hours (Fig. 6.1). Three of the clinics scheduled three daily dispensing periods, so that medication was available during the morning, afternoon, and evening; two of the clinics had only two dispensing periods, and one had one long continuous dispensing period from 6:15 a.m. to 6:00 p.m.

The reason most of the clinics have discrete periods for medication is to facilitate patient scheduling and control. It is less disruptive and otherwise efficacious to have patients adhere to a definite schedule for medication. This schedule is arranged with the patient to promote or facilitate his rehabilitation, as when a schedule is arranged to facilitate a patient's employment. In addition, definite medication schedules enable the counseling and medical staff to more readily contact patients when these services are needed.

With respect to the number of daily hours of dispensing, three of the six clinics were open to dispense methadone 8 hours or more per day. The remaining three clinics were open for dispensing for 4.0, 4.75 and 5.5 hours per day. There was, then, considerable variation in the dispensing hours at the clinics. In this regard, it should be noted that the clinic that dispensed methadone continuously for 12 hours had a sizable patient population and an automated dispensing procedure.

With respect to weekend dispensing schedules, all six programs were open on Saturdays, and four were open on Sundays as well. Typically, the clinics were open for 3 to 4 hours during weekend mornings.

Hours for Counseling and Provision of Medical Services

As might be expected, counseling and other services were usually scheduled for the regular weekday hours. Specifically, the six programs had the following weekday schedules for counseling, respectively: 8:00 a.m. to 6:00 p.m.; 9:30 a.m. to 5:30 p.m.; 9:00 a.m. to 6:30 p.m.; 7:00 a.m. to 6:00 p.m.; 7:30 a.m. to 4:30 p.m.; and 6:15 a.m. to 6:00 p.m. There were minor variations of these daily hours in some clinics, e.g., when there were weekly staff meetings or other treatment-related activities. In addition to this weekday schedule, three programs provided counseling hours on Saturday mornings and one had counseling sessions Sunday mornings as well.

In general, the scheduling of services to patients in methadone maintenance programs is organized around the provision of methadone. The hours scheduled for dispensing methadone establish a framework for the delivery of most services to patients. The provision of counseling and medical services is usually coordinated with the dispensing hours for the convenience of both patients and staff.

Methadone Dispensing Practices at the Six Programs

The dispensing practices of individual programs and patients' compliance with these procedures provide crucial information about two aspects of methadone maintenance treatment. First, dispensing practices document the distribution of methadone doses, the number of take-homes allowed, and other aspects of this medication procedure. Second, patients' weekly medication schedules establish a viable means for measuring attendance inasmuch as accurate records are kept of each methadone dose dispensed or missed. Therefore a patient's or program's missed medication rate is the obverse of their attendance rate. The extent of patient attendance is an important measure of both individual compliance and program performance; attendance also is a measure of the amount of treatment provided by a program.

The importance of the dispensing function in methadone maintenance programs is dictated by the reality that all patients in methadone maintenance treatment are prescribed a daily oral dose of methadone, and this medication schedule obtains 7 days a week, 365 days a year. As a consequence, not only is the regular consumption of a prescribed dose of methadone a hallmark of this treatment modality, but the dispensing function provides a framework for the entire operation of the program.

Although patients in outpatient methadone maintenance therapy are scheduled to receive this medication 365 days per year, all of these dosages are not commonly consumed at the clinic, as some patients are allowed to take home prepared doses for use when they are not scheduled to attend the clinic. Patients are often allowed take-home doses after they have been in treatment for several months, become stabilized on an appropriate dose regimen, and otherwise progress in treatment. Patients who are allowed one or more take-home doses per week are also required to attend the clinic for on-site consumption and monitoring during the remaining days of the week. The number of earned take-homes (excluding Sunday medication if the clinic is closed) a patient receives is an indication of his treatment status, although programs (as well as cities and states) differ in their take-home policies.

Weekly Scheduled Attendance for Methadone Medication

Three main features characterize patient attendance at methadone maintenance programs. First, there are strict mandated weekly schedules of attendance for all patients. Second, patient schedules are individually determined, so each patient's attendance or take-home status for each day of the week is predetermined. Third, patients' schedules are continuously in effect 52 weeks a year. Each of these features of outpatient methadone maintenance treatment is discussed before turning to the relevant research findings about patients' attendance at the six clinics.

Each methadone maintenance program has a mandated weekly attendance schedule for its entire census. This schedule is based on the need to dispense oral methadone to all patients on a daily basis. These attendance (or dispensing) schedules are mandated and strict in that every patient has an assigned schedule that dictates his attendance status every day of the week. This schedule is strict in that it is scrupulously checked, and absences are flagged and recorded and checked; repeated absences are cause for dismissal.

Each patient is assigned a definite attendance schedule, which is changed as his status or progress in treatment changes. A patient's attendance and dosage schedule are similar in that both are individually determined and both tend to reflect patients' treatment status or progress.

TABLE 6.1. Weekly Scheduled Attendance for Methadone Maintenance Medication: 1928[a] Patients at Six Clinics.

	Attendance per week (%)			
Program	1–2 days	3–4 days	Daily[b]	Absolute[c]
1	0.0	<0.1	99.9	73.3
2	18.2	18.2	63.7	44.5
3	13.9	9.5	76.6	67.2
4	1.3	3.1	95.6	69.3
5	5.8	7.7	86.5	78.1
6	14.4	20.2	65.4	32.6
Total	10.3	12.4	77.3	54.4

[a]The census of patients recieving methadone was slightly higher than the methadone maintenance census, as the former includes a few who have begun detoxification.
[b]Daily refers to attendance at least 5 days per week.
[c]Absolute refers to attendance every day the clinic is open.

The fact that attendance requirements are continuous for 52 weeks of the year is a third feature of these outpatient programs. The extent of social control exercised by drug abuse treatment programs that mandate attendance requirements (or dispensing schedules) for their entire patient census 365 days a year is considerable. How these attendance requirements work out in practice is the next topic.

Research Findings About Attendance

Most methadone maintenance patients are required to attend their clinics for medication on a daily basis. At the six clinics, 77.3 percent of the 1928 patients were scheduled to attend at least five times a week (Table 6.1). Of these daily attendees, most were scheduled to attend on weekend days as well. If absolute attendance is defined as attending the clinic every day it is open for dispensing, 54.4 percent of the patients had such "absolute" attendance schedules.

Although daily attendance was required for over three-fourths of the patients, 22.7 percent of the census were scheduled to attend less frequently: one to four times per week (Table 6.1). Of these 473 patients, more than two-thirds attended 2 or 3 days per week; generally, these patients came for medication on Mondays, Wednesdays, and Friday or Mondays and Thursdays. Only two of the six programs scheduled any patients for medication once a week.

As with many other aspects of methadone maintenance treatment, it was found that dispensing practices among the six programs varied considerably. Three of the programs scheduled daily attendance for more than 86 percent of their patients (i.e., 99, 96 and 87 percent), whereas the other three scheduled this attendance for fewer patients (i.e., 77, 65, and 64 percent of the census). These differences in attendance were more marked with respect to absolute rates of attending; four of the programs required that two-thirds or more of their patients attend the clinic every day it is open in order to obtain their medication. In contrast, two programs did not require this continual or absolute attendance of most patients; only 33 and 44 of their patients were scheduled to attend on weekends as well as weekdays.

It should not be inferred from the forgoing discussion that a restrictive attendance schedule is desirable and a more liberal attendance policy undesirable. Such an assumption would be unwarranted, as there is a positive association between number of take-home doses allowed (i.e., less restrictive attendance requirements) and successful outcome measures. Although analysis of the association of treatment services with treatment outcome is undertaken in a later chapter, it is pertinent to note that more highly scheduled attendance is not necessarily efficacious.

With regard to the research findings about patients' attendance, it is necessary to differentiate between scheduled attendance and actual attendance. Both are important. Scheduled attendance refers to the number of times per week patients are assigned to attend; actual attendance refers to the extent to which they adhere to these schedules. Actual attendance rates are the obverse of the missed medication rates. The latter rates refer to the percent of patients who missed one or more methadone medications during a week.

Doses Dispensed On-Site and as Take-Home Medication

Another perspective of dispensing practices at the programs is afforded by a tabulation of the total number of methadone doses scheduled as on-site or as take-home medications. For the 1928 patients at the six programs, 13,496 doses of methadone were scheduled for dispensing during the week. Of these doses, 10,365 were to be consumed at the clinic, and 3131 were prepared as take-home doses. Thus, 76.8 percent of the methadone was prepared for oral consumption at the clinics and 23.2 percent as take-home doses.

There was considerable variation in dispensing practices among the programs with respect to scheduling on-site or take-home medication for patients. At one program 92.4 percent of the weekly doses were scheduled for consumption at the clinic and only 7.6 percent as take-home doses. Conversely, at another clinic 69.7 percent of the methadone doses were prepared for on-site consumption, with 30.3 percent of the doses prepared for dispensing as take-home bottles of liquid methadone. Two programs prepared take-home doses for all patients on Sundays when these clinics were closed.

Although three-fourths of the methadone doses were consumed on-site under face-to-face observation of the dispensing nurse (or pharmacist), some take-home doses were allowed for almost one-half of the 1928 patients. Thus 45.5 percent of the patients were permitted one or more earned take-homes* during the week; this number often involved one or two weekend doses.

Differences among the six programs in their dispensing practices with regard to earned take-home methadone were striking. Four programs did not dispense take-home doses of methadone to most of their patients; the percentage of patients without earned take-homes at these four clinics were 78.8, 73.2, 67.2, and 67.2, respectively. Conversely, most of the patients at two of the programs (67.4 and 54.8 percent) were allowed one or more earned take-homes. The principal reason for these marked variations in dispensing practices was due to different rationales or orientations about methadone maintenance treatment. Programs that adhered to a long-term maintenance policy allowed more take-home medication.

Missed Medication Rates

The extent to which patients missed their scheduled methadone doses during the week was ascertained for each of the programs. These missed medication rates were derived from the active pharmacy records as part of the comprehensive confidential on-site data collection effort.

It was found that 84.2 percent of the 1928 patients had perfect attendance during the week as they met their weekly medication schedules. Conversely, 15.8 percent of the patients missed one or more scheduled appointments for their prescribed methadone dose (Table 6.2). Variations among the six programs were notable. The number of patients at each clinic who missed one or more medications ranged from 1.8 to 26.8 percent; thus weekly absences were 15 times higher at one clinic than another. Higher missed medication rates were associated with more absolutist attendance policies.

Lastly, with respect to missed medication rates, it is pertinent to note that most patients who were absent missed one or two doses during the week, so the percentages of the total doses missed was considerably less than the percentage of patients involved. Consequently, 95.1 percent of the 13,493 doses scheduled were successfully dispensed. This figure of 95.1 percent, then, is equivalent to an average daily attendance rate.

Doses of Methadone Dispensed to 1928 Patients

Each patient in methadone maintenance treatment is prescribed an individual dose to be taken on a daily basis. This dosage is determined by the

*Earned take-homes are methadone doses dispensed to patients for consuming at home on days when the clinic is open.

TABLE 6.2. Weekly Methadone Doses Scheduled and Missed: Six Programs, 1928 Patients

Program	Doses scheduled (Total no.)	Percent of doses (n = 13,493)		Patients with earned take-homes[b] (%)	Missed doses (%)	
		On-site	Take-homes		Patients	Doses
1	1,596	92.4	7.6	26.8	19.7	5.5
2	1,967	73.5	26.5	54.8	1.8	0.3
3	1,404	83.1	16.9	32.8	0.9	2.3
4	1,596	79.9	20.1[a]	32.8	26.8	7.7
5	>2,000	77.6	22.4[a]	22.2	24.1	7.8
6	>2,000	69.7	30.3	67.4	14.1	5.0
Total	13,496	76.8	23.2	45.5	15.8	4.9

[a]These two programs were closed on Sundays, so all patients received take-home methadone on this day. Data in this column include these Sunday take-homes. Conversely, [b]earned take-homes exclude these Sunday required doses.

physician or other treatment staff at each program on the basis of patient need, progress in treatment, and program policy. Considerations that influence the dosage policy of methadone maintenance programs include the dictates or recommendations of federal, state, and local governments, previously established dispensing practices at each clinic, and pertinent knowledge available to the director and relevant staff about effective clinical doses.

Tabulation of the doses of methadone dispensed to 1928 patients at the six clinics reveals a considerable spread in the frequency distribution (Table 6.3). Some patients received a daily dose of 5 mg of methadone and

TABLE 6.3. Methadone Dose Distribution to 1928 Patients

Methadone dose (mg)		Total patients No.	%
0–9		40	2.1
10–19		131	6.8
20–29		191	9.9
30–39		256	13.3
40–49		310	16.1
50–59		307	15.9
60–69		274	14.2
70–79		189	9.8
80–89		198	10.3
90+		32	1.7
Total		1928	100.0
Mean dose	47.3		

others a daily dose of 95 mg. Most patients, however, were prescribed doses between 30 and 69 mg (59.5 percent were in this dosage range); the mean dose dispensed to these 1928 patients was 47.3 mg. With respect to lower and higher doses dispensed, 18.8 percent of the patients received doses below 30 mg, and 21.8 percent had doses of 70 mg or higher.

The main factor contributing to the considerable variation in the dosages prescribed to the 1928 patients is differences in dispensing policies among the programs: Some programs adhered to a low dose methadone maintenance policy, whereas others believed in average doses; and one dispensed relatively high doses of methadone to most patients.

The variation in methadone doses dispensed to patients at each of the clinics is depicted in Figure 6.2. Two of the programs, A and B, are low dose in orientation with 82 and 51 percent of their patients, respectively,

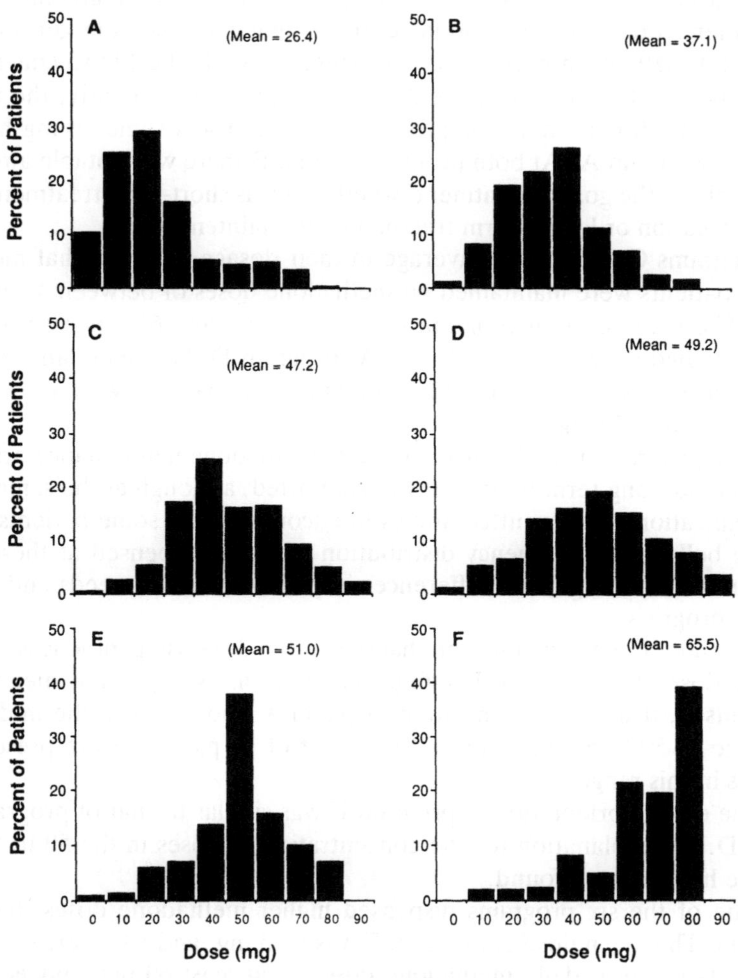

FIGURE 6.2. Dose distribution in six methadone maintenance programs.

receiving less than 40 mg of methadone daily. Three other programs (C, D, E) dispensed average doses of methadone to most patients, with 67, 61, and 78 percent, respectively, receiving doses between 40 and 80 mg. Lastly, one program (F) had a higher dose orientation, as 39.1 percent of its patients were prescribed doses of 80 mg or more. Dose-dispensing practices at each of these programs are reviewed next.

Program A had a decidedly low dose methadone orientation with 81.5 percent of its patients on a daily dose of 39 mg or less; moreover, almost one-half of these patients (44.1 percent) had daily doses of 19 mg or less. Only 18.4 percent of the patients were prescribed methadone doses of 40 mg or more.

Program A, with a mean methadone dose of 26.4 mg, had the lowest average daily dose dispensed. This low dose policy was fostered by local administration and supported by the director of the program.

Program B was also low dose in orientation, with more than one-half of its patients prescribed methadone doses of 39 mg or less. A larger proportion of its patients, however, were dispensed doses in the 40 to 59 mg range (37.7 percent) than at program A (9.7 percent); consequently, the mean methadone dispensed at this program (37.1 mg) was some 10 mg higher than at program A. At both programs A and B there was notable ambivalence about the goal of treatment: whether it was short-term treatment and detoxification or longer-term treatment and maintenance.

Programs C and D were average in their dosage policy in that most of their patients were maintained on methadone doses of between 40 and 80 mg. The mean dose at program C was 47.2 mg, and 66.9 percent of the patients had doses of 40 to 79 mg. At program D the mean daily methadone dose was 49.2 mg, and 61.2 percent of the patients were prescribed doses of 40 to 79 mg.

Both programs C and D had a general methadone maintenance orientation in that long-term treatment was supported, although at the same time detoxification was permitted and even encouraged for some patients. The more bell-shaped frequency distribution of doses dispensed at these two programs reflects general differences in patients' clinical needs and treatment progress.

Program E had average methadone dose dispensing practices and a mean dose of 51.0 mg. Although program E was average in its mean dose dispensed, it had a concentration of patients who received the midrange dosage of 50 to 59 mg; almost 40 percent of its patients were prescribed doses in this range.

The dosage orientation at program E was similar to that of programs C and D. An explanation for the concentration of doses in the 50 to 59 mg range has not been found.

One of the six programs dispensed higher methadone doses than the others. The mean dose at program F was 65.5 mg. and 80.1 percent of the patients received daily methadone doses of at least 60 mg. Indeed, 39.2 percent of the patients received 80 mg or more as a daily dose.

The dosage orientation at program F was toward higher doses of methadone. Both long-term treatment and a methadone maintenance orientation were evident; detoxification was not promoted as a therapy or treatment objective.

Further Findings and Comments About Dispensing Practices

Given the marked variation among programs in terms of the hours open for dispensing, a separate analysis of this variable was undertaken. It was found that there was a lack of association between the number of hours that programs were open and their attendance rate.

With regard to methadone dosage, it was found that patients who received lower doses were more likely to be absent and miss their medication ($p < .001$). Also, as might be expected, patients who missed their methadone medication were prescribed fewer take-home doses ($p < .001$). Somewhat surprisingly, there was not a significant association between patients' dose and length of stay in treatment (i.e., years in treatment); this finding probably reflects the pervasive impact of definite dosage policy at most programs.

In addition to the findings about methadone doses dispensed at the six clinics compiled from the active dispensary records, patients were asked about satisfaction with their current methadone dose. In a separate analysis of 490 male patients, 66.6 percent responded that their methadone dose was satisfactory, 27.4 percent held it was too low, and 6.0 percent stated it was too high.

When reviewing the attendance and dispensing practices at the six programs, an important monitoring and triage function of the dispensing nurses was noted. In their daily contact with the patient population, members of the dispensing staff commonly perform numerous tasks: They monitor and record each patient's daily attendance and medication, observe him consume his methadone, dispense scheduled take-home doses, collect empty take-home bottles, supervise urine collection, collect fees, answer patients' questions, reply to patients' complaints or requests for further service (e.g., change in dosage, need for medical care), dispense other prescription drugs (23 percent receive other medication), provide such over-the-counter items as vitamins or stool softeners, check patients for signs of alcohol or other intoxification (withhold methadone if necessary), and arrange appointments with the counseling, medical, or administrative staff.

Urinalysis

Methadone programs commonly require that patients provide urine samples to designated clinic staff once a week. These samples may be collected at scheduled or unscheduled (i.e., random) days, depending on clinic policy. In addition to regularly scheduled urine samples, patients may be required to provide additional specimens if continued drug abuse or other problems are suspected or evident. In the latter instances, it may be deemed necessary to obtain "observed" urine specimens. In this situation, a staff member is present to observe the patient while urinating. The purpose of obtaining observed urine specimens is to prevent falsification of urinalysis by the patient; as by substitution of someone else's urine for his own.

Collected urine specimens are commonly sent to commercial laboratories for analysis to detect the presence of specific illegal drugs (e.g., heroin, cocaine, barbiturates, PCP, amphetamines) as well as methadone. Absence of methadone in a sample indicates that a patient is not taking his prescribed take-home dose.

Urinalysis is an important part of methadone maintenance treatment because it affords an objective means of monitoring patients' abstinence from or involvement in drug abuse. Urinalysis is not only an important adjunct to counseling, it provides a monitoring and assessment function for the entire program.

Counseling Services

Ten Counseling Services

It was found that the counseling services available at the six programs could conveniently be classified under ten headings (Table 6.4): (1) case management; (2) social service liaison; (3) intake assessment; (4) individual counseling sessions; (5) brief contacts; (6) group therapy; (7) family counseling or therapy; (8) psychological assessment; (9) specialized vocational counseling; and (10) education classes. The first two of these services involved the management of records and services. The remaining eight services involved seeing patients in order to provide direct counseling services.

Case Management

The principal monitoring function of the counselor is directed toward those patients who have been assigned to him and for whom he has special responsibility—his caseload. After a patient has been added to the caseload, the counselor is responsible for developing and implementing an ongoing treatment plan, monitoring compliance and progress, and documenting the delivery of services. This function of *case management* involves maintenance of an active folder or jacket of information about each patient's history, present needs, and treatment status. Case management also involves joint conferences in which a patient's treatment status is

TABLE 6.4. Counseling Services Available at the Six Programs in 1985 and 1986

Type of service	1	2	3	4	5	6
Case management and referral						
Case management	■	■	■	■	■	■
Social services liaison	■	■	■	■	■	■
Direct care: seeing patients						
Intake assessment	○	|	|	○	○	■
Individual sessions	■	■	■	■	■	■
Brief contacts	■	■	■	■	■	■
Group therapy	■	■	■	○	|	|
Family therapy	■	■	|	|	○	|
Psychological assessment	■	○	○	■	○	○
Specialized services						
Vocational counseling	○	|	○	|	■	■
Education classes	○	■	■	○	■	|

■ = both years; | = either 1985 or 1986; ○ = neither year.

reviewed by his designated counselor along with other staff in order to obtain additional advice and supervision about the most appropriate course of treatment to follow.

Case management also involves recommending or implementing social service liaison and referrals for patients. These outside services include assistance for welfare, legal, and medical problems. The counselor's job includes making arrangements for the delivery of various community services to the patients and monitoring both patient and agency compliance.

Because he is responsible for tracking patients' progress in treatment and coordinating the provision of services (dispensing, medical, administrative, and counseling services) the counselor becomes both an advocate and a disciplinarian for patients who misbehave in the clinic, who get arrested, or otherwise become enmeshed in the recurrent problems associated with their addiction. He is an advocate when he represents patients before others (a treatment team or disciplinary authority); he is a disciplinarian when he sits in judgment or imposes sanctions on patients.

Direct Services Provided By Counselors

Although case management is an important function that counselors perform in methadone maintenance programs, the core role of drug abuse counselors is to provide direct services to patients. This face-to-face interaction with patients includes (1) intake assessment of new patients; (2) individual counseling sessions; (3) brief contacts; (4) group therapy; (5) family counseling; and (6–8) psychological assessment, vocational counseling, and education classes. These types of counseling are described next and their availability at the six programs noted.

Obtaining required information from patients at intake was a responsibility of counselors at three programs, whereas at three others the task was undertaken by other staff. In the latter regard, some programs had an intake worker whereas others assigned this task to various administrative staff. Although the amount of information obtained from patients during the intake procedure differed considerably among the programs, common data elements included demographic items, drug abuse and criminal history, family and employment status, and current treatment needs. A physical examination by the medical staff was another required aspect of the admission process.

Individual counseling sessions are the hallmark of the counselors' role in methadone maintenance programs. All six programs provided individual counseling services to their patients. During these biweekly sessions, patients meet with their assigned counselors to discuss ongoing problems (e.g., employment, recent arrest, illness), current treatment progress (attendance, clean urine specimens), and related topics. The content of the counseling sessions varies according to individual needs and circumstances as well as the patient's time in treatment. At these sessions, counselors endeavor to establish rapport with patients, assist them in understanding and complying with clinic rules and procedures, and encourage and support them in establishing a more stable and legitimate way of life.

Typically, counselors focus on the need to curtail drug abuse and to seek suitable employment. The approach of counselors differs considerably depending on their own and their program's treatment policy. Some counselors stress behavior modification and social rehabilitation, whereas others emphasize resolution of psychological problems. Some counselors are didactic in their interaction with patients and stress the need for compliance with clinic rules, whereas others are more interested in how the patient is coping in the community. The lack of uniformity in the content of counseling sessions is due, then, to both differing needs of patients and the different treatment objectives of the programs.

Another type of service counselors provide are brief, informal contacts that occur on an occasional or as-needed basis. Patients stop by to see their counselors to ask a question, report on a job contact, say hello, or complain about some aspect of their treatment. Sometimes counselors initiate these contacts, as when a patient has been absent or has had a positive urine test. At other times patients seek their counselors to obtain advice or complain. These brief contacts are important, as they provide continuity to the counselor–patient relationship. Brief contacts occurred in all six programs, but their frequency differed.

Group therapy is a special type of treatment in which one or more counselors (or other staff) assemble a suitable group of patients for a supervised and cathartic discussion of their individual problems. To be most effective, group therapy requires specially trained and experienced therapists. Because most programs do not have such specialized staff, less-dynamic group meetings are held by the counseling staff. Some group sessions were held at five of the six programs studied (Table 6.4).

Family therapy or counseling is also a specialized type of psychosocial treatment. In this case a patient's family or household members become the focus of counseling. Again, special professional training and experience are required if this intervention is to be effective. Furthermore, because this therapy involves assembling family members at the clinic on a regular basis (along with the patient), family therapy is difficult to accomplish at busy, understaffed methadone maintenance clinics. For these reasons, family therapy was not consistently available at most of the clinics. Five of the six clinics did, however, provide some family or couples counseling during 1 of the 2 years studied.

Psychological assessment of patients was available at two of the six clinics. This assessment was commonly undertaken by counselors who used one or more standard instruments to assess patients' psychological status.

The availability of specialized vocational and educational services at the six programs was limited. Designated vocational services were consistently available at only two of the programs, and these staff members were often untrained for special vocational assessment, counseling, or placement of patients: In this regard, it should be noted that the provision of specialized vocational counseling is different from the more informal advice offered by counselors in their individual sessions.

The availability of education at the programs was also limited. Only three of the programs consistently offered education classes to their patients.

Availability of Counseling Services: Year to Year Consistency

It is pertinent to review the findings about the presence, or absence, of the various counseling services at the six programs during the 2-year period of intensive study in order to document the services that were and were not regularly available. When measuring the treatment output of programs, it is necessary to differentiate between the occasional availability and the consistent availability of the particular services.

Case management, social liaison, and referral services were consistently available at all six clinics. Indeed, given the fact that counselors at the programs are continually involved in coordinating and documenting the delivery of treatment services, it seems unnecessary to pursue further this record-keeping and management role of counselors. It is, however, important to recognize that case management is a crucial aspect of the counseling role, as it facilitates the delivery of various services to designated patients.

With regard to direct care services provided by counselors at the programs, only two of these services were consistently available at all six programs: individual sessions and brief contacts (Table 6.4). The remainder of the counseling services were not consistently available at all six programs. Intake assessment by counselors was consistently available at only one program; group counseling was consistently available at three programs, and both family therapy and psychological assessments were available at only two of the six programs.

A review of the data on counseling service at the six programs reveals that only two of the six enumerated direct care services were consistently available at the six programs (individual sessions and brief contacts). The remaining services—intake assessment, group therapy, family counseling, psychological assessment—were not consistently available at the programs.

Percentage of Patients Who Receive Various Counseling Services

To ascertain that certain counseling services are present or available at methadone maintenance programs is only a first step in determining how much treatment is provided at these programs because some of these services are accessible to only a few patients or are infrequently provided to all. Therefore it is necessary to ascertain how many patients receive specific types of counseling on a regular basis. Measuring the output of services to the entire program census provides a comprehensive basis for further analysis, whereas a mere enumeration of available services establishes only that these services are extant. Indeed, the term "availability" is often a misnomer in that few patients are able to utilize many of the services that are extant at the programs.

The counseling services that are regularly provided to most patients at the six methadone maintenance programs are case management, individual sessions, and brief verbal contacts. The remaining counseling services, however, are not provided to most of the patients on a regular monthly basis (Table 6.5). The extent to which each of the ten enumerated counseling services was provided to patients at the six programs on a monthly basis is discussed next.

All of the patients at the six programs received case management from their counselors on a regular monthly basis. Thus a record review established that counselors recorded treatment data about their patients on a regular basis. Although the timeliness, completeness, and integration of the record data varied among the programs, this counseling function was fulfilled for the entire census. A smaller percentage of patients were involved in such case management functions as social service liaison or referrals outside the program.

Intake assessment of new patients was a responsibility that was not delegated to counselors at most of the programs. Intake assessment did, however, occur at the six programs, but it usually involved other staff. Thus intake assessment was not a major responsibility of counselors; further-

TABLE 6.5. Patients (n = 1909) Receiving Ten Types of Counseling Services During Past 30 Days

Counseling services	Patients receiving service (%)	Comment
Case management	100	From record review at program
Social services liaison	5–10	Estimate from output
Intake assessment	—	Applies to admissions
Individual sessions	91–95	From patient reports
Brief contacts	50–75	Estimate from clinic observation
Group therapy	21.1	From output data
Family therapy	2.2	From output data
Psychological assessment	—	Frequency data not collected
Vocational counseling	2.5	From output data
Education classes	5.6	From output data
Others: home visits, recreational activities, letters	7.1	From output count

more, it involved few patients on a monthly basis, as it occurred only once during the process of admission.

Almost all patients at the six programs had individual sessions with their designated counselors on a regular basis. Commonly these sessions occurred twice a month. In those few cases when patients were not seen by a counselor during the month, it was due to a delay in assignment following admission, staff vacancies, or similar reasons. These instances were exceptions, however. Regular individual counseling sessions supported with case management were recognized by both staff and patients as the foundation and core of the rehabilitation process.

Counselors brief contacts with patients were a frequent occurrence at all six programs. Although we were able to compile data on the number of such contacts that occurred on a weekly basis at the programs, it was not feasible to ascertain how many patients had and did not have such contacts. Therefore the percentage figure about contacts presented in Table 6.5 is only an approximation.

Group counseling sessions were provided to one-fifth (22 percent) of the patients at the six programs in 1985. This type of counseling was consistently available at three of the programs, available sometimes at two programs, and completely unavailable (i.e., absent during both years) at one program. Further information about the provision of group counseling services is presented later.

Although family therapy was sometimes available at five of the six programs (Table 6.4), the percentage of patients who received this form of treatment was low (i.e., 2 percent). The same low rate of coverage applied to psychological assessment, but the exact percentage of patients covered during a month was not determined.

Specialized vocational or educational services were not provided to most of the patients at the six programs. As noted previously, vocational counseling was consistently available at only two programs, and education classes were conducted at three programs. Neither of these counseling services touched more than 90 percent of the patients. Indeed, only 2.5 percent of the 1909 patients were involved in vocational education, and only 5.6 percent were involved in education classes during the 30-day period of study. (These figures refer to counseling or rehabilitative services provided at the programs. The figures do not include cases in which outside referral was made for vocational counseling or cases in which patients attended classes elsewhere. In both instances, few patients obtained such outside services.)

It is pertinent to note that some additional services were provided to patients or their families by counselors at the six programs. These variegated additional services included home visits, writing letters for patients, sponsoring recreational events, and similar activities. Seven percent of the patients at the six programs received these additional services on a monthly basis.

A special comment is relevant about the crisis intervention services provided at the programs. Although it was not feasible to quantify the number of crises that occurred at the clinics and to classify the types of episodes involved, it was evident that the counseling, medical, and administrative staffs were continually involved in providing crisis intervention for patients in their programs. It was found that counselors provided various types of crisis intervention for patients with acute needs at all of the programs. Patients' crises involved a multitude of problems: suicide attempts, acute depression, auto accident, arrest, fear of gang violence, rape, assault, bereavement, loss of place to live, discharge from program, recognition of HIV positivity, end of welfare payments for family, and so forth. Although some type of crisis intervention was available at the programs during the day when counselors were at work, the six programs differed in their planning for crises. Some had only limited arrangements to deal with patients' crises, whereas others had designated counselors regularly assigned at all times to provide crisis intervention.

Finally, with respect to counseling services, it should be noted that two of the six programs provided aftercare services for patients who had left treatment. Aftercare services, then, were not commonly available at most programs.

Weekly Provision of Counseling at the Six Programs

It was found that three distinct types of direct care service (brief contacts, individual sessions, group sessions) constituted the preponderance of counseling provided to patients at the six programs. How frequently each of these counseling services was provided to patients at the six programs

TABLE 6.6. Weekly Frequency of Three Counseling Services Provided to 1,874 Patients at Six Methadone Maintenance Programs

Program	Brief contacts (no.)	Individual sessions (% of patients. seen)	Group counseling (% of patients seen)
1	>300	62.7	12.5
2	218	52.5	21.5
3	273	57.9	39.7
4	199	48.6	—
5	137	51.3	100.0
6	>300	28.4	0.4
Total	2345	46.4%	21.1%

was determined in order to ascertain the overall amount of services provided at each program.

On a weekly basis, the 57 counselors at the six methadone maintenance programs engaged in 2345 brief contacts (or mini face-to-face meetings) with their patients, conducted 897 individual counseling sessions, and met with 408 patients in group sessions. Thus with regard to frequency of contact between counselors and patients, the brief contacts accounted for 64.3 percent of the counselor–patient interactions, individual sessions accounted for 24.6 percent of the interactions and group sessions accounted for 11.2 percent of the counseling services (Table 6.6).

The role of brief contacts in the treatment process is difficult to assess for a number of reasons. To begin with, this aspect of counseling has been taken for granted and therefore ignored insofar as documentation and assessment is concerned. Most brief conversations between program staff and patients are not documented, as they occur as part of the ongoing treatment process and are mostly unplanned.

These brief encounters, which include conversations about clinic and rehabilitative issues, are significant as they provide continuity to the treatment process. This continuity is not only important to patients' progress in treatment, but the interaction and communication that occurs during these brief exchanges is a major means whereby the management and coordination of treatment services is effected.

It is pertinent to note that the original program data collection plan did not include measurement or consideration of brief contacts. Their significance was realized only during the on-site observation of program operations that preceded the first comprehensive output measurement.

Regularly scheduled private sessions in which a counselor confers individually with each patient on his caseload are a foundation of long-term methadone maintenance treatment. In these individual sessions, patients' complaints and progress are discussed and, as feasible, suitable courses of action are planned. Inasmuch as these sessions are commonly scheduled twice a month, counselors confer with some one-half of their caseload every week. Four of the six programs were similar in terms of the percentage of patients seen in individual sessions per week (from 49 to 58 percent): However, at one program 63 percent of the patients were seen per week, whereas at another only 28 percent were seen in individual sessions.

The third major type of counseling service provided at the programs was group sessions. Typically, one or more counselors conducted these specialized meetings with some 6 to 12 patients. These meetings were usually convened to address specific needs, e.g., alcoholism, cocaine abuse, or health problems. Therefore the sessions tended to be topical rather than psychodynamic in content. These sessions usually lasted 60 to 90 minutes.

Several further comments are pertinent about the group sessions. First, it is important to note that these sessions involved only one-fifth of the patients. Second, the sessions were specialized as to topic and therefore varied greatly in content from time to time and program to program. Third, the sessions tended to supplement individual sessions in that regular individual counseling continued before, during, and after the occurrence of the group sessions. It is worth noting that one program used group sessions as a temporary substitute for individual sessions because of staff shortages, and another did not provide group sessions at all.

Caseloads; Duration and Content of Individual Sessions

The mean caseload of full-time counselors at the six programs was 41.2 patients (Table 6.7). Thus the average counselor provided case management and direct care to more than three dozen patients, but this average figure obscures the considerable differences in caseloads among the programs. Although three of the programs had a mean caseload of fewer than 40 patients, three had higher figures, and two of the three had mean caseloads of more than 50 patients (56.3 and 63.7, respectively).

Similar variations among the programs were found with respect to the mean number of individual sessions provided per week. Thus the mean number of individual sessions held by counselors was 17.0 per week, but this mean varied from 14 to 32 per week at the six programs. In general, programs with larger caseloads had more sessions per counselor, as might be expected.

The duration of individual counseling sessions at the programs varied considerably more than the content of the sessions. Thus the mean length of all counseling sessions was 37.3 minutes, but it varied from 22 to 56 minutes at the programs. Conversely, the content of these counseling sessions was devoted to rehabilitation issues about two-thirds of the time at all of the programs; the range in each program's mean percentage of time that these sessions addressed rehabilitation (contrasted with program compliance issues) was only 60 to 72 percent. The counselors, then, appeared to be dealing with similar topics at the six programs in their individual

TABLE 6.7. Duration and Content of Individual Counseling Sessions at the Six Programs

Program	Caseload[a] (Mean no. patients)	Weekly sessions (mean no./ counselor)	Length of sessions (min)	Content of sessions	
				Compliance	Rehabilitation
1	41.6	26.1	55.6	34.7	65.3
2	32.1	13.7	31.5	28.4	71.6
3	28.2	13.8	41.1	33.6	66.4
4	39.7	20.3	47.5	30.3	69.7
5	63.7	32.0	22.5	40.5	59.5
6	56.3	14.1	23.0	37.9	62.1
Total	41.2	17.0	37.3	34.0	66.0

[a]Mean number of patients for counselors with full caseloads (1985).

counseling sessions, although the time allocated to individual counseling sessions at the programs differed considerably.

In a separate analysis of counselors' weekly work tasks at the six programs, it was found that they spent 39 percent of their time seeing patients, 31 percent in case management and other office work, 12 percent at staff meetings, and 18 percent at such other tasks as urine monitoring, switchboard duty, and similar duties. The proportion of time counselors at the six programs spent seeing patients varied from a mean of 47.3 to 32.3 percent.

Medical Services

Medical Staff at the Six Programs

The medical staff at these six methadone maintenance programs can be divided into three groups: (1) physicians; (2) nurse practitioners and physicians' assistants; and (3) dispensing nurses or pharmacists. All programs had at least one part-time physician, but five of the six had two part-time physicians. In 1985 these six programs were served by 11 physicians (Table 6.8). The actual amount of coverage provided by physicians at the programs varied from 9.2 hours per week at one program to 34.4 hours per week at another, or 0.23 full-time equivalent (FTE) to 0.86 FTE). The mean amount of time physicians were at the six programs per week in 1985 was 22.5 hours (0.56 FTE). The total physician coverage for the 1,874 patients at the six programs was the equivalent of slightly more than three full-time physicians, an FTE figure of 3.37.

Three of the programs were served by physicians' assistants (PAs) or by a nurse practitioner (NP). One program had two full-time PAs, and the other two each had less than one-third coverage by a PA or an NP.

All but one of the programs had coverage by dispensing nurses; the

TABLE 6.8. Weekly Medical Services Provided to 1,874 Patients by Physicians at Six Methadone Maintenance Programs (1985)

Program	Physicians (no.)	% Full time, by FTE	Referrals[a] (no.)	Patients treated[b] (no.)	Hypothetical pts. treated during week/FTE MD	Treated during week (% of census)
1	2	0.86	2	65	75.6	25.6
2	2	0.29	*a*	8	27.6	3.1
3	2	0.23	2	19	82.6	8.7
4	2	0.69	3.5	36	52.2	13.8
5	1	0.50	8.5	45	90.0	20.0
6	2	0.80	6.5	35.5	44.4	5.4
Total	11	3.37	22.5	208.5	61.9	11.1

[a]There were no referrals to outside facilities by physicians at this program during the designated week, but there was a follow-up visit to a patient at a local hospital.

[b]Patients treated in week includes referrals.

program without dispensing nurses had coverage by pharmacists. Nurses comprise the largest category of medical staff at the programs, with a total of 21 registered nurses and licensed practical nurses. Each of the five programs with dispensing nurses had three to six nurses on staff. For these five programs, there was a mean of 3.48 FTEs of nurse coverage.

Medical Services Provided at the Six Programs

When considering the provision of medical services in these methadone maintenance programs, it is efficacious to delineate the roles of the three staff groups and then to analyze each with respect to the type and amount of treatment they provided to patients.

MEDICAL SERVICES PROVIDED BY PHYSICIANS

The role of the 11 physicians in the six methadone maintenance programs was generally similar except that 2 of the 11 were program directors and therefore had extensive administrative duties. [There was a change in directors at two of the programs during the study period that affected this figure. By late 1986 only one of the directors was a physician.] When analyzing the provision of services by these two physicians, an appropriate proportion of their time has been allocated to treatment and administration.

All 11 of the physicians provided medical care to patients in the methadone maintenance programs. Although the nature of this care varied somewhat from program to program, depending in part on individual medical specialty and program orientation, in general the physicians provided medical coverage through case reviews and consultation with other staff, physical examinations, and direct patient care, as well as by making referrals to outside medical facilities. Other services occasionally provided by physicians included psychiatric evaluation and therapy, advice about rehabilitation including legal and family problems, and medical education of various kinds. The percentage of physicians' time devoted to seeing patients varied considerably among the programs; sometimes this percentage was above 80 percent, whereas in others it was below 40 percent.

When analyzing the extent of medical services provided by physicians in the six programs, marked differences in the amount of treatment provided were noted (Table 6.8). Physicians in some programs treat eight times more patients per week than did those in others; the number of patients treated by physicians per week ranged from 8 to 65. Similarly, there were variations in the percentage of the patient census seen by physicians in the programs on a weekly basis, from a high of 25.6 percent of the patient population to a low of 3.1 percent.

These marked differences in the amount of medical services provided by physicians in the programs were partly due to variation in staffing. When differences in the number of patients treated is calculated with regard to hypothetical FTEs, this variation is greatly reduced. The number of patients which would be seen per FTE physicians per week ranged from 27.6 to 90.0, four of the programs treated more than 50 patients per week on this hypothetical basis.

Three points require comment with regard to the medical services provided by physicians at these programs. First, and most significant, is that there are vast differences in the medical coverage available and provided by physicians: Eight times more patients are seen by physicians in some programs than in others. With respect to programs with lesser coverage, only 3 to 5 percent of the patients are seen by physicians during a week.

Second, with regard to the treated prevalence figures based on FTE physicians (Table 6.8), it is important to note that these estimates are hypothetical in the sense that none of the programs, in fact, employs a full-time physician or has the equivalent of this extent of physician coverage (i.e., one FTE) on their staff. Therefore this calculation only estimates the number of patients who would be seen at each program per physician if they had a full-time physician or equivalent coverage. (This qualification applies only to the FTE estimates in Table 6.8; in the remainder of the table the actual weekly output of physicians' services is tabulated.)

Third, it is important to note that the major reason patients in some programs do not receive more care by physicians is that there are extraordinary differences in the staffing patterns in these methadone maintenance programs. It has been found that some programs have three times more coverage (FTE 0.23 versus 0.86) by physicians than others and that, in general, there are major variations in the amount of medical services available and provided by each of the three types of medical staff.

Services Provided by Physicians' Assistants and Nurse Practitioners

The three PAs and the NP were devoted principally to providing general medical care. These medical services included intake and other physical examinations, reviewing recommendations for methadone dosage change (as well as for other medication), making referrals both within and outside the program, and similar duties. In general, these staff members worked closely with the physicians. With respect to output of medical services, the four PAs–NP treated 138 patients per week, which constituted 55.6 patients per FTE.

It is pertinent to note that only three of the six methadone maintenance programs had either PAs or NPs on their staff. Furthermore, these highly trained medical staff were in full-time status at only one program.

Medical Services Provided by the 21 Nurses

The principal role of nurses in most of the programs was to dispense methadone to patients. In the five programs that employed nurses for this purpose, 47 to 78 percent of their time was devoted to this task. At the same time, most of the dispensing nurses also provided other treatment to patients at the clinics. During the 1985 output week of measurement, these nurses provided additional medical service to 288 patients. The nurses, then, commonly had a dual treatment role in the programs: dispensing methadone and providing medical care.

The dispensing role of the nurses usually involved continuous dose preparation, record keeping, taking attendance, urine specimen scheduling, and similar tasks. Sometimes the nurses also collected urine specimens and fees from patients on a daily basis.

The second role of nurses was to provide general medical care. In this role, nurses screened patients for alcohol or other intoxication, provided liaison to physicians and other staff, gave medical advice and education to patients, and otherwise assisted patients in numerous ways. Although the role of nurses in particular programs varied somewhat, in most cases they fulfilled both the dispensing and the treatment roles. As might be expected, the treatment role of the nurses was less intensive than that of the physicians or PAs–NPs, but it was more continuous as the dispensing nurses usually saw a designated list of patients on a daily basis for medication.

In three of the five programs that had dispensing nurses, these staff members saw 20 to 29 patients per FTE; in the other two programs the nurses saw five or six patients per FTE. Corresponding differences in the percentage of patients seen by nurses were observed at the six programs. The three programs that had a high number of patients seen by nurses (programs 2, 3, and 4) also had high percentages of patients seen per week: from 30 to 43 percent of the patient census. In the other two programs, the nurses treated fewer than 5 percent of the patients per week (Table 6.9).

With respect to output of medical services, the nursing staff served fewer

TABLE 6.9. Medical Services Provided by Dispensing Nurses at Five Methadone Maintenance Programs During Designated Week in 1985

	Dispensing nurses		Dispensing time and other functions		General medical services provided by nurses			
						Patients seen		
Program	No.	FTE	% Time dispensing[a]	Collects urines	No. of referrals	No.	Per FTE	Treatment provided (% Total patients seen during week)
1	3	2.64	78	Yes	6.0	16.5	6.3	4.4
2	4	3.80	47	No	7.0	78.0	20.5	29.9
3	5	3.25	60	No	16.5	94.5	29.1	43.3
4	3	2.60	50	No	12.0	74.5	28.7	33.3
5	6	5.13	76	No	12.5	24.0	4.7	3.5
Total	21	17.42	—	—	54.0	287.5	16.5	16.3

[a]The percent time dispensing is the median figure for the staff in each program.

patients than the PA–NP staff per FTE (16.5 versus 55.6), but this situation was to be expected as the nurses had a major dispensing role along with their medical care role. The role of the pharmacists was primarily to dispense methadone; they provided few other services to patients.

TOTAL MEDICAL SERVICES PROVIDED PER WEEK

To ascertain the overall medical services provided to patients in these six methadone maintenance programs, the enumeration of services provided by physicians, PAs or NPs and dispensing nurses were combined (Table 6.10). From this tabulation, it may be seen that there are still considerable variations in the provision of medical care. First, the number of patients seen per week by the medical staff varied from 36 to 185 at the six programs. Although this figure involved some duplication (as a few patients are seen by more than one type of medical staff), it does reflect the number of treatment events and is a rather accurate enumeration of the extent of medical services provided on a weekly basis.

Second, it is relevant to compare the provision of services when the medical staff are standardized. As before, the number of patients treated per FTE has been calculated, and when the figures are treated in this manner (Table 6.10) some of the prior differences dissipate. Although the number of patients seen in the six programs per full-time staff varies from 9.7 to 38.5, in five of the six programs each full-time staff treat 22 to 38 patients per week. Therefore the main reason for marked differences in treatment services provided was that some programs have more treatment staff than others.

Third, analysis of the provision of treatment services can be undertaken with respect to the percentage of the patient population seen per week by

TABLE 6.10. Patients Seen by the Total Medical Staff of Each Program During a Designated Week in 1985

	Total medical staff				
Program	No.	By FTE	Patients treated during week[a]	Patients seen per FTE	Percent of patient census seen during week by medical staff
1	5	3.5	81.5	23.3	21.7
2	7	4.4	96.0	21.8	36.8
3	8	3.7	116.5	31.5	53.4
4	5	3.7	36.0	9.7	13.8
5	4	3.1	119.5	38.5	53.3
6	10	7.9	184.5	23.4	26.9
Total	39	26.3	634.0	24.1	33.4

[a]The number of patients seen by the total medical staff in each program per week was determined by summing the enumeration for the physicians, the physicians' assistants, nurse practitioners and dispensing nurses. There is some overlap in the combined figures for each program, but the sum indicates the number of treatment episodes or medical contacts.

the medical staff. These figures show notable differences among the six programs. The proportion of patients who received medical services on a weekly basis at the six programs ranged from 14 to 53 percent. Thus patients in some methadone programs are four times as likely to receive medical services as those in others.

Review of Medical Services Provided

A review of the findings pertaining to the provision of services by the medical staff at the six programs lends support to four major conclusions. First, it was found that there were marked differences in both the number and type of medical staff who serve these methadone programs. Some programs have almost continuous daily medical coverage by physicians, whereas others have only part-time coverage on certain days and no coverage on others. Some programs have highly qualified full-time PAs or NPs, but most do not. Most, but not all, of the programs have nurses. One program had pharmacists, but five did not. Notable differences in the medical staff available to provide treatment were thus evident.

Second, we found that there were comparable variations in the medical services provided patients in the six programs. In one program, fewer than 5 percent of the patients saw a physician during the week, whereas in another 25 percent or more saw a physician. Similar variations among the programs in the frequency of treatment provided by the entire treatment staff were documented.

Third, it was found—as might be expected—that the weekly output of medical services to patients was related to the number and type of available staff. This finding is important, as it indicates that the available medical staff (even though often limited) is actively engaged in providing treatment to patients who are in need of medical care. It is not that these services are neither sought nor provided. Rather, the findings indicate that there is a pressing need for additional medical treatment in these programs. This conclusion is based on the output data as well as record reviews and on-site observation of clinic operations.

Lastly, from an evaluation perspective, this description of the treatment services by the medical staff is only a first step in determining the effectiveness of treatment. The next step is to investigate whether the provision of these and other treatment services in methadone maintenance programs are related to patient improvement and successful rehabilitation. For example, do the type and duration of treatment affect patient outcome? Before turning to the topic of patient change or improvement as a result of treatment, it is pertinent to review the output findings from 1985 to 1986 and consider the issue of year to year stability in the provision of treatment services at the six programs studied.

Year to Year Change in the Provision of Treatment Services

Two comprehensive on-site measurements of treatment services output were undertaken to assess the feasibility of the measures employed as well as to obtain information about how consistently services were provided to patients from year to year. Initially, during the planning stage of the project, attention was focused on the reliability of treatment domain measurements, as standard instruments were not available and the feasibility of obtaining numerous new measurements was unknown (e.g., missed medication rate, counselor turnover rate, staff–patient demographic concordance). Once the first treatment domain data collection effort was successfully completed, however, it was evident that most of the planned measures of service delivery could be obtained, and that, consequently, comparisons between the treatment and rehabilitation services provided in 1985 and 1986 were feasible. Although it was recognized that trend inferences drawn from only two time periods had limitations, the second treatment domain measurement (of 1986) proved to be both methodologically and substantively valuable.

Evaluation Methodology

With respect to evaluation methodology, the second data collection effort at the programs provided a means of obtaining repeat measurements of the entire treatment domain, which enabled the reliability of various measures to be determined and particular variables revised, supplemented, or

TABLE 6.11. Change in Dispensing Practices from 1985 to 1986: Mean Dose and Take-homes[a]

	Mean dose			Percent of patients with earned take-homes		
Program	1985	1986	Change in year	1985	1986	% Change
1	33.9	37.1	+3.2	23.6	26.8	+3.2
2	66.9	65.5	−1.4	58.2	54.8	−3.4
3	47.2	51.0	+3.8	34.4	32.8	−1.6
4	27.3	26.4	−0.9	47.9	32.8	−15.1
5	50.2	47.2	−3.0	29.0	22.2	−6.8
6	48.1	49.2	+1.1	63.2	67.4	+4.2
Total	46.0	47.3	+1.3	47.8	45.5	−2.3

[a]Data for 1985 refer to 1,898 patients; data for 1986 refer to 1,928 patients; see Table 6.1[a] note.

dropped. In addition to these methodological considerations, the second program data collection effort also made it possible to measure year to year change in the provision of services at each of the programs and to obtain comparable data about other aspects of the treatment domain.

To assess stability or change in the year to year delivery of treatment services at the six methadone maintenance programs, five comparisons between 1985 and 1986 outcome findings were undertaken. The first two comparisons refer to dispensing practices and the other three to the provision of counseling services. All five comparisons refer to change in the provision of treatment services.

Methadone Dosage

The mean dose of methadone dispensed to patients at each of the six programs remained stable between 1985 and 1986, although there was a wide range in mean dosage among the programs (Table 6.11). In the latter regard, the mean dose dispensed at each of the six programs in 1985 varied from a high of 66.9 mg to a low of 27.3 mg; in 1986 the mean doses ranged from 65.5 to 26.4 mg. The highest dose program in 1985 was also the highest dose program in 1986; so too with the lowest dose program—it was the same for both years. The rank order of mean dosages at the six programs was similar at the extremes, but there was some change in rank among those at the middle dose range (i.e., 47–52 mg) as there were only minor differences between them.

The year to year variation in the mean dose of methadone dispensed at each of the six programs was minimal. The difference in the mean doses dispensed during 1985 and 1986 was less than 4 mg at all six programs. Furthermore, no trend in the direction of this year to year change was evident; the mean dose was slightly higher in 1986 at three programs, but it was slightly lower at the other three.

These findings about the methadone dose prescribed at the programs in both 1985 and 1986 indicate that there is considerable stability in these practices at the six programs. It seems evident that the dosages dispensed at the programs reflects each program's dosage policy, whatever it may be, and that this policy does not usually change from year to year.

Take-home Privileges

Another relevant change measure of dispensing practices is the percent of patients at each program who had take-home medication privileges (take-homes refer to earned take-homes) in 1985 and 1986. As was found with respect to mean dosage, the range in values among the six programs on this measure was considerable. In 1985, there were 63 percent of the patients at one program who had take-homes, whereas at another only 24 percent had take-homes. In 1986 the range was similar, with 67 percent of the patients having take-homes at one program but only 22 percent at another. The rank order for the two programs with the highest percent of patients with take-home methadone was the same both years, but there was some year to year variation in the ranks of the remaining programs.

The year to year change in the percentage of patients who had take-homes was minimal at five of the six programs. At these five, the change in percentage of patients with take-homes from 1985 to 1986 was less than 10 percent; at one program there was a 15 percent decline in the percentage of patients with take-homes: from 48 percent to 33 percent.

With respect to the direction of the change in the percentage of patients allowed take-home doses, there was a decrease in this percentage at four programs and an increase at two. This year to year change was minimal, as noted, in all but one of the programs.

It was found, then, that the percentage of patients at the methadone programs who were prescribed take-home doses was generally stable from year to year, but that there was evidence of a decrease in this percentage with take-homes at one program. Again, the findings support the conclusion that it is the policies of individual programs that determine dispensing practices and that these policies are, with exceptions, stable from year to year.

Counseling Service Changes

The provision of counseling services at the six programs was found to be less consistently available and stable in delivery from year to year than the dispensing practices. This greater variation in counseling services was notable with respect to the availability of various services and the extent to which available services were provided.

Considerable change occurred in the availability of counseling services at the six programs between 1985 and 1986. (Table 6.4) This change is most evident with respect to four of the six types of direct care counseling service and the two types of specialized service. Six of the eight types of direct care or specialized services were not consistently available at these six programs during 1985 and 1986. These six services were intake assessment, group counseling, family therapy, psychological assessment, vocational counseling, and education classes.

At one of the six programs intake assessment was consistently done by counselors. At the remainder, it was either not done at all by counselors during either year (three programs) or done only in 1986 by counselors (two programs). There was, then, an increase in this service performed by counselors at two programs in 1986 compared with 1985. Although intake assessment is often not a function of counselors (it is done by other staff)—and therefore this service is elsewhere available at the programs—the shifting of this function indicates change in the delivery of services.

A considerable reduction in the availability of both group and family counseling occurred between 1985 and 1986. Group counseling was discontinued at two programs during the year, and three programs dropped family therapy during the year. Conversely, there was no change among the programs between 1985 and 1986 in regard to the availability of psychological assessment, although only two programs provided this service both years.

There was a change in the availability of vocational and educational services at the programs between the 2 years. One program dropped vocational counseling, but another added it during the year. Hence there was change in the availability of vocational counseling at two programs during the 1985–1986 year, but by the end of 1986 this service was still available at three programs as had been the case in 1985.

The availability of educational services decreased at the programs between 1985 and 1986, as one program discontinued this type of specialized service. At the end of 1986, three programs had special education available for patients and three did not.

Once the year to year availability of specific counseling services at each of the programs had been ascertained (i.e., whether each type of service is present or absent at each of the programs), it became feasible to measure the frequency of provision of these services to patients during both years. Two such measures of the annual stability of counseling services were derived. One measure was *change* in the percent of patients seen per week in individual sessions at each program from 1985 to 1986. In 1985 counselors at four of the programs conducted individual sessions with approximately one-half of their patients per week (i.e., 48.6, 51.3, 52.5, and 57.9 percent). At the remaining two programs, counselors held individual sessions with 62.7 and 28.4 percent of their patients, per week in 1985.

By 1986 the percentage of patients seen per week in individual sessions at the six programs differed considerably. The rank order of programs by percent seen varied greatly from 1985. The percent of patients seen by their counselors in a week changed from 11 percent to 31 percent at five of the programs; and at two of the five there was a decline of 17 percent and 31 percent; while at three programs there was in increase of counseling of 11 to 13 percent of patients seen. The percentage of patients seen in individual sessions per week was stable from year to year (i.e., a change of less than 5 percent) in only one program.

In addressing the effectiveness of drug abuse treatment services, there are three approaches to consider. The first approach is to ascertain which specific services are being provided to patients at designated programs. This determination involves identification and classification of the treatment and rehabilitation services which are available at each program on a regular basis. Next an enumeration of how frequently each of these services are provided is relevant; this enumeration includes both total "output" of the program as well as percent of patients receiving each service. In this chapter the treatment and rehabilitative services provided at six methadone maintenance programs have been considered from this perspective.

Overview of Measurement and Assessment

To summarize the treatment and rehabilitation provided at the six programs, 35 measures were derived. These 35 variables supplement the 54 treatment domain measures described in the previous chapter. Together, then, the 89 variables measure the entire treatment domain. (The 89 variables are listed in Appendix A).

The 35 variables that summarize the services provided at the methadone maintenance programs refer to dispensing practices, counseling services, urinalysis, and medical services. These variables, then, are for the most part identical to or derived from the research findings already presented in this chapter, except that they include combination measures and special assessments of services.

In recapitulating the scope of measurement afforded by the 35 variables, these variables can be classified into four somewhat distinct aspects of the treatment and rehabilitative services provided at the programs.

1. Presence or absence of specific services at each program
2. Number or percent of patients who receive a specific service per week or month
3. Content of the specific service provided
4. Assessment of the adequacy of the treatment provided

The first dimension of output measurement refers to whether specific services are available at the programs. These measures have been discussed in this chapter. Examples include such services as family therapy or education classes.

The second dimension of output measure refers to the number or percentage of patients who receive designated services per week or month; these variables have also been discussed. With regard to the third dimension, somewhat less attention has been focused on the content of the services provided. But relevant measures include dosage and the duration of counseling sessions.

Quality of Care Assessement

The last dimension of output—which has not been discussed—involves assessment of the adequacy of the treatment or rehabilitation provided at each program. The eight measures derived were (1) the number of secondary types of counseling services provided at each program (variable 74, Appendix A); (2) assessment of the overall adequacy or quality of counseling services (variable 85); (3) assessment of the adequacy or quality of medical care provided (variable 86); (4) assessment of the psychiatric coverage provided (variable 87); (5) assessment of the referral services provided (variable 88); (6) compositive measure of the overall adequacy or quality of medical care provided (variable 89); (7) director's treatment effectiveness (variable 20); and (8) the management and coordination of treatment services (variable 44). The last two measures were discussed in Chapter 5.

Most of the eight assessments was independently made, except the medical care composite score, which was a summation of three measures and the composite score of the director's effectiveness which was also a summation of three measures. The assessment of counseling services provided was a measure of the quality and adequacy of these services at each program. The rating of the medical services was an assessment of the amount of service provided and its quality. The frequent lack of medical services was a principal reason for assessing lesser adequacy and quality of services as (there is no adequacy or quality if a service is not commonly available) as occurred for example, with respect to psychiatric or referral services.

Conclusion

Treatment Provided

The completion of two intensive on-site data collection efforts at the six programs afforded the substantive means for measuring and evaluating the treatment and rehabilitative services provided to the methadone maintenance patients. With regard to the output of services, it was found that most of the programs were open 7 days a week, 365 days a year to provide treatment to their addict patients. Daily attendance at these outpatient clinics was compulsory, except that some patients who had progressed in treatment were permitted to skip one or more visits per week; when not scheduled to attend the clinic, patients were given take-home doses of methadone to maintain their proper level of medication. More than three-fourths of the patients (77.3 percent) were required to attend their respective clinics at least 5 days a week. Indeed, 54.4 percent of the 1928 patients were scheduled to attend the programs every day that it was open, including weekends. Daily dispensing was equated with compulsory daily attendance at these programs.

The extent to which patients complied with their scheduled attendance at the clinics was also ascertained. It was found that 84.2 percent of the 1928 patients had perfect weekly attendance, and 15.8 percent missed one or more of the oral doses of methadone. For the entire week, 95.1 percent of the 13,493 doses scheduled were dispensed; the missed medication rate for the week was 4.9 percent. Therefore daily attendance at the programs was high—over 95 percent.

The dosage of methadone prescribed for all patients enrolled at the six programs was recorded. It was found that there were considerable differences among the programs in this regard. Three programs dispensed average doses of methadone to their patients (mean dose 45–55 mg), two dispensed lower doses (25–40 mg), and one program dispensed higher doses (mean dose over 60 mg).

All patients at the programs were required to submit to regular urinalysis in order to check for the use of illicit drugs as well as to verify compliance with their consumption of methadone take-homes. These urinalysis results afforded an objective means whereby the staff could monitor patients' compliance with the treatment goal of abstinence from drug abuse.

The extent to which ten types of counseling service were available at each of the programs was ascertained in 1985 and then again in 1986. It was found that four of the ten types of counseling services were consistently available: case management; social service liaison or other referral; individual counseling sessions; and brief face-to-face contacts. Six types of counseling services were not consistently available at the six programs: intake assessment, group counseling, family therapy, psychological assessment, vocational counseling, and education classes. With regard to direct care, then, the principal counseling services provided were individual sessions and brief, "as needed" contacts between counselor and patient.

The percentages of patients at the programs who were provided each of these ten types of counseling services were ascertained from the on-site data collection. The pertinent findings about direct care services regularly provided by counselors were as follows: Most patients attended individual counseling sessions twice a month, and most patients also had one or more additional brief contacts with their counselors. About one-fifth of the patients received group counseling during the month. Fewer than 6 percent of the patients attended educational classes, and fewer than 5 percent received family therapy or vocational education.

Counselor' caseloads as well as the duration and content of individual counseling sessions were studied inasmuch as these regular face-to-face individual sessions with patients are the keystone of the counseling process in methadone maintenance programs. It was found that the mean caseload of counselors was 41.2 patients, that the counselors held individual sessions with their patients twice a month, that these sessions lasted some 40 minutes, and that rehabilitation was the focus of these sessions (two-thirds of the time), although program compliance issues were also addressed (about one-third of the time).

Medical Services Provided

The medical staff at the six programs was only a fraction of the size of the dispensing or counseling staff. Therefore the treatment provided by the 11 part-time physicians (3.4 FTEs) and the four PAs or NP was considerably less; fewer patients were seen on a weekly or monthly basis. It was found that, overall, at the six programs 11.1 percent of the patients were treated by a physician on a weekly basis, and the total medical staff provided some treatment to more than one-third of the patients at the programs on a weekly basis. The small medical staff was, then, busy in the provision of medical services to the addict patients. In this regard there were marked differences among the programs in the amount of medical services provided (13 to 53 percent of patients seen per week); these variations reflected the fact that some programs had considerably more medical staff than others.

Evaluation of Services Provided

In addition to collecting data at the programs about the treatment and rehabilitative services provided to patients, these services were also evaluated. These assessments included measures of the availability of specific services, the number or percent of patients treated, content of specific services, and the adequacy or quality of care provided.

These assessments of specific services (e.g., psychiatric coverage) or types of service (e.g., counseling or medical care) were either objective or comparative. Thus determining which types of counseling services were available at each program was an objective enumeration—each of the services either was or was not available at each of the programs and, if available, the frequency of provision could be ascertained. Conversely, rating the adequacy of the overall counseling or medical services was a comparative measure; the program with the most adequate counseling services was rated high on this service, and a program with less adequate service was rated low on this variable.

Effectiveness of Treatment and Rehabilitative Services

In addressing the effectiveness of drug abuse treatment services, there are three approaches to consider. The first approach is to ascertain which specific services are being provided to patients at designated programs. This determination involves identification and classification of the treatment and rehabilitation services which are available at each program on a regular basis. Next an enumeration of how frequently each of these services are provided is relevant; this enumeration includes both total "output" of the program as well as percent of patients receiving each service. In this chapter the treatment and rehabilitative services provided at six methadone maintenance programs have been considered from this perspective.

A second approach to determining the effectiveness of treatment services is to study the effect of these services on patients as they progress in treatment and rehabilitation. If treatment services are effective, patients should improve as they receive more of these services during the course of treatment. Moreover, the length of stay in treatment should produce successful patient outcome if the treatment is effective. This approach is investigated in the next chapters, which consider the effect of treatment on patients' drug use and criminal behavior.

A third approach to addressing the effectiveness of drug abuse treatment services is to analyze the relative effect of these services on patient outcome when compared with other factors. For example, is the provision of services more important than program factors (i.e., other treatment domain elements, such as staff or administration) or prior patient characteristics in effecting successful patient outcome in methadone maintenance treatment? This third approach is the topic of a later chapter.

7 Reduction in Drug Abuse During Methadone Maintenance Treatment

The extent to which addict patients' drug abuse is reduced or eliminated during methadone maintenance treatment is a crucial issue inasmuch as this modality was established to interdict patients' dependence on illicit opiate use. From this perspective, then, methadone maintenance is effective to the extent that it minimizes or eliminates drug abuse. Three corollary questions, however, also need to be addressed.

Issues and Plan of Analysis

The first question pertains to the distinction between opiate and nonopiate drugs. Should methadone maintenance be considered effective if it reduces opiate abuse? Or should its effectiveness be judged on the basis of reduction in nonopiate drug abuse as well? When addressing this question, two points seem pertinent. The first observation is that methadone maintenance was established to combat illicit opiate use (particularly heroin use), and therefore it should be evaluated according to this criterion. The second point is that its effectiveness in reducing other types of drug abuse also needs to be investigated. If control of heroin addiction is accompanied by a reduction of other types of drug abuse as well, so much the better. If not, further intervention may be indicated.

The second question pertains to rehabilitation, or the nonpharmacological aspects of treatment. It should not be assumed that methadone maintenance treatment is exclusively or primarily a pharmacological intervention. The rehabilitative aspects of this treatment were emphasized by Dole and Nyswander from the beginning, and the regimen of rehabilitating heroin addicts has been clearly set forth. Therefore it should not be inferred that the reduction in particular types of drug abuse that occur during treatment are necessarily the result of methadone. Other aspects of the treatment process (e.g., counseling, medical services, urinalysis, attendance) also affect a reduction in drug abuse among patients.

A third question to be addressed concerns whether it is the reduction in drug abuse during or after treatment that should constitute the criterion of effectiveness. Is methadone maintenance effective if it reduces or eliminates drug abuse among patients who stay in treatment? Or is it effective only if patients who leave treatment continue to abstain from drugs? One answer is that methadone maintenance is effective to the extent that it reduces or eliminates drug abuse among patients who continue in outpatient treatment and who continue to receive appropriate services; in this sense, outpatient methadone maintenance treatment is similar to medical and psychiatric regimens that provide continuous long-term outpatient medication or other appropriate services to patients with chronic illness. Still, whatever treatment outcome criterion is selected (and there need not be only one), it is scientifically efficacious to investigate both the reduction in drug abuse that occurs during treatment and that which occurs (or does not occur) after treatment is terminated. In this chapter, attention is directed toward the reduction in drug abuse that occurs during methadone maintenance treatment. The question of what occurs to patients after they leave methadone maintenance treatment is addressed in Chapter 8.

The research findings pertaining to the reduction, or change, in drug abuse that occurs during methadone maintenance treatment can conveniently be analyzed with respect to three data sets (1) the reduction in abuse of specific drugs which occurs by patients' time in treatment; (2) the annual reduction in drug abuse; and (3) the reduction in intravenous drug abuse. Taken together, these three analyses provide a comprehensive assessment of how effective these six methadone maintenance programs were in reducing patients' illicit drug abuse. Each of these three sets of findings are presented and discussed. First, however, it is relevant to review findings pertaining to patients' pretreatment drug abuse prevalence in order to establish baseline figures for specific drugs of abuse.

Pretreatment Drug Abuse Prevalence

Following the onset of illicit drug abuse which usually took place during their teenage years, 97 percent of these 617 males used heroin on a daily basis (Table 7.1). Dependence on opiates was the predominant aspect of their drug abuse history, as they had had 11.2 years of regular heroin use and this was supplemented by the use of other opiates; 29.6 percent were regular users of other opiates, and they had 8.9 mean years of such use.

In addition to their history of opiate addiction, these patients also regularly abused an assortment of nonopiate drugs. The two most common other drugs were marijuana and cocaine, which were regularly abused by, respectively, 69.4 and 46.6 percent of the addicts. In both cases the drugs were regularly used for many years (10.5 years for marijuana and 5.8 years for cocaine). Regular use was defined as use of a drug at least three times a week for a year or longer.

TABLE 7.1. Drug Abuse History of 617 Male Methadone Maintenance Patients: Years of Regular Abuse

Drug of abuse	No. of valid cases	Regular users[a] No.	Regular users[a] %	Mean years of use for positives
Heroin	608	590	97.0	11.2
Other opiates	609	180	29.6	8.9
Barbiturates	609	141	23.2	4.5
Other sedatives	609	202	33.2	5.5
Cocaine	610	284	46.6	5.8
Amphetamines	609	143	23.5	3.1
Cannabis	612	425	69.4	10.5
Hallucinogens	597	89	14.9	2.9
Inhalants	608	32	5.3	2.8
Alcohol to intoxication	609	305	50.1	8.5

[a]Those with one or more years of regular use of each drug.

Next in lifetime prevalence were other sedatives (e.g., Valium, Quāālude), which were used by 33.2 percent of the patients, followed by amphetamines (23.5 percent) and barbiturates (23.2 percent). With regard to mean years of regular use, these three classes of drugs were used for 5.5 to 3.1 years each. Hallucinogens and inhalants were the least frequently abused drugs. Hallucinogens were regularly abused in the past by 14.9 percent of the addicts and inhalants by only 5.3 percent.

Use of alcohol to intoxification on a regular basis was common within this addict population: 50.1 percent reported 1 year or more of such abuse, and their mean duration of regular alcohol use to intoxification was 8.5 years.

Although the drug abuse history of these methadone maintenance patients is extensive, it should not be inferred that most are indiscriminate polydrug abusers. Prior research has established that most opiate addicts pursue definite patterns of drug use over the years and that heroin remains as their principal drug of choice.[1] Whether this preference for opiates will be replaced by a preference for cocaine remains to be seen.

Reduction in Drug Abuse During Methadone Maintenance Treatment

Reduction of Drug Abuse by Patients' Length of Stay in Treatment

The 617 addict patients who were interviewed during late 1985 at six methadone maintenance programs were a stratified representative sample of the 1874 patients in these clinics. There were 126 new admissions, 346 average-stay patients, and 145 long-term patients. These three cross-sectional cohorts of patients afforded a means of analyzing patient differences in drug abuse by time already spent in treatment. As noted, face-to-face interviews employing the Addiction Severity Index (ASI) and Part II questions were utilized to measure such change.

The extent to which drug abuse among these patients decreased during methadone maintenance treatment is tabulated in Table 7.2. As expected, the extent of opiate use among the admission sample was high, with 66.7 percent reporting heroin use during the past 30 days and 15.1 percent reporting use of other opiates. Inasmuch as most of those patients came directly from "the street" and the remainder from jail, other incarceration, or treatment, the admission sample was still in transition from various stages of their addiction status to stabilization on methadone.

With respect to nonopiate use, the admission sample—or at least a major portion of it—was simultaneously involved in the abuse of these drugs. Thus 46.8 percent had used cocaine during the past 30 days, 48.4 percent had used marijuana, 38.9 percent had used alcohol to intoxication, and 31.8 percent had used sedatives other than barbiturates. In sum, these new admissions were significantly involved in nonopiate drugs prior to admission.

Patients who were in treatment for 0.5 to 4.5 years reported a markedly lower prevalence of drug abuse. With respect to the use of heroin, 23.1 percent reported continued use, but such use was only for 6.2 days per month. Use of other opiates similarly declined from 15.1 percent (of admission sample) to 8.1 percent of the average-stay sample. For nonopiate drug use, there also was a general decline in the percent who used these drugs. There was not, however, a significant decine in marijuana use (48.4 versus 47.7 percent), and the overall frequency of use per month for those who continued to abuse specific nonopiate drugs did not decline in most cases.

The long-term impact of methadone maintenance therapy and rehabilitation is evident in the decreased extent of drug abuse among those in treatment for 4.5 years or more. Among these 145 patients, both opiate use and nonopiate use has almost ceased (with the exception of cannabis and alcohol abuse). Thus 92 percent of these patients reported no use of heroin and 97 percent reported no use of other opiates. For nonopiate drugs, 96 percent or more reported no use of barbiturates or amphetamines, and 83 percent were not using cocaine. Somewhat higher rates persisted for marijuana use (37.2 percent) and alcohol use to intoxification (29.7 percent).

Annual Reduction of Drug Abuse Among Methadone Maintenance Patients

The annual change in drug abuse among the 386 patients of the in-treatment sample is presented in Table 7.3. These patients were first inter-

TABLE 7.2. Frequency of Opiate and Nonopiate Drug Use During the Past 30 Days for Three Treament Cohorts of Methadone Maintenance Patients

Drug of abuse	Admission sample (up to 0.49 years) (n = 126)			Average stay sample (0.50–4.49 years) (n = 346)			Long-term sample (4.5+ years) (n = 145)		
	No.	%	Mean days	No.	%	Mean days	No.	%	Mean days
Heroin	84	66.7	18.7	80	23.1	6.2	11	7.6	11.1
Other opiates	19	15.1	10.9	28	8.1	7.5	5	3.5	15.0
Barbiturates	5	4.0	9.0	6	1.7	5.7	4	2.8	15.0
Other sedatives	40	31.8	8.1	73	21.1	11.2	21	14.5	14.7
Cocaine	59	46.8	13.3	95	27.5	9.0	25	17.2	6.3
Amphetamines	7	5.6	2.9	14	4.1	5.0	3	2.1	11.0
Cannabis	61	48.4	15.4	165	47.7	16.7	54	37.2	13.8
Hallucinogens	0	0.0	0.0	0	0.0	0.0	0	0.0	0.0
Inhalants	0	0.0	0.0	0	0.0	0.0	0	0.0	0.0
Alcohol to intoxication	49	38.9	11.4	114	33.0	11.2	43	29.7	7.8

Reduction in prevalence by time in treatment was significant at the 0.01 level for all drugs abused (i.e., excluding hallucinogens and inhalants) except cannabis. Mean days of drug use refers to those who used each drug during the past 30 days.

TABLE 7.3. Annual Change in Drug Abuse for 386 Methadone Maintenance Patients

Drug	% Using drug, past 30		Frequency of use for positives (Mean days of use), past 30		Frequency of use change: 1985–1986: Significant Change
	1985	1986	1985	1986	
Heroin	19.7	16.3	11.3	9.6	NS
Other opiates	5.4	6.2	8.2	6.6	NS
Barbiturates	1.6	3.1	14.2	8.6	NS
Other sedatives	17.1	14.8	11.4	11.6	NS
Cocaine	21.0	24.4	8.5	9.9	NS
Amphetamines	2.3	1.6	3.6	7.5	NS
Cannabis	42.2	37.3	15.8	13.0	Decline in use; $p = < 0.01$
Alcohol to intoxication	31.6	29.5	9.2	10.6	NS

viewed while in treatment during late 1985 and then reinterviewed during late 1986 while still in treatment. The prevalence and frequencies of their drug use for 1985 and 1986 refer to the number of days of use of each drug during the past 30 days. These data were obtained from patients' responses to the standard ASI items pertaining to current drug use.

The in-treatment sample of 386 males had been in methadone maintenance treatment an average of 45 months at the time of their first interview in 1985. Although this sample included some new admissions, most of the patients had been in treatment for 3 years or more. Therefore their prevalence of current drug abuse was already reduced from preadmission levels. Only two drugs (excluding alcohol) were used by as many as 20 percent of the patients, i.e., cocaine and marijuana, which were used respectively by 21.0 and 42.2 percent of the patients in 1985.

The changes in drug abuse that occurred among the 386 patients between 1985 and 1986 were minimal. Although there were minor declines in the number of patients using five of the eight common drugs of abuse, these changes were not significant except for the decline in marijuana use. Similarly, the frequency of days of use per month for those who used each of the eight classes of drugs varied only slightly from 1985 to 1986. These findings indicate only slight year to year change in drug abuse prevalence among the small number of patients who abused these drugs. Still, there was evidence of a reduction in the use of one drug, cannabis.

The annual changes in drug abuse prevalence at each of the six programs were similar to the overall findings for the six programs combined. Patients' prior length of treatment and low rates of drug abuse in 1985 were conducive to lack of significant change by 1986 for most drugs at most of the programs. Still, there was a significant decline in marijuana use at two programs and a significant decline in heroin use at a third. Consequently, drug abuse did decline at three of the six programs concomitantly; there was no significant increase in drug use at any of the programs.

Reduction of IV Drug Abuse During Methadone Maintenance Treatment

A separate analysis of how intravenous drug abuse and needle-sharing practices were affected by methadone maintenance treatment was undertaken. The extent to which methadone maintenance programs reduce intravenous drug abuse has particular significance in the AIDS era as active intravenous drug users are a high risk population. Although considerable literature exists pertaining to the effectiveness of methadone maintenance treatment,[2,3] most of the studies cited do not refer to the reduction of intravenous drug use as an outcome variable.

The findings pertaining to current intravenous drug use and needle-sharing practices were obtained from the second face-to-face interviews with 506 patients during late 1986. The second interviews were conducted at the six clinics or in the community if the patients had left treatment. There were 399 interviews obtained from patients still in treatment and 107 interviews obtained from patients who had left treatment. Of the in-treatment sample, seven patients reported no history of intravenous drug use, three interviews were classified as invalid on the basis of standard ASI criteria (i.e., three or more invalid scales), and one patient did not provide answers about his history of intravenous drug use. With these 11 cases removed, the in-treatment sample consisted of 388 patients. The out-of-treatment sample is discussed in Chapter 8.

In the second face-to-face interview, each patient was asked about the type and frequency of injections during his last period of intravenous drug use; this period was defined as the month preceding his last injection of illicit drugs. Information was obtained on the number of days per month of both intravenous use and needle sharing. Days per month of intravenous drug use were measured for two reasons: (1) This procedure was used during prior research,[4] which indicated that recall was facilitated by the days-per-month schema; and (2) the procedure reduced the distortion introduced by high values, such as persons who injected 200 or more times a month. (Other researchers have used the total number of injections per month as a measure of frequency.[5] Both of these measures of frequency have advantages and limitations. Indeed, the two procedures are supplementary in that each provides particular data sets.)

The present analysis is focused on intravenous drug use rather than on needle-sharing behavior because needle-sharing frequency responses obtained from addicts tend to underestimate the extent of this practice. This underreporting occurs because addicts tend to define needle sharing in a restricted sense. For example, they include needle sharing only when it occurs with strangers but not with partners or spouses. Beyond this point it is worth noting that intravenous drug use is fundamentally a group activity. Heroin addicts commonly receive their first shot—their "wings"—from another addict and continue to participate in the social relationships (including sharing drugs, needles, and works) that accompany the life of heroin addiction.[6] Thus needle sharing can be viewed as a corollary of intravenous drug use.[7] It remains to be determined to what extent this close association between intravenous drug use and needle sharing can be altered during the AIDS era through specialized treatment, education, and other prevention efforts.[8,9]

Last Period of Intravenous Drug Use for Patients in Treatment

When the 388 patients were asked the month and year of last intravenous drug use, 18.6 percent gave a date that preceded their current treatment, 17.8 percent gave a date that coincided with their admission, 21.9 percent gave a date that occurred after they had entered treatment, and the remaining 41.8 percent reported intravenous drug use the past year (Table 7.4). This last group included those who reported use during the past year but not during the past month (12.9 percent) as well as those who reported use during the past month (28.9 percent).

The overall findings with regard to the effectiveness of methadone maintenance treatment in reducing intravenous drug use are depicted in Figure 7.1. All of the addicts under study were prior intravenous drug users; hence the 100 percent prevalence shown refers to the last addiction period that preceded their current treatment. Prevalence of intravenous drug use at admission was 81 percent, as some addicts were incarcerated or in other treatment before their current admission. During their admission period, the intravenous drug use prevalence dropped from 81 to 63 percent. This decline continued during long-term treatment but at a lesser rate. After 4 years of outpatient methadone maintenance the prevalence of intravenous drug use was reduced to 29 percent. In sum, then, intravenous drug use was reduced by 71 percent from their prior addiction status.

These patients showed considerable variation as to when and under what circumstances they stopped their intravenous drug use, or if they had given it up at all. When considering the point at which cessation of intravenous drug abuse occurred (if it occurred), it is pertinent to note that all of this in-treatment sample had been in treatment for at least a year and most had been in treatment for several years. At the time of the second interview in 1986, the mean time in treatment was almost 4 years.

Analyzing further at what point during the treatment process intravenous drug use ceased, attention focused on patients' last period of such use. With respect to those who stopped intravenous drug use earliest (group A, Table 7.4), it was found that 72 patients had stopped before their current treatment began. These patients commonly entered treat-

TABLE 7.4. Frequency of IV Drug Use and Needle Sharing During Patients' last IV Use Period[a] for 388 Male Patients in Methadone Maintenance Treatment

		(1) Patients in each status		(2)	(3)	(4) Needle[b] sharers during last period		(5)
Group	Treatment status at last IV use	No.	%	For each group: mean months in treatment	IV use (mean days per month)	No.	%	Needle-sharing days per month (for positives)
A	Before current treatment	72	18.6	52.5	20.9	31	47.0	11.1
B	At admission (2-month period)	69	17.8	35.5	25.2	33	49.3	15.1
C	During treatment	85	21.9	66.2	10.1	20	34.5	8.2
D	Last year (11 months)	50	12.9	33.8	8.5	5	13.9	4.4
E	Current IV use—*last month*	112	28.9	35.0	11.2	29	29.9	7.5
Total		388	100.0	45.0	14.9	118	36.4	10.6

[a]Last intravenous drug use period is the month preceding each patient's last injection of illicit drugs.

[b]Needle sharing during most recent period of IV drug use. Needle-sharing frequency data were available for 324 subjects. Column 4 calculations are based on these patients.

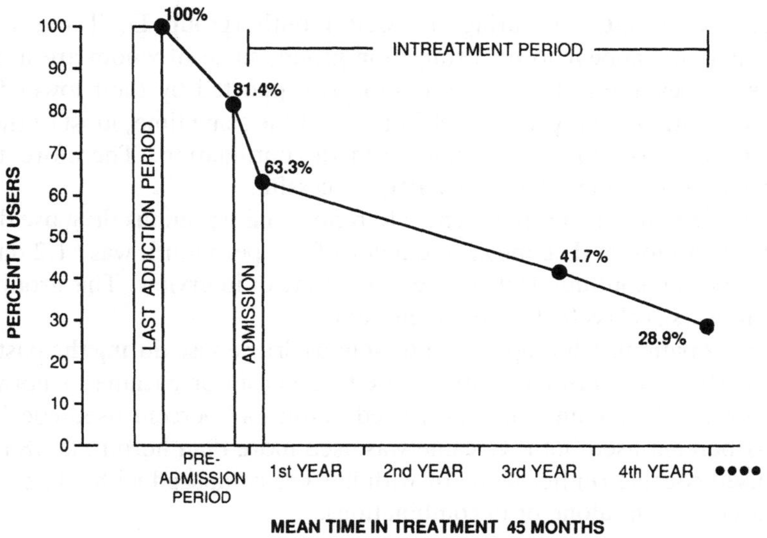

FIGURE 7.1. Impact of methadone maintenance treatment on intravenous drug use for 388 male methadone patients in six programs.

ment from other programs or from jail. It is significant that these patients did not relapse to intravenous use *at all* during the 53 mean months of their current treatment despite the fact that their prior frequency of use was high: 21 days per month. This group can be classified as treatment successes with respect to discontinuation of intravenous drug use and concomitant needle sharing.

Almost one-fifth of the patients (group B, Table 7.4) gave up their intravenous drug use at the time of admission (i.e., 1 month before or after admission). This finding establishes that methadone maintenance treatment can stop intravenous drug use rapidly among some heroin addicts. This cessation of such use persisted over the entire 36-month period during which these patients underwent treatment. As with the previously described group, the frequency of prior intravenous drug use was high: 25 days per month. This group of addict patients also can be classified as treatment successes.

Another one-fifth of the patients ceased intravenous drug use after admission to treatment (group C, Table 7.4). Cessation of intravenous use for this group was gradual over the years. With regard to last frequency of intravenous use, these patients had markedly lower use rates (10 days per month) than the preadmission or admission groups; this lower frequency of intravenous use may reflect the partial effect of treatment. Because these patients ceased intravenous use while in treatment, they too can be considered successes.

Some 13 percent of the patients reported intravenous drug use during the past year but not during the past month (group D, Table 7.4). These patients appear to be a transition group, some of whom are in the process of cessation. This interpretation is supported by their lower frequency of intravenous drug use (8.5 days). At the same time, most of these patients have yet to achieve long-term discontinuation. Therefore this group can be considered as only partly successful.

Of the 388 patients in treatment, 112 reported intravenous drug use during the past month. The mean frequency of use per month was 11.2 days; some reported continuous daily use to the time of interview. This group of current users is classified as treatment failures.

The 112 patients who reported intravenous drug abuse during the past 30 days in 1986 were primarily injecting either heroin or cocaine or both of these drugs: 22 percent commonly used heroin, 47 percent used cocaine, and 31 percent used both. Cocaine was used more than heroin, as 78 percent used cocaine (either alone or with heroin) compared with 53 percent who used heroin (alone or in combination).

Extent of Needle Sharing Among the Five Patient Groups

Of the 324 male patients for whom relevant data were available, 118 reported that they had shared needles during their last period of intravenous drug use. Although the percentage of patients who shared needles was higher before treatment (Table 7.4, groups A and B) than after methadone maintenance treatment was begun (groups C, D, and E), this difference was not statistically significant.

Treatment did, however, have an effect on the frequency of needle sharing. The frequency of needle-sharing days was significantly lower for sharers whose last intravenous use occurred after admission (groups C, D, and E) than for the admission or preadmission groups (A and B); $t = 4.689$, $df = 177.1$ using separate group variances, and $p < 0.001$.

To recapitulate, 36.4 percent (n = 118) of 324 patients had shared needles during their last or current period of intravenous drug use. Of these needle sharers, 64 had stopped this practice before or during admission, 20 stopped during treatment, 5 had stopped at least temporarily for the past month), and the remaining 29 continued to share needles. This last group—active needle sharers—constituted 9 percent of the patients in treatment.

Differences Among the Six Programs in Reducing IV Drug Use

At the outset of this evaluation project in 1984, it was anticipated that the six methadone maintenance programs selected for study would vary somewhat in program characteristics and in the delivery of treatment services, even though the original selection procedure was designed to exclude inadequate programs. It was not anticipated, however, that such marked and persistent differences among the programs as occurred would be found. During our first comprehensive on-site evaluation of the programs, we were surprised to find wide variations in the type, frequency, and quality of treatment provided to patients at the six programs. These findings about treatment domain differences have been presented in previous chapters. Given these findings about program differences, the question arose as to whether comparable differences existed with regard to the effectiveness of particular programs in reducing intravenous drug abuse.

The six methadone maintenance programs were found to vary greatly in their effectiveness of reducing intravenous drug use among patients in treatment (Table 7.5). The most striking finding is the wide range in the proportion of patients at the various programs who were current intravenous drug users—from 9.8 percent to 57.1 percent. Four of the programs were reasonably effective, with intravenous drug use stopping among 75 to 90 percent of their patients. In two programs, however, more than 56 percent of the patients were still injecting drugs.

Collateral program differences were also found with respect to when intravenous drug use ceased. In one program 38 percent of the patients stopped use at admission, whereas in two others only 4 to 8 percent did so. Significantly, there was a high positive association between success at admission and success in keeping patients from current use (Spearman rank correlation 0.9429, $p<0.05$). Again, it is revealing that four of the programs affected use at admission for a sizable portion of their patients (14 to 38 percent) whereas two programs affected fewer than 8 percent.

These considerable differences in program effectiveness were unexpected. Although we had anticipated that there would be minor variation in outcome due to program differences, we thought that the dominant influence on treatment success would be such patient characteristics as length of addiction, employment history, prior criminality, and severity of psychiatric symptoms. This expectation was not substantiated by the research findings. Instead, it was found that program variables were of paramount importance in reducing intravenous drug usage. This topic is investigated further in Chapter 11.

Discussion

From the present findings, it is evident that there is a decrease in the abuse of both opiate and nonopiate drugs during methadone maintenance treatment. This decline is most apparent and consistent with respect to heroin use—fewer than 8 percent of long-term patients were using heroin. A decline in most nonopiate drug use from pretreatment levels also occurred, but use of marijuana and alcohol consumption to intoxication continued at

TABLE 7.5. Differential Effects of Treatment Programs: Last IV Drug Use by 388 Male Patients in Six Methadone Maintenance Programs

Treatment[a] program	Sample (No.)	Last Period of IV use: % reporting last use during each period					Not current IV users (%)
		Before treatment	At current admission	While in treatment	During past year[b]	Current month	
A	82	18.3	37.8	28.0	6.1	9.8	90.2
B	62	30.6	17.7	21.0	12.9	17.7	82.3
C	65	27.7	13.8	24.6	15.4	18.5	81.5
D	64	18.8	17.2	23.4	15.6	25.0	75.0
E	66	10.6	7.6	12.1	13.6	56.1	43.9
F	49	2.0	4.1	20.4	16.3	57.1	42.9
Total	338	18.6	17.8	21.9	12.9	28.9	71.1

[a]The six programs have been ordered from high to low according to their prevalence of IV drug use; these letter designations do not correspond to those of other tables.

[b]This column refers to IV use during the past year but does not include the past month.

a high level. The fact that the incidence of opiate and nonopiate abuse continued to decline with length of time in treatment (even after 4 years or more) is significant, as it indicates that such long-term stay is effective.

Several observations are germane regarding the issue of the continued use of opiate and nonopiate drugs during methadone maintenance treatment. First, patterns of drug abuse that obtain during treatment tend to be a function of the drug abuse history.[1] Patients who were regular users of amphetamines, cocaine, or marijuana were predisposed to continue such use during treatment. Similarly, those who had no history of such abuse were less likely to begin. The point to be made is that a history of drug abuse is an important determinant of current use, even when the patient is in treatment.

Second, when setting treatment goals and objectives in drug abuse treatment programs, it is important to establish priorities based on realistic goals. With respect to priorities, the issue arises as to whether all drugs of abuse (and routes of administration) are to be regarded as equally injurious. Should emphasis be focused on reducing cocaine use rather than marijuana smoking? What about intravenous drug use and needle sharing? The point is that it is unrealistic to hold that all drug abuse among these patients can be eliminated inasmuch as it has never been accomplished with any sizeable population of opiate addicts. Because this goal of complete abstinence is unobtainable for most confirmed heroin addicts, the question arises as to what constitutes realistic goals. An answer to this question is provided by perusal of the present research findings, which indicate the extent of reduction in specific types of drug abuse that occur (and do not occur) among patients in methadone maintenance programs. Complete abstinence from all drugs is most uncommon, but overall reduction can be effected.

Several observations about the 71 percent reduction of intravenous drug use during methadone maintenance treatment are pertinent. Although this overall reduction is notable, it may nonetheless be disturbing to find that 29 percent of the patients reported intravenous drug use during the past month. In this regard, for many patients intravenous drug use continued at a reduced frequency from pretreatment levels; thus it was reduced but did not cease. The difficulty of stopping drug use completely among long-term heroin addicts has been consistently noted since this drug was introduced during the early 20th century. Indeed, it has been said that no treatment programs exist that can take most opiate addicts off of opiates.[10] Still, it is important to note that intravenous drug use ceased for most of the ex-addicts who remained in outpatient treatment for a year or more. This fact establishes that cessation of intravenous drug use can be achieved for most patients who remain in methadone maintenance treatment. At the same time, one should not ignore the reality that many heroin addicts do not voluntarily seek treatment and many who do fail to remain in treatment sufficiently long for rehabilitation to occur.

It is a major finding of this evaluation that some methadone maintenance programs are markedly more effective than others in reducing intravenous drug use among their patients. This finding takes on added significance after it has been demonstrated that the more effective programs can be identified and described and, furthermore, that effective and ineffective programs did not differ with regard to patient characteristics.[11] These findings suggest that treatment effectiveness in reducing drug abuse among patients in outpatient methadone maintenance programs is largely a function of treatment domain factors or elements.

Conclusion

A review of the drug abuse history of 617 male patients in methadone maintenance treatment revealed that most of these patients had been regular abusers of opiates and other drugs since adolescence. Against this background, there was a marked reduction in both opiate and nonopiate drug abuse after admission to treatment. In this regard, it was found that length of stay in treatment was related to patients' reduction in drug abuse. Heroin use rapidly declined after admission and continued to decrease after 2 years or more in treatment. There was also a reduction in other types of drug abuse, but this decline in nonopiate drug abuse was more varied and inconsistent. These findings support the efficacy of long-term methadone maintenance treatment in reducing or eliminating drug abuse.

With regard to the special issue of the reduction of intravenous drug abuse during methadone maintenance treatment, it was found that this modality of treatment is also effective in reducing intravenous drug use by heroin addicts: 71 percent of a sample of 388 patients who remained in treatment at six programs had stopped intravenous drug use; and most had refrained completely from such use for 1 year or more.

Marked variation in treatment effectiveness was unexpectedly found among the six methadone maintenance programs with respect to the reduction of drug use among their patients. Current intravenous drug use varied among the programs, from less than 10 percent of the patients at one program to more than 57 percent of the patients at another. These findings demonstrate not only that marked differences in effectiveness exist, but that some programs operate at high levels of effectiveness.

References

1. Ball JC, Corty E, Erdlen DL, Nurco DN (1986) Major patterns of polydrug abuse among heroin addicts. In Harris LS (ed): NIDA Research Monograph 67: Problems of Drug Dependence, 1985: Proceedings of the 47th Annual Scientific Meeting. Rockville: US Health and Human Services, pp 256–262

2. Cooper JR, Altman F, Brown BS, Czechowicz D (eds) (1983) Research on the Treatment of Narcotic Addiction: State of the Art. NIDA Treatment Research Monograph Series. Rockville: US Department of Health and Human Services
3. Tims FM, Ludford JP (eds) (1984) Drug Abuse Treatment Evaluation: Strategies, Progress, and Prospects. NIDA Research Monograph 51, A RAUS Review Report. Rockville: US Health and Human Services
4. Nurco DN, Cisin IH, Balter MB (1981) Addict careers. II. The first ten years. Int J Addict 16:1327–1356
5. Marmor M, Des Jarlais DC, Cohen H (1987) Risk factors for infection with human immunodeficiency virus among intravenous drug abusers in New York City. AIDS 1:39–44
6. Novick DM, Klan I, Kreek MJ (1986) Acquired immunodeficiency syndrome and infection with hepatitis viruses in individuals abusing drugs by injection. Bull Narcotics 38:15–25
7. Des Jarlais DC, Friedman SR, Strug D (1986) AIDS and needle sharing within the IV-drug use subculture. In Feldman D, Johnson T (eds): The Social Dimensions of AIDS: Methods and Theory. New York: Praeger, pp 111–125
8. Des Jarlais DC, Friedman SR (1987) HIV infection among intravenous drug users: epidemiology and risk reduction AIDS 1:67–76
9. Friedman SR, Des Jarlais DC, Sotheran JL, et al (1987) AIDS and self-organization among intravenous drug users. Int J Addict 22:201–219
10. Ball JC (1972) On the treatment of drug dependence, Am J Psychiatry 128:107–108 (editorial)
11. Corty E, Ball J (1987) Admissions to methadone maintenance: comparisons between programs and implications for treatment, J Subst Abuse Treat 4:181–187

8
Follow-up Study of 105 Patients Who Left Treatment

Attention is focused in this chapter on 105 patients who left the six methadone maintenance programs after their first interview and who were reinterviewed in the community a year later. Before discussing the findings from this follow-up study, it is pertinent to address the issue of retention in methadone maintenance treatment.

Rates of Retention in Treatment

Determination of retention rates for patients in drug abuse programs is essential for evaluation because it is necessary to know how many patients are stabilized or otherwise rehabilitated after admission and how many drop out or leave treatment. Treatment cannot be considered effective if a patient leaves shortly after admission or is asked to leave because of noncompliance with clinic rules.[1]

Of the 1874 patients attending the six methadone maintenance programs during late 1985, there were 617 males selected for longitudinal study—approximately 100 patients from each program. These program samples consisted of new admissions as well as a random selection of all patients in treatment at each program for 6 months or longer.

To calculate meaningful retention rates, each of the program samples was classified by patients' length of prior treatment. Three cohorts of patients were designated: new admissions, average length of stay patients, and long term stay patients. New admissions were the patients who enrolled in these programs during late 1985.[2] The average length of stay patients had been in treatment for 6 months to 4.5 years at the time of interview in 1985. The long term stay patients had been in continuous treatment in these six programs for 4.5 to 20.0 years.

Retention rates at the programs selected for study were related to patients' time in treatment—the longer patients stayed in methadone maintenance treatment, the higher was the retention rate. Only 38 percent of the new admissions were still in treatment a year later. Conversely, 63 percent of the average stay patients and 84 percent of the long-term stay patients were still in outpatient methadone maintenance treatment during late 1986.

The association between length of stay and retention rates was similar at the six programs (Table 8.1). With regard to new admissions, none of the programs was able to retain as many as half of their patients for 12 months. Furthermore, the 1-year retention rates at the programs were similar; five of the six rates varied only between 33 and 44 percent. Similar retention rates have been reported in national studies.[3,4]

Almost two-thirds of the average stay patients remained in treatment during the designated year, and, again, these rates were similar at five of the six programs. From 62 to 72 percent of the patients were retained at five of the programs; only at program M were one-half (50 percent) of the average stay patients still in treatment a year later.

Almost 85 percent of the long term stay patients remained in treatment from 1985 to 1986. As with the other cohorts, most of the programs had similar retention rates. Thus, 75 to 95 percent of the long-term patients remained in treatment at five of the six programs, and even at program M more than two-thirds of the long-term patients remained in treatment.

It is noteworthy that the relation of retention rates to length of treatment was consistent in all six of the programs studied. In each of the programs, retention rates were lowest among new admissions, markedly higher among average length of stay patients, and highest among long-term stay patients.

Follow-up of Patients Who Left Treatment

Follow-up Procedure in the Three Cities

As discussed in the prior section, some one-third of the 617 male methadone maintenance patients left treatment during the year after their 1985 interview. Of the patients who left, 107 were followed up and interviewed in households, on "the street," in jail, or at other locations in the community. These follow-up interviews were undertaken by the same experienced field staff from the Institute for Survey Research who had completed the first interviews in 1985. The field procedures employed in locating and interviewing the addict respondents in New York City, Philadelphia, and Baltimore were based on knowledge derived from previous follow-up studies of opiate addicts in the United States.[5–11]

The standard follow-up version of the Addiction Severity Index (ASI) was employed in these field interviews, and this instrument was supplemented by Part II questions on posttreatment drug use, needle-sharing practices, incarceration, and other pertinent items. More than 98 percent of the subjects who were contacted in 1986 agreed to be reinterviewed.

TABLE 8.1. One-Year Retention Rates in Six Methadone Maintenance Programs

Program	Patients in sample (no.)	New admissions		Avg. stay in treatment		Long-term patients		Retention of all patients	
		No.	% Stayed	No.	% Stayed	No.	% Retention	No.	%
M	95	20	25.0	64	50.0	11	72.7	45	47.4
N	107	12	33.3	58	72.4	37	94.6	81	75.7
O	105	36	41.7	49	69.4	20	75.0	64	61.0
P	105	14	42.9	63	61.9	28	78.6	67	63.8
Q	100	18	44.4	58	65.5	24	79.2	65	65.0
R	105	26	38.5	53	62.3	26	92.3	67	63.8
Total	617	126	38.1	345	63.2	146	84.2	389	63.0

Note: Data refer to the number of patients who remained in treatment between the fall of 1985 and the fall of 1986. Average length of stay patients were in treatment for 6 months to 4.5 years prior to 1985; long-term patients were in treatment 4.5 years or longer.

Two of the 107 follow-up interviews were deemed invalid by ASI criteria; the follow-up sample of valid cases was, then, 105 male addicts.

The 105 after treatment follow-up interviews took place in the respective three cities in which the addicts lived. With respect to location, 55 of the dropouts were interviewed in households or "on the street," 11 were interviewed in jail, and the remaining 39 were located and interviewed in such places as drug treatment programs and welfare agencies.

The out-of-treatment sample who were interviewed constituted 48 percent of those patients who had left treatment. They were not, however, a strict random sample of the out-of-treatment cohort at each program because funding limitations restricted the scope and completion rate of the follow-up. Therefore the follow-up was partly a sample of convenience obtained from successive random samples drawn from each program's out-of-treatment patients. Nonetheless, in a comparison of those who were followed up and interviewed with those who were not followed indicated that there were no significant differences between those two cohorts[12,13] in demographic or prior addiction characteristics. Differences between the follow-up sample of 105 and the 399 patients who remained in treatment are discussed later.

Reasons for Leaving Methadone Maintenance Treatment

In the follow-up interviews, the 105 ex-patients were asked why they had left methadone maintenance treatment. Their answers were found to constitute five general reasons or circumstances (Table 8.2). First, 22 percent of the ex-patients reported that they had been detoxified and completed treatment at the programs. Thus about one-fifth of the former patients left methadone maintenance treatment because their treatment was completed.

A second reason for leaving the programs they attended in 1985 was to transfer to another drug abuse treatment program. Sixteen of the follow-up sample left because of transfer. The programs they transferred to included detoxification and other methadone maintenance treatment, and there was some minor involvement with other modalities.

A third reason for leaving methadone maintenance treatment was because of arrest and incarceration. This reason applied to 11 of the 105 ex-patients.

A fourth reason patients left treatment was for disciplinary infractions or noncompliance with program procedures. This group included six patients who were discharged for numerous positive urinalysis results. Other common reasons for disciplinary discharges were drug sales, fighting, and absenteeism.

A fifth general reason given for leaving methadone maintenance treatment was that they "just dropped out." This catch-all explanation applied to one-third of the 105 patients. Included in this rubric were seven subjects who said that they dropped out because the program was too expensive

TABLE 8.2. Reasons for Leaving Methadone Treatment

Reason for leaving	Patients who left No.	%
Treatment completed (detoxified)	23	21.9
Transferred to other treatment	16	15.2
Arrest and incarceration	11	10.5
Discharged by program	21	20.0
Dropped out voluntarily	34	32.4
Total	105	100.0

(programs charge up to $50 a week for treatment), three who had specific complaints about the program (conflict with a counselor, schedule problems, and "unhappy at program"), two who reported problems with methadone (it "disagreed with my medical problem" and "bowels adversely affected"), and three miscellaneous reasons.

In sum, then, one-fifth of the patients had left methadone maintenance treatment because their treatment had been completed. The remainder dropped out on their own volition, transferred to other drug abuse treatment, were involuntarily discharged, or were arrested and incarcerated.

Addiction Status Since Last Methadone Maintenance Treatment

Each former patient's posttreatment addiction history was obtained in the face-to-face follow-up interview. In this interview, each ex-patient was asked how many weeks he had spent addicted, not addicted, incarcerated, or in treatment elsewhere since leaving the designated methadone maintenance program; the average time since leaving was 7 months.

Since leaving methadone maintenance treatment, these 105 ex-patients spent 23 percent of their time addicted, 29 percent of their time in drug treatment programs (mostly other methadone maintenance programs), 11 percent of their time in jail or hospitals (mostly in jail), and 37 percent of their time not addicted (Table 8.3). These data refer to total weeks accumulated in these statuses by all 105 patients and obscure the fact that most ex-patients moved from one status to another during this posttreatment period. Thus 51 percent of these ex-patients spent weeks on the street when they were not addicted to opiates, and 39 percent spent weeks on the street when addicted; another 39 percent of the 105 males had obtained further methadone treatment, and 9 percent entered other drug abuse treatment. Lastly, 19 percent of the ex-patients had spent time in jail since leaving the six programs, and 18 percent had been hospitalized.

TABLE 8.3. Number of Weeks in Each Status Since Leaving the Six Methadone Maintenance Programs, 105 Ex-patients

Patient status	Total weeks in each status	Percent of pts. with this status	Percent of weeks in each status
On street, addicted	758	39.0	22.8
On street, not addicted	1239	51.4	37.3
In jail	304	19.0	9.2
In hospital	58	18.1	1.8
In other MM treatment	846	39.0	25.5
In other drug treatment	117	8.6	3.5
Total	3322	—	100.0

Note: Mean time since leaving the designated methadone maintenance (MM) programs was 7.2 months.

Relapse to IV Drug Use After Treatment

The extent to which the out-of-treatment sample of 105 subjects relapsed to intravenous drug abuse provides a summary measure of their after-treatment drug abuse experience. To obtain pertinent information on this topic, each former patient was asked to state the month of his last intravenous drug use as well as the frequency of such use and the needle-sharing practices associated with it. The responses tabulated in Table 8.4 and depicted in Figure 8.1 indicate that relapse to intravenous drug use among the out-of-treatment subjects was common and that it increased with time out of treatment. There was evidence of a quick return to intravenous drug use for almost one-half of the sample, as 46 percent relapsed within 1 to 3 months after leaving treatment. This rate of relapse increased to 58 percent among those out of treatment 4 to 6 months and increased further to 73 percent among those out of treatment 7 to 9

TABLE 8.4. Relapse to IV Drug Use Among 105 Patients After Methadone Maintenance Treatment

Months since treatment	Patients who left treatment (no.)	Relapse to IV drug use since leaving: %	Relapse to IV drug use since leaving: Mean days of IV use/month
1–3	12	45.5	15.9
4–6	34	57.6	14.4
7–9	31	72.7	9.9
10–12+	28	82.1	14.1
Total	105	67.6	14.5

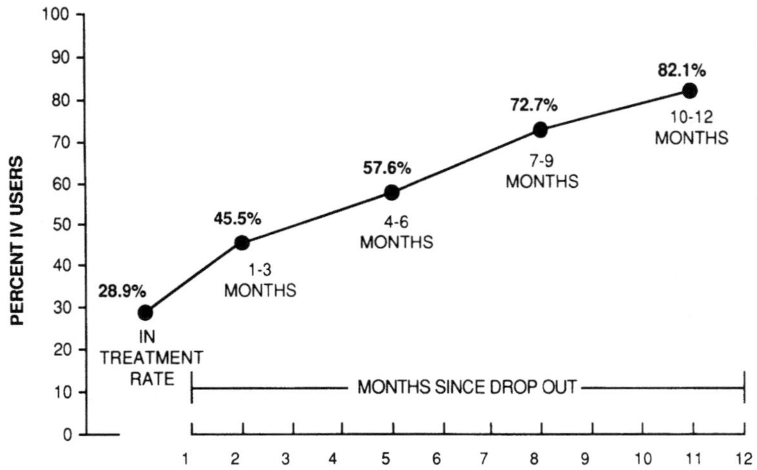

FIGURE 8.1. Relapse to intravenous drug use after methadone maintenance treatment for 105 male patients who left treatment.

months. The highest relapse rate was found among those out of treatment 10 to 12 months: 82 percent had relapsed to intravenous drug use.

Although most of the patients who left methadone maintenance treatment had relapsed to intravenous drug abuse by the time of follow-up, not all did so. The question then arises as to what extent do patients remain abstinent after completion of treatment and detoxification. Answers to this question are important because they could shed light on the conditions that lead to the successful termination of treatment.

Of the 105 male patients who were followed up after leaving methadone maintenance treatment, 23 had successfully completed treatment prior to departure. (Most of those who left, as noted, dropped out or were discharged for noncompliance with program policy.) The 23 who completed treatment were gradually detoxified prior to discharge and otherwise deemed by the treatment staff to be ready to become drug-free and independent of program support. These 23 patients were, then, the group considered most likely to remain drug-free in the community.

By the time of follow-up interview in the community, the 23 former patients who had completed treatment could be classified into three groups on the basis of their addiction status. The first group of nine addicts had relapsed to intravenous drug abuse since leaving treatment; seven of the nine were current users, and two had relapsed but had not used intravenous drugs during the past 30 days. The second group consisted of seven patients who had already returned to drug abuse treatment; all but one of these seven had been readmitted to methadone maintenance treatment, commonly different programs from those they left since 1985. The third group of seven ex-patients had not relapsed to intravenous drug use after completing their methadone maintenance treatment. This last group of former patients are designated "cures" to emphasize their nonaddiction status in the community, even though this attribution is provisional because they have been out of treatment less than 1 year.

The posttreatment addiction history of the 23 patients who completed treatment is tabulated in Table 8.5. During the 8 months since completion of treatment, 14 of the 23 had relapsed to intravenous drug use, and 10 of the 14 were current intravenous drug users (i.e., during the 30 days prior to interview). As noted previously, the frequency of relapse was related to time out of treatment, which varied from 2 to 12 months; the mean months since treatment was 7.8 months.

Somewhat surprisingly, the length of methadone maintenance treatment

TABLE 8.5. Follow-up History of 23 Patients Who Completed Methadone Maintenance Treatment

ID	Months since last IV use	Months in MMT	Since MMT			Current status
			Months	IV use	Past 30 days	
1	0	13	11	+	+	Active—street
2	24	19	5	0	0	Cured
3	0	37	16	+	+	DFT
4	68	48	5	0	0	Cured
5	0	3	9	+	+	MMT
6	2	15	6	+	0	MMT
7	0	41	10	+	+	Active—street
8	0	164	4	+	+	Active—street
9	0	43	2	+	+	Active—street
10	0	12	11	+	+	Active—street
11	0	29	7	+	+	Active—street
12	4	13	10	+	0	Nonactive—street
13	14	7	6	0	0	Cured
14	23	46	8	0	0	Cured
15	14	9	5	0	0	MMT
16	11	7	6	0	0	MMT
17	0	7	7	+	+	MMT
18	5	15	12	+	0	Nonactive—street
19	65	60	5	0	0	Cured
20	13	4	9	0	0	Cured
21	26	21	6	0	0	Cured
22	4	15	7	+	0	MMT
23	0	10	12	+	+	Active—street
Total	21.0	27.7	7.8	14	10	Cured = 7 (30.4%)

Abbreviations: ID, patient identification number; MMT, methadone maintenance therapy; DFT, drug-free treatment.

Note: Former patients who have not used intravenous drugs since leaving treatment are termed "cured." This classification is provisional, as most have been at risk (i.e., out of treatment) for only 6 months.

provided to these 23 patients prior to discharge varied markedly, from 3 to 164 months. Although 70 percent of the patients had been in treatment for 12 months or longer (one-half of them for 2 years or more), 30 percent had had less than 12 months of outpatient treatment. It is surprising that these short-term periods should be considered by the program staff as sufficient for the completion of treatment.

The seven patients who were designated "cures" at the time of follow-up interview were distinct from the remainder of the treatment-completed group in two ways. First, with regard to their posttreatment history these ex-patients had not relapsed at all to intravenous drug use since leaving treatment. Second, it was found that they had not engaged in such drug use for some 3 years. These patients had, then, stopped intravenous drug use as a consequence of treatment, and this cessation continued after they completed treatment. Of particular note is the finding that five of seven ex-patients who remained cured to the time of follow-up interview had stopped their intravenous use of drugs when they were admitted to methadone maintenance programs years before. The mean time between last intravenous drug use and follow-up interview was 33 months. Thus those patients who were able to resist relapse in the community after completion of methadone maintenance outpatient treatment had previously been able to stop intravenous drug use while in treatment in these same communities. In this sense, posttreatment success in relapse prevention was a continuation of treatment success.

Discussion

Comparison of Follow-Up Subjects With Those Who Remained in Treatment

To determine if the follow-up sample of 105 males were different from the 388 patients who remained in treatment through 1986, the two groups were compared. Analysis of pretreatment characteristics revealed that the two groups were similar (Table 8.6). The out-of-treatment sample did not differ significantly from the in-treatment sample with respect to age at onset of opiate addiction, length of heroin addiction, race, years of education, number of prior drug abuse treatments, or years in prison.

The two groups were found to differ with respect to three variables. The follow-up males had less work experience prior to methadone maintenance treatment: Only 29 percent of the follow-up subjects were employed full time during the 3-year period prior to treatment compared with 53 percent of the in-treatment patients who were employed during this period. The out-of-treatment group were also slightly younger than the in-treatment group: 35.6 years versus 38.3 years. Finally, the 105 follow-up subjects had spent about one-half as much time in their prior methadone maintenance

TABLE 8.6. Pretreatment Characteristics of 493 Male Methadone Maintenance Patients: In-treatment and Dropout Samples

Patient characteristics	Total (n = 491)	In treatment (n = 386)	Dropouts (n = 105)	Significance (p)
Age at onset of opiate addiction (mean years)	18.9	18.7	19.7	NS
Duration of heroin addiction (mean years)	11.2	11.4	10.3	NS
Prior treatments for drug abuse (mean no.)	3.5	3.2	4.3	NS
Race (%)	39.6	41.5	32.4	NS
Schooling (mean years)	11.6	11.6	11.9	NS
Preadmission employment (% full time prior 3 years)	45.5	53.3	29.4	<0.05
Time in prison (mean years)	2.5	2.3	3.1	NS
Age at second interview mean years	37.7	38.3	35.6	<0.05
Duration in current (or past) treatment (months)	40.5	45.0	24.0	<0.05

programs as the in-treatment sample from these same programs (24 versus 45 months). Thus the follow-up males were slightly younger, were less likely to have been employed prior to treatment, and spent less time in their last methadone treatment than patients who remained in treatment.

Similarities and Differences Among Follow-Up Patients at the Six Programs

The retention rates by time in treatment were similar for five of the six programs. The program with the lowest retention rates (i.e., for admissions, average stay, and long term stay patients) is also lowest with respect to such other outcome criteria as percent of patients who are current intravenous drug users while in treatment and percent who have positive urine tests.

The reasons for patients leaving treatment did not differ appreciably among the six programs. Dropping out of treatment was the principal reason for leaving at each of the programs, and only one-third or fewer of the patients who left at each of the programs had completed their treatment.

The most notable differences among the patients who left treatment from the six programs had to do with current addiction status. The number of follow-up subjects from the six programs who were current intravenous drug users were as follows: 29, 35, 41, 43, 60, and 75 percent, respectively. Significantly, the two programs with the highest percentage of current users among the follow-up subjects (60 and 75 percent) were the same programs that had the highest populations of current intravenous drug users among patients still in treatment. These results indicate that there is a carry-over of drug abuse from treatment to posttreatment behavior in the community. The same carry-over phenomenon was evident among the seven cured subjects in that they had abstained from intravenous drug use while in treatment and continued this abstinence after treatment. These findings about cures should be cautiously regarded, however, owing to the small number of patients involved.

Conclusion

Although methadone maintenance treatment was found to be effective for patients who remained in treatment for 1 year or more, this condition did not obtain for patients who left treatment: 82 percent of the patients who left treatment relapsed to intravenous drug use within 1 year.[14]

Investigation of the conditions under which patients leave methadone maintenance programs revealed that only 22 percent had left after successful completion of their detoxification and rehabilitation; and of these 23 patients, only 7 refrained from intravenous drug use by the time of follow-up. Most of the patients who left did so because they were dissatisfied with the program or because they were discharged for noncompliance with the treatment regimen.

How to increase the retention rate in drug treatment programs remains an unresolved issue. Still, the present findings provide pertinent data about several aspects of this problem. First, it should be noted that one-half of the follow-up sample obtained further drug abuse treatment during the following 8 months, which indicates that a desire for treatment persists even among those who drop out. To what extent these and other patients would profit from more specialized or intensive treatment is not known. It seems likely that an expansion and intensification of available services—such as group counseling, psychiatric coverage, and vocational education—would increase patient retention. In this regard, developing new models of methadone maintenance might be efficacious. Programs that meet the minimal needs of stable patients with steady employment (e.g., early dispensing hours) could be established as well as those that address the special needs of such populations as the aged, handicapped, and pregnant patients.

A second observation is that the considerable switching from one methadone maintenance program to another that occurs supports the need to develop a more integrated and comprehensive citywide treatment system. Such an expanded network could offer more diverse and specialized types of drug treatment programs as well as facilitate appropriate transfers and referrals. Such planning should take into acount the enduring dynamics of the life course of opiate addiction that this follow-up study substantiates: Long-term treatment is indicated, relapse is frequent, and cure is uncommon.

References

1. Cooper JR, Altman F, Brown B, Czechowicz D (eds) (1983) NIDA Treatment Research Monograph Series: Research on the Treatment of Narcotic Addiction: State of the Art. (ADM) 83–1281 . Rockville: US Department of Health and Human Services
2. Corty E, Ball JC (1987) Admissions to methadone maintenance: comparisons between programs and implications for treatment, J Subst Abuse Treat 4:181–187
3. Hubbard RL, Marsden ME, Rachal JV, et al (1989) Drug Abuse Treatment: A National Study of Effectiveness. Chapel Hill: University of North Carolina Press
4. United States General Accounting Office (1990) Methadone maintenance: some treatment programs are not effective; greater federal oversight needed. In: GAO Report to the Chairman, Select Committee on Narcotics Abuse and Control, House of Representatives (March). Washington, DC: US Government Printing Office
5. Ball JC, Pabon DO (1965) Locating and interviewing narcotic addicts in Puerto Rico. Sociol Soc Res 49:401–411
6. Vaillant GE (1966) A twelve-year follow-up of New York narcotic addicts. I. The relation of treatment to outcome. Am J Psychiatry 22:727–737
7. O'Donnell JA (1969) Narcotic Addicts in Kentucky. USPHS Publication 1881. Washington, DC: US Government Printing Office
8. Ball JC (1975) Sample selection in American follow-up studies of drug abusers. In Bostran H, Larsson T, Ljungstedt N (eds): Drug Dependence—Treatment and Treatment Evaluation. Skandia International Symposia, 1974. pp 221–231
9. McGlothlin WH, Anglin MD (1981) Long-term follow-up of clients of high and low dose methadone programs, Arch Gen Psychiatry 38:1055–1063
10. Maddux JF, Desmond DP (1981) Careers of Opioid Users. New York: Praeger
11. Nurco DN, Cisin IH, Balter MB (1981) Addict careers. II. The first ten years. Int J Addict 16:1327–1356
12. Ball JC, Lange WR, Myers CP, Friedman SR (1988) Reducing the risk of AIDS through methadone maintenance treatment, J Health Soc Behav 29:214–226
13. LaPorte C (1989) Personal communications
14. Bespalec, DA (1974) Relapse rates after treatment for heroin addiction. J comm Psychiatry 2, pp 85–87

9
Prevalence and Change in Psychiatric Symptomatology Among Methadone Maintenance Patients

Investigating the prevalence of psychiatric factors among drug abusers has been a subject of study in the United States for more than 50 years.[1] Most of the early studies focused on opiate addicts, as they comprised the principal population of drug abusers at risk for hospitalization or imprisonment. Pescor's study of the clinical records of 1036 addicts hospitalized at Lexington during 1936–1937 referred primarily to opiate abusers.[1] Pescor's analysis was followed by a succession of other studies that also investigated personality factors and psychopathology among opiate abusers.[2,3,4]

There has been a renewed interest in studying the prevalence of psychiatric disorders among drug abusers.[5–9] In this regard, the Addiction Severity Index (ASI) has been extensively employed to measure the prevalence of psychiatric symptoms among methadone maintenance patients.[10] This instrument contains a 22-item scale that provides information about each subject's psychiatric status. Specifically, the subject is asked if he has suffered from seven psychological symptoms: serious depression; serious anxiety; hallucinations; difficulty in understanding, concentrating, or remembering; trouble controlling violent behaviors; thoughts of suicide; and suicide attempts (Table 9.1). In each instance, the subject is asked if he has ever experienced the symptom (i.e., lifetime prevalence) and if it has occurred during the past 30 days. In addition, the subject is instructed not to include symptoms that are a result of drug or alcohol use.[11]

The ASI composite psychiatric severity score is composed of items that indicate the subject's current psychiatric status. These items refer to the number of symptoms endorsed for the past 30 days, if the subject took psychotropic medication during this period, the number of days during the past 30 that the subject experienced any serious psychological or emotional problems, his rating of how bothered he has been by these problems, and, finally, how important it is to him to receive treatment for these psychological problems.[12]

An abridged version of this chapter is to be found in Corty E, Ball JC, Myers CP (1988) Psychiatric symptomatology in methadone maintenance patients. *Journal of Consulting and Clinical Psychology* 56:776–777.

TABLE 9.1. Lifetime and Recent Prevalence of Psychiatric Symptoms Among Male Methadone Maintenance Patients (1985)

	Percent with symptom	
Psychiatric symptoms	Lifetime	Past 30 days
Serious depression	48.3	16.6
Serious anxiety	51.7	22.9
Hallucinations	8.6	2.3
Difficulty understanding, concentrating, remembering	28.0	16.6
Trouble controlling violent behavior	24.9	7.9
Thoughts of suicide	15.3	3.5
Suicide attempt	8.5	0.4
Had one or more symptoms	68.4	35.4

Valid cases = 567.

Lifetime Prevalence of Psychiatric Symptoms

Of the 567 male patients for whom relevant ASI and other data were obtained, more than two-thirds (68.4 percent) reported having experienced one or more of these seven psychiatric symptoms in their lifetime. The most prevalent symptom reported was serious anxiety, which was experienced by 51.7 percent of the patients. This symptom was followed by serious depression, which had a lifetime prevalence of 48.3 percent. Two other psychiatric symptoms were experienced by some one-fourth of the patients: serious difficulty in understanding, concentrating, or remembering and trouble controlling violent behavior. Next with respect to lifetime prevalence, 15.3 percent of the patients reported suicidal thoughts, and 8.5 percent had attempted suicide; 8.6 percent of the patients reported that they had had hallucinations.

The number of symptoms experienced during their lifetime varied from none to seven. As noted, 68.4 percent reported one or more symptoms, and 31.6 percent reported none. One symptom was reported by 15.7 percent of the males, two symptoms by 21.3 percent, three symptoms by 13.1 percent, four symptoms by 8.5 percent, and five or more symptoms by 9.9 percent of the patients.

Recent Psychiatric Symptoms

With regard to the presence of these same seven symptoms during the past 30 days, 35.4 percent of the 567 patients reported one or more symptoms. Again, as with lifetime prevalence, serious anxiety was the most common symptom with 22.9 percent reporting this problem during the past 30 days. The two next most prevalent symptoms were serious depression and serious difficulty in understanding, concentrating, or remembering, each reported by 16.6 percent of the patients. The remainder of the symptoms were each experienced by fewer than 8 percent of the patients.

During the past 30 days, 35.4 percent of the patients reported having experienced one or more of these psychiatric symptoms, and 64.6 percent reported no such symptoms. Almost 16.0 percent reported having experienced one symptom, 10.2 percent two symptoms, 5.8 percent three symptoms, 2.5 percent four symptoms, and 1.2 percent five or more symptoms.

Psychiatric Severity Composite Scores by Time in Treatment

The mean psychiatric severity composite score for the 567 patients at the time of the first interview T_1 was 0.12, with a standard deviation of 0.18. A cross-sectional analysis of these scores by patients' length of stay in treatment (LOS at T_1), controlling for age, was not significant ($r = .015$). Thus, there was no relation found between the length of time these patients had been in methadone maintenance treatment and their current psychiatric symptomatology.

Analysis of Psychiatric Severity Among Those Who Left Treatment

Before discussing the longitudinal findings pertaining to change in psychiatric composite scores, it is pertinent to note several findings about patients who left treatment after the first interview in 1985. A separate analysis of the patients who left treatment after T_1 was undertaken to compare those who were reinterviewed at T_2 and those who were not. The two groups were compared with respect to ten dependent variables in a discriminant function analysis; these variables were age, time in treatment at T_1, crime days last summer, and the seven ASI composite scores. No significant differences were found. Therefore the left-treatment patients who were interviewed at T_2 were deemed to be representative of the entire left-treatment group insofar as these ten measures are concerned.

An additional comparison was undertaken with respect to those patients who left their methadone maintenance programs after T_1 because their treatment was completed and those who dropped out. Again, discriminant function analysis was employed; the dependent variables were age, length of stay in treatment (LOS), the seven ASI composite scores at T_2, percent of T_1 to T_2 time spent in other drug abuse treatment, and the number of crime days per week during the recent summer. No significant differences in these measures between these two groups of patients were found. Therefore for the longitudinal analysis of patients' psychiatric severity scores, the left-treatment sample is considered as one group.

Longitudinal Analysis of Change in Psychiatric Severity

A detailed analysis of ASI psychiatric severity scores among 446 patients who were interviewed twice was undertaken to measure change during this 1-year period. In this analysis, new admission patients were restricted to those interviewed shortly after admission as well as in treatment patients who provided the required data sets for this comparison.

The 446 patients consisted of two groups. (1) 353 patients who were in continuous methadone maintenance treatment at the six programs during the 1985–1986 period of study; and (2) the 93 patients who were at these six programs at the time of the first interview but not at the time of the second interview; this second sample was reinterviewed after they left treatment. The 93 patients consisted of the follow-up sample of 105 patients described in Chapter 8 less 12 for whom the requisite data were lacking.

The mean psychiatric severity scores of the two samples of patients at the time of their first and second interviews are presented in Table 9.2. These findings also indicate the extent (or lack) of change in psychiatric severity scores by length of time in treatment at T_1.

A perusal of the data presented in Table 9.2 reveals that there was little change in patients' psychiatric severity composite scores between T_1 and T_2. Morever, as indicated from the cross-sectional analysis of T_1 findings, there was no significant effect of length of stay in methadone maintenance treatment on patients' psychiatric severity composite scores.

The next step in the analysis was to investigate the factors associated with the T_2 psychiatric severity scores. A significant negative correlation ($r = -.13$, $p < .01$) was found between T_2 psychiatric severity scores and percent of time from T_1 to T_2 that the 446 patients had been in their designated methadone maintenance programs. The more time that patients spent in treatment over the past year, the lower (i.e., the better) was their psychiatric composite score.

It is necessary, however, to investigate this correlation further in order to take into account other factors that might affect the T_2 psychiatric composite score. Therefore a multiple regression analysis was undertaken. In the first step, T_1 psychiatric composite score, age, length of stay, and percent of time from T_1 to T_2 that those who left the six programs spent in other treatment programs were entered as dependent variables. In the next step, the percent of time from T_1 to T_2 that patients had been in their designated programs was entered. By this procedure "baseline" variables were covaried to ascertain the association between the amount of methadone maintenance treatment attained over the past year and T_2 psychiatric severity.

The first step of the multiple regression yielded a significant $R = .44$, $F(4.442) = 26.54$, $p < .001$. Two variables—T_1 psychiatric composite score and percent of time spent in treatment at other programs—made significant contributions to the equation; their respective B weights were .42 and .11. In the second step, adding the percent of time over the past year

TABLE 9.2. ASI Psychiatric Severity Composite Scores for 446 Methadone Maintenance Patients at T_1 and T_2

Sample	No.	Mean composite scores (SD) at various times during methadone maintenance treatment				
		<1 mo	6–11 mo	1.0–1.9 years	2–4.9 years	>5 years
Continuous treatment (T_1 and T_2)		n = 31	n = 24	n = 84	n = 113	n = 101
At T_1 Mean Psychiatric Composite Score	353	0.08 (0.15)	0.09 (0.21)	0.12 (0.18)	0.10 (0.17)	0.10 (0.16)
At T_2 Mean Psychiatric Composite Score	353	0.06 (0.12)	0.10 (0.20)	0.10 (0.17)	0.12 (0.18)	0.10 (0.16)
Left treatment after T_1		n = 28	n = 18	n = 15	n = 27	n = 5
At T_1 Mean Psychiatric Composite Score	93	0.11 (0.15)	0.12 (0.21)	0.20 (0.23)	0.11 (0.15)	0.09 (0.15)
At T_2 Mean Psychiatric Composite Score	93	0.16 (0.17)	0.12 (0.20)	0.12 (0.15)	0.15 (0.19)	0.17 (0.18)

Abbreviations: T_1 and T_2, the times of the first and second interviews, respectively.

Note: The psychiatric severity composite score can range from 0 to 1. Higher scores indicate a greater degree of psychiatric symptomatology. The score is based on patients' problems during the past 30 days.

spent in treatment at the designated programs did not explain a significant additional amount of variance. Thus, patients' psychiatric composite scores at T_2 were most strongly related to their psychiatric composite scores at T_1 and, to a lesser extent for those who left the six programs, the amount of treatment received in other programs between T_1 and T_2.

Discussion

To recapitulate, it was found that patients' duration of treatment at the six methadone maintenance programs had no effect on their psychiatric status as measured by the psychiatric severity composite score of the ASI. From the first ASI interview, no relation was found between patients' length of treatment and their current psychiatric severity. From the longitudinal analysis, it was found that patients' psychiatric composite score at T_2 was most evidently related to their comparable score at T_1. Patients' length of stay in these six programs during the T_1–T_2 year did not affect their psychiatric status.

Other studies[13,10] of patients in methadone maintenance programs have found that treatment leads to a decrease in reported psychiatric symptoms. In addition, the severity of patients' psychiatric disorder at admission has been found to be related to follow-up status.[14,15] The present research findings do not substantiate these earlier findings about the significance of psychiatric status in drug abuse treatment outcome.

Two comments are relevant with respect to considering these differences in research findings about the role of psychiatric severity in the treatment of addict patients. The first comment refers to differences in treatment provided.

The prevalence of psychiatric symptoms among patients at the six programs in New York City, Philadelphia, and Baltimore was lower than that reported elsewhere: 64.6 percent of the 567 patients studied reported that they did not experience any psychiatric problems during the prior 30 days; their psychiatric severity composite score was therefore zero. With regard to patients admitted at T_1, more than 61 percent of this cohort also had a psychiatric composite score of zero. In sum, then, the extent of psychiatric impairment among the 567 methadone maintenance patients studied was found to be lower than that previously reported.

With regard to the role of methadone maintenance in reducing psychiatric severity among addict patients, the present ASI findings do not support such an interpretation. Rather, the lack of change in psychiatric status found among the patients studied seems consistent with the treatment provided at these six programs. Well over 90 percent of the patients did not receive psychotherapy during the study period. Therefore given the absence of relevant treatment it is not surprising that their psychiatric status did not change while these patients were in methadone maintenance treatment.

References

1. Pescor MJ (1943) A statistical analysis of the clinical records of hospitalized drug addicts. Public Health Reports, Supplement 143. Washington, DC: US Government Printing Office, pp 1–30
2. Chien I, Rosenfeld E (1957) Juvenile narcotics use. In: Law and Contemporary Problems. Durham: Duke University of Law 22:52–68
3. Pickens RW, Heston LL (eds) (1979) Psychiatric Factors in Drug Abuse. New York: Grune & Stratton
4. Kleber HD, Gold MS (1978) Use of psychotropic drugs in treatment of methadone maintained narcotic addicts. In Kissin B, Lowinson JH, Millman RB (eds): Annals of the New York Academy of Sciences: Recent developments in chemotherapy of narcotic addiction. New York: New York Academy of Sciences, pp 81–98
5. O'Brien CP (1987) Treatment research. In: Drug Abuse and Drug Abuse Research: The Second Triennial Report to Congress from the Secretary. Rockville: US Department of Health and Human Services
6. McLellan AT, Childress AR, Griffith J, Woody GE (1984) The psychiatrically severe drug abuse patient: methadone maintenance or therapeutic community? Am J Drug Alcohol Abuse 10:77–95
7. Lehman AF, Myers CP, Corty E (1989) Assessment and classification of patients with psychiatric and substance abuse syndromes. Hosp Community Psychiatry 40:1019–1025
8. Woody GE, Luborsky L, McLellan AT, O'Brien CP (1983) Psychotherapy for opiate addicts: does it help? Arch Gen Psychiatry 40:639–645
9. Senay EC (1989) Methadone maintenance. In: Treatments of Psychiatric Disorders. Task Force Report of the American Psychiatric Association. Washington, DC: APA, 2:1342–1430
10. McLellan AT, Luborsky L, O'Brien CP, et al (1986) Alcohol and drug treatment in three different populations: is there improvement and is it predictable? Am J Drug Alcohol Abuse 12:101–120
11. McLellan AT, Luborsky L, O'Brien CP (1980) An improved diagnostic evaluation instrument for substance abuse patients: the addiction severity index. J Ner Ment Dis 168:26–33
12. McGahan PL, Griffith JA, Parente R, McLellan AT (1982) Composite Scores from the Addiction Severity Index. NIDA Project DA02554 and the Veteran's Administration. Unpublished report on the construction of ASI composite scores
13. McLellan AT, Luborsky L, O'Brien CP, et al (1982) Is treatment for substance abuse effective? JAMA 247:1423–1428
14. McLellan AT, Luborsky L, Woody GE, et al (1983) Predicting response to alcohol and drug abuse treatments: role of psychiatric severity. Arch Gen Psychiatry 40:620–625
15. Rounsaville BJ, Kosten TR, Weissman MM, Kleber HD (1986) Prognostic significance of psychopathology in treated opiate addicts: a 2.5 year follow-up study. Arch Gen Psychiatry 43:739–745

10
Reduction of Crime Through Methadone Maintenance Treatment

When studying the effectiveness of outpatient methadone maintenance treatment, it is relevant to consider whether crime is reduced consequent to this treatment, as crime is a major component of the deviant and self-destructive way of life associated with contemporary heroin addiction in the United States.[1,2] Therefore reduction or elimination of crime is an important aspect of successful rehabilitation. Thus the extent to which crime is reduced during treatment in methadone maintenance programs is a measure of the success of the programs. Conversely, if methadone programs do not reduce crime, do not curtail or eliminate intravenous drug use, and otherwise are unable to change and rehabilitate patients, they cannot be considered successful.

The extent to which drug abuse treatment reduces crime among patients concerns not only the programs involved but society as well, as it is the community outside the treatment programs that is beset by the vast volume of crime committed by heroin addicts. Therefore any reduction in criminality within this population is advantageous to the neighborhoods and cities where addicts live. For it is now established that drug abusers constitute a major segment of the offending population in most metropolitan areas.[3,4,5]

When addressing the question of whether methadone maintenance treatment reduces crime among patients in treatment, it is efficacious to formulate specific questions for determination.

1. To what extent are the participation in crime and the frequency of offenses committed by heroin addicts reduced or stopped after they enter methadone maintenance treatment?
2. How soon after admission is crime reduced?
3. Does treatment reduce criminality generally or only "drug related crime"?
4. What effect does long-term methadone maintenance treatment have on the reduction or elimination of crime by patients?
5. Do particular programs differ in their effectiveness in reducing patients' criminal behavior?

Measurement of Crime Among Heroin Addicts

Before delineating the lifetime and annual prevalence of crime among these heroin addicts and then assessing the reduction that occurred during and after treatment, it is pertinent to recapitulate how these crime data were obtained. First, the pretreatment history of each patient was classified as to addiction, nonaddiction, and prison time periods; the last addiction period that preceded admission was identified as a particular period for measurement in order to ascertain crime rates during the most recent period of active addiction. The rationale for this classification and its implementation has been described in detail elsewhere.[6]

In brief, information pertaining to patients' prior and current criminality were obtained directly from each patient by means of confidential face-to-face interviews. Specially trained interviewers from outside the clinic were employed for this purpose, and the interview schedules were immediately removed from the clinic upon completion. Most of the patients were interviewed twice (once during late 1985 and again a year later) so there were repeat measures of their criminal behavior. In this regard, detailed information was obtained about the frequency of crime committed during six specific time periods: (1) lifetime arrests; (2) last addiction period prior to admission; (3) the summer prior to admission; (4) admission period; (5) after 6 months in treatment; and (6) after 1 year or more in treatment. The detailed interview data obtained from each patient about his past and current criminal behavior was supplemented by clinic data, urinalysis reports, and other records. Further information about the interview instrument and data collection procedure employed was presented in Chapter 2.

Pretreatment Criminality of Addict Patients

The 617 methadone maintenance patients from New York City, Philadelphia, and Baltimore had, for the most part, a long history of criminality prior to treatment. The extent and nature of their prior criminality can be ascertained from their lifetime arrest history and, more cogently, from the offenses committed during the addiction period that preceded their current admission to methadone maintenance treatment.

Lifetime Arrests of the 617 Male Addicts

The number and type of arrests experienced by the addicts prior to their first interview in 1985 is tabulated in Table 10.1. The 617 male addicts reported 4723 adult lifetime arrests. Of these males, 86.2 percent had been arrested; 13.8 percent reported no arrests. There were 8.9 mean arrests for those with one or more arrests.

The most common reason for arrest was involvement in the drug busi-

TABLE 10.1. Lifetime Adult Arrests for Male Addicts, by Type of Arrest

Arrest for	Total arrests		Persons with arrest type		Mean arrests—for positives (no.)
	No	%	No	%	
Shoplifting	766	16.2	194	31.5	3.9
Parole violation	493	10.4	186	30.2	2.7
Drug offenses	1409	29.8	378	61.5	3.7
Forgery	127	2.7	77	12.5	1.6
Weapons offenses	324	6.9	178	28.9	1.8
Burglary	756	16.0	232	37.7	3.3
Robbery	324	6.9	144	23.4	2.3
Assault	325	6.9	152	24.7	2.1
Arson	16	0.3	11	1.8	1.5
Rape	9	0.2	9	1.5	1.0
Homicide	39	0.8	33	5.4	1.2
Other offenses	135	2.9	76	12.4	1.8
Total	4723	100.0	—	86.2	8.9

Note: 85 addicts reported no arrests; thus 86.2 percent had one or more arrests. The mean number of arrests for those who were arrested was 8.9. There were 616 valid cases.

ness, mostly sale of drugs—29.8 percent. Next in frequency were arrests for shoplifting, burglary, and parole violation, which, respectively, accounted for 16.2, 16.0, and 10.4 percent of the 4723 arrests. The next three most frequent types of arrest were for assault, robbery, and weapons offenses, each of which accounted for 6.9 percent of the total arrests. The remainder of the arrests involved forgery, arson, rape, homicide, and other nondrug offenses, which together accounted for 7 percent of the total arrests. Finally, arrests for a variety of offenses classified as "other offenses" constituted 2.9 percent of the total arrests.

The arrest participation rate (i.e., percent arrested for a specific type of crime) was high for 8 of the 11 types of crime enumerated. The crime for which the largest number of addicts were arrested were drug offenses: 61.5 percent of the addicts had one or more such arrests. Next in frequency of participation was burglary, with 37.7 percent of the addicts involved in this type of arrest. Third and fourth in participation rates were shoplifting and parole violation with, respectively, 31.5 and 30.2 percent of the addicts arrested for these crimes. Next in order of arrest participation rates were weapons offenses (28.9 percent), assault (24.7 percent), robbery (23.4 percent), and forgery (12.5 percent). The three remaining designated types of arrest, (arson, rape, and homicide) involved, respectively, 1.8, 1.5, and 5.4 percent of the addicts.

As might be expected, these addicts also had a considerable history of penal incarceration prior to their current treatment: 66 percent had been incarcerated and 36 percent had spent 2 years or more in prison. These findings about prior incarceration are similar to those reported from national surveys of drug abuse treatment programs.[7]

Although the arrest and incarceration data provide an overview of the lifetime criminality of these heroin addicts, these figures grossly underestimate the day-to-day offenses in which the addicts are engaged because fewer than 1 percent of the crimes addicts commit result in arrest.[8] Therefore the detailed information obtained from the addicts in confidential interviews about their regular criminal behavior when "on the street" provides a more accurate and meaningful account of their criminality.

Annual Extent of Criminality Among the 617 Addicts

The annual frequency of 14 types of offenses for the 617 male addicts is tabulated in Table 10.2. These data refer to the most recent period of addiction prior to treatment when these males were "on the street" and regularly using opiates. Addiction periods commonly last about 2 years, but the offense rates have been annualized to facilitate analysis.

During their last period of addiction, the male addicts committed 293,308 offenses on an annual basis. This horrendous "volume" of crime

TABLE 10.2. Annual Offense Rates for 617 Male Addicts During Their Last Addiction Period

Offense type	Annual offienses		Addicts in each type		Mean offenses per year—positives (no.)
	No.	%	No.	%	
Auto theft	2,363	0.8	36	6.0	65.6
Store theft	35,211	12.0	212	35.2	166.1
Other theft	12,505	4.3	99	16.5	126.3
Burglary	12,408	4.2	136	22.6	91.2
Robbery	6,752	2.3	82	13.6	82.3
Forgery—prescriptions	8,935	3.0	80	13.3	111.7
Forgery—Checks	5,247	1.8	58	10.0	90.5
Fencing stolen property	32,429	11.1	194	32.9	167.2
Pimping	15,075	5.1	50	8.3	301.5
Numbers racket	36,645	12.5	183	30.3	200.2
Con games	17,756	6.1	107	17.8	165.9
Loan sharking	5,353	1.8	32	5.3	167.3
Assault	2,353	0.8	43	7.2	54.7
Drug business	96,930	33.0	347	57.6	279.3
Other crime	3,346	1.1	19	3.1	176.1
Total	293,308	100.0	—	80.5	601.0

Note: 118 addicts reported no crime during their last addiction period; thus 80.5 percent reported specific offenses. The mean number of different types of crime (of the 14 types listed above) committed by those who engaged in crime during this period (488 of 606) was 3.6. The number of valid cases was 606.

amounted to a mean of 601.0 offenses per year for those who reported criminal behavior. Of the 606 addicts with relevant data, 118 reported that they were not engaged in crime during their last addiction period. Thus 80.5 percent of the addicts reported that they had engaged in crime during this period, and each provided detailed information about the types and frequencies of the offenses he had committed.

The four most frequent types of offenses committed during their last addiction period were theft from stores, fencing stolen property, involvement in the numbers racket, and drug business crime. The 35,211 store theft offenses accounted for 12.0 percent of the total annual offenses. Fencing stolen property was similar in frequency, with 32,429 offenses, or 11.1 percent of the total annual offenses. Numbers racket crime was slightly more common, with 36,645 offenses of this type, or 12.5 percent of the total. The most frequent type of crime was involvement in drug distribution (mostly selling), with 96,930 such offenses; this type of crime constituted 33.0 percent of the total 293,308 annual offenses.

Four other types of crime were next in frequency, each with more than 12,000 offenses per year. They were theft of property other than from stores (e.g., mailboxes, cars) with 12,505 offenses, burglary with 12,408 offenses, pimping with 15,075 offenses, and con games with 17,756 offenses.

The six remaining common types of crime committed by the addicts were forgery of prescriptions with 8935 offenses, robbery with 6752 offenses, loan sharking with 5353 offenses, forgery of checks with 5247 offenses, auto theft with 2363 offenses and assault with 2353 offenses. In addition to the 14 common types of offenses there were 3346 miscellaneous offenses that were classified as "other crime."

Individual criminal careers of the addicts were analyzed to ascertain whether their crime was diffuse and changeable or focused and specialized on a few types of crime. The extent of addicts' specialization in particular offense types is shown in Table 10.2. For 13 of the 14 types of crime (excluding the "other crime" category) it was found that only a minority of addicts were involved in each type; the exception was drug business crimes in which 57.6 percent of the addicts were engaged. With the exception of drug business, then, most of the addicts did not, as a group, engage in any single type of crime. Most did, however, engage in several types of crime on a specialized basis. Although only a small proportion of addicts engaged in any one type of crime (excepting drug sales), they did so at a high rate. Consequently, the frequency of offenses per year for most types of crime was high for those who committed each of these offenses. For 9 of the 14 types of crime, the mean annual offense rate for those who pursued each of these specific types was more than 100 offenses per year. Because most addicts specialized in one to four types of crime, their overall mean offense rate is several times this figure. As noted, the mean annual offense rate for those who engaged in crime was 601.0 offenses.

Crime-Days Per Year at Risk When Addicted

To measure and portray the addicts' day-to-day involvement in crime on an annual basis more cogently, it is efficacious to determine the number of days per year they are involved in crime. This measure of criminality, crime-days per year, has the advantage of facilitating a ready conceptualization of a population's involvement in criminality, as it enumerates the days per year an individual is engaged in crime and the number of days per year he is not engaged in crime. Thus if the mean crime-days per year for a sample of addicts is 238, we know that on average they engaged in crime 238 of 365 days of the year and did not engage in crime for the other 127 days. In addition to ready comprehension of the extent of individual involvement in crime, the crime-days measure controls for outlier cases of high frequency that occur in studies of high risk populations. Further information about the development and use of this measure has been reported elsewhere.[9]

Offenses and Crime-Days Per Year for 617 Addicts When Addicted

It is necessary to ascertain the number of offenses individual addicts commit on an annual basis and to determine the number of days they spend in these criminal pursuits because the frame of reference of the individual is indispensable when analyzing criminal behavior. This focus on individual participation rates and the frequency with which they commit offenses is a corollary of considering aggregate offense rates. After establishing the extent and nature of crime in a given population, the question arises as to how many offenders are involved in crime on a daily, weekly, or less frequent basis. Compilation of the frequency distribution of the number of crimes committed on an individual basis is crucial to an in-depth analysis of criminal behavior.[10]

The number of offenses that each of the 617 males committed per year when addicted and the number of days per year they were engaged in crime (i.e., crime-days per year) are depicted in Table 10.3. With respect to offenses, 488 addicts (80.5 percent) reported that they engaged in crime during the designated year, and 118 (19.5 percent) reported they did not engage in crime during the year.

For the 80.5 percent of the addicts who engaged in crime during their last addiction period, their annual number of offenses varied from 1 to 3588. The mean number of offenses committed by these 488 addicts per year was 601.0 offenses (Table 10.2), so that most were continually engaged in crime. Only 41 of the 488 addicts who engaged in crime (8.4 percent) reported fewer than 100 offenses per year. Indeed, 59.0 percent of the addicts reported more than 365 offenses per year.

The number of crime-days amassed by the addicts per year during their last addiction period is also presented in Table 10.3. Of the 600 addicts who provided valid data, 469 (78.2 percent) reported that they engaged in

TABLE 10.3. Offenses and Crime-Days per Year for 617 Addicts When Addicted

No. of crime events	Offenses per year: No. of addicts	Offenses per year: %	Crime-days per year: No. of addicts	Crime-days per year: %
0	118	19.5	131	21.8
1–99	41	6.8	22	3.7
100–199	45	7.4	68	11.3
200–299	29	4.8	40	6.7
300–399	98	16.2	339	56.5 (range 0–365)
400–499	50	8.3	—	—
500–599	27	4.5	—	—
600–699	30	5.0	—	—
700–799	45	7.4	—	—
800–899	24	4.0	—	—
900–999	16	2.6	—	—
1000–1999	75	12.4	—	—
2000–3588	8	1.3	—	—
Total	606	100.0	600	100.0
Mean	484.0		237.5	

Note: There were 606 valid cases for offense data and 600 cases for crime-days data.

crime, and 131 (21.8 percent) reported that they did not. The 2.3 percent difference between the number of addicts reporting no offenses and those reporting no crime-days during the year is a result of slight underreporting of crime-days due to a briefer baseline enumeration period for this measurement (i.e., only weeks, rather than weeks, months, and the entire year).

The range in crime-days per addicted year for the 600 addicts was from 0 to 365. The preponderance of those who committed crime did so repeatedly. The mean number of crime-days for the 469 males who committed crime was 303.9 crime-days per year; furthermore, 339 of those who committed crime (72.3 percent) were involved in crime 300 or more days per year.

Analysis of these crime-day findings reveals that there are three general groups of addicts with respect to annual criminal involvement: (1) 21.8 percent who are not actively engaged in crime (possession or use of drugs were not included as criminal behavior); (2) 21.7 percent who were engaged in crime but not on a daily basis (i.e., 1 to 299 crime-days); and (3) the majority (56.5 percent) who were engaged in crime for 300 days or more per year when addicted.

The crime-days data also provide a means for determining the amount of time addicts spend engaged in crime. With respect to the three groups identified above, the no-crime group did not spend time actively engaged in crime. Conversely, the other two groups were involved in crime most of the days when they were "on the street" and addicted. Specifically, these

469 males were engaged in crime 83 percent of the year; on average, they committed crimes 304 of 365 days per year when addicted.

Reduction in Crime During Methadone Maintenance Treatment

Overall Reduction in Crime

The reduction of criminal activity among the 491 addicts who had been in methadone maintenance treatment for 6 months or more was analyzed. This group of 491 patients consisted of the entire 1985 cohort of 617 males less 126 new admissions. These 491 patients, then, were a representative sample of patients enrolled in these six programs 6 months or longer.

There was a marked reduction in criminality among the 491 male addicts after they entered the six methadone maintenance programs. This reduction in crime was evident in a decline in the number of aggregate offenses as well as a decrease in individuals' participation in crime (Table 10.4).

TABLE 10.4. Reduction in Annual Offenses and Participation Rates After Stabilization in Methadone Maintenance Treatment: 491 Male Patients.

	Pretreatment: Last addiction period		In treatment 6 months or longer		Percent reduction	
Offense	No. of offenses	No. of addicts	No. of offenses	No. of patients	No. of offenses	Persons (%)
Auto theft	2,253	30	260	3	− 88.5 %	− 90.0
Store theft	29,631	177	3,028	31	− 89.8	− 82.5
Other theft	10,195	81	720	9	− 92.9	− 88.9
Burglary	10,713	116	1,452	14	− 86.5	− 87.9
Robbery	5,286	70	656	9	− 87.6	− 87.1
Forgery—prescription	8,193	66	912	14	− 88.9	− 78.8
Forgery—check	3,929	46	528	8	− 86.6	− 82.6
Fencing	27,577	162	4,220	33	− 84.7	− 79.6
Pimping	13,044	41	3,156	11	− 75.8	− 73.2
Numbers racket	29,299	147	15,520	81	− 47.0	− 44.9
Con games	14,123	87	2,940	17	− 79.2	− 80.5
Loan sharking	4,469	27	1,236	10	− 72.3	− 63.0
Assault	2,081	39	196	8	− 90.6	− 79.5
Drug business	78,548	284	15,264	80	− 80.6	− 71.8
Other crimes	3,017	17	15	4	− 99.5	− 76.5
Total	242,358		50,103		− 79.3	
Percent in crime		81.7		33.8		58.6

Note: The 491 patients comprise the entire 1985 cohort of 617 male addicts less 126 new admissions.

TABLE 10.5. Reduction in Crime by Time in Methadone Maintenance Treatment

		With crime		Mean crime-days		
Time in treatment	No. of pts.	No.	%	Past 30 days	For year	Per year for positives
Admission period	126	47	37.3	5.8	69.3	185.8
1 Year	148	33	22.3	2.4	28.3	126.9
2 Years	83	14	16.9	1.8	21.1	125.1
3 Years	67	8	11.9	1.0	12.4	103.9
4 Years	43	8	18.6	2.7	32.1	172.5
5 Years	39	8	20.5	2.7	32.6	158.9
6 Years or more	110	12	10.9	1.2	14.5	132.9
Total	616	130	21.1	2.7	32.1	152.1

The total number of crime-days for the 616 addicts in 30 days was 1646.0; for the year it was 19,752.2 crime-days.

Crime was also found to decrease by length of outpatient treatment: Patients in long-term treatment had substantially lower crime rates (Table 10.5). Although some patients were unable to stop their criminal behavior after stabilization in methadone maintenance treatment, crime rates among patients in all six programs were reduced from pretreatment levels.

Reduction in Aggregate Offense and Participation Rates

The overall reduction in offenses committed by the 491 male heroin addicts after admission to methadone maintenance treatment is tabulated in Table 10.4. Their pretreatment crime refers to annual offenses and participation rates during their last addiction period. The in-treatment offense data refer to annual offense and participation rates for these same 491 addicts after 6 months or more of outpatient methadone maintenance attendance.

There was a marked decline in all 15 types of offenses among the 491 patients after they were admitted to methadone maintenance programs and stabilized in their treatment regimen. The overall reduction in the number of offenses committed per year from the last addiction period to stabilized treatment was 79.3 percent—from 242,358 offenses per year to 50,103 offenses per year (Table 10.4). Although the annual number of offenses decreased by more than 80 percent for 10 of the 15 types of offense (i.e., auto theft, store theft, other theft, burglary, robbery, prescription forgery, check forgery, fencing stolen property, assault, and "other offenses"), it decreased less for such organized types of crime as drug business, pimping, loan sharking, con games, and, especially, involvement in the numbers racket. These findings indicate that it was more difficult for the addicts to terminate their involvement in organized crime than to eschew more independent criminal behavior. Although these variations in offense rates of particular types of crime are important to note, the finding of principal significance is that there was a reduction of almost 80 percent in the amount of crime committed by addicts after they were stabilized in methadone maintenance treatment.

The reduction in the number of individuals who engaged in each of the 15 types of offense was generally similar to the reduction in the aggregate number of offenses committed. There was an 88.5 percent reduction in auto theft (from 2253 offenses during the last addiction period to 260 offenses when in treatment) and a 90.0 percent reduction in the number of individuals engaged in this type of crime (from 30 to 3).

When analyzing the reduction in the number of individuals involved in particular types of crime, it is pertinent to note wherein the greatest absolute decline in criminal participation occurs. The greatest reduction in participation in crime occurred with respect to drug business offenses—declining from 284 addicts involved in drug business crime during the last addiction period to only 80 involved while in treatment. Other types of crime in which there was a reduction in participation by 100 or more individuals were store theft, burglary, and fencing stolen property.

Among the 491 addicts, 81.7 percent were engaged in some type of crime during their last addiction period. After 6 months or longer in outpatient treatment, only 33.8 percent of these same 491 patients were involved in crime. In sum, almost one-half of the addict patients involved in crime gave up crime completely after stabilization in methadone maintenance treatment, although a sizable minority did not. This point raises the issue of the effect of time in treatment.

Reduction in Crime by Time in Treatment

The 617 patients who were interviewed during late 1985 were a cross-section of the 1874 patients in treatment at these six programs in New York City, Philadelphia, and Baltimore. Therefore it was feasible to compare pretreatment crime rates (i.e., last addiction period) with current crime rates based on time in treatment, as most of these patients had been in continuous outpatient attendance for 1 year or more.

It was found that crime committed by addict patients was substantially reduced during the course of methadone maintenance treatment and that (with qualifications to be noted) the longer outpatient treatment was continued the lower were the crime rates (Table 10.5, Fig. 10.1). Thus, mean crime-days per year decreased from 237.5 crime-days at the last addiction period prior to treatment to 69.3 crime-days during the admission period. This 70.8 percent decline in aggregate crime-days was followed by further declines during the first, second, and third years of outpatient treatment. Mean crime-days per year during the first year of treatment (i.e., 6 months to 1.49 years) was 28.3, during the second year it was 21.1, and during the third year it was 12.4. The crime rate was higher among patients in treat-

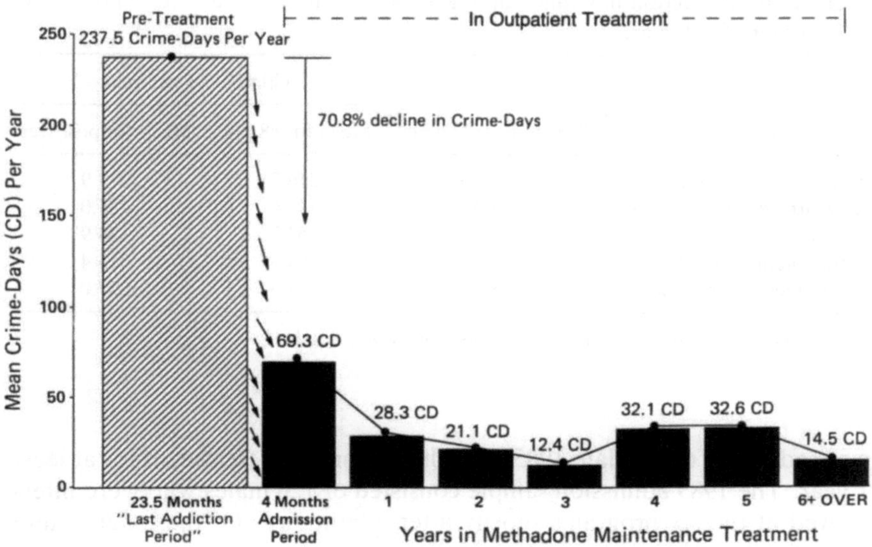

FIGURE 10.1. Reduction in crime by years in methadone maintenance treatment.

ment 4 or 5 years (32.1 and 32.6 mean crime-days per year, respectively) but declined again among the 110 patients in treatment for 6 years or more to 14.5 crime-days per year. The mean crime-days per year for these latter 110 patients in treatment for 6 years or longer, decreased by 93.9 percent from the pretreatment rate of 237.5 crime-days per year during the last addiction period. Long-term treatment, then, was associated with the lowest crime rates. (Figure 10.1)

When comparing the seven time-in-treatment cohorts (i.e., admissions and years 1 to 6) with respect to criminality, it is relevant to consider variations in such variables as age and last addiction period crime rates for the cohorts. The mean ages for the seven cohorts were 33.8, 34.9, 36.9, 37.5, 38.7, 38.7, and 40.1 years, respectively, for the admission through year 6 cohorts. The mean offense rates for these seven cohorts during their last addiction period were, respectively, 404.3, 466.6, 537.8, 576.0, 460.6, 385.4, and 541.6 offenses per year. With respect to both age and pretreatment criminality, these factors were either only tangentially related (in the case of age) or unrelated (in the case of pretreatment crime) to the decrease in crime that occurred during successive years of outpatient methadone maintenance treatment.

Reduction in Crime Among 48 Admissions

To ascertain the year-to-year effect of treatment on a specific group of patients it is pertinent to trace the change in crime rates among patients who

TABLE 10.6. Reduction in Crime Among 48 New Admission Patients Who Stayed in Treatment for 1 year.

		Crime-days per year	
Time period	% committed crimes	Mean for 48 pts.	Mean for positives
Last addiction period	77.3	216.3	279.9
Pretreatment, 4–6 months	50.0	143.0	286.0
Admission period	35.4	52.7	148.9
In treatment, 6 months	43.8	94.3	215.4
In treatment, 12 months	25.0	64.3	257.0

Note: There were 44 valid cases for the last addiction period.

were admitted during late 1985 and who remained in treatment for at least 1 year. The 1985 admission sample consisted of 126 males who were interviewed at the six programs shortly after admittance. Of these 126, there were 48 still in treatment at the same programs during late 1986, and they were reinterviewed by the same professional interviewers.

From the two face-to-face confidential interviews, six principal data sets were obtained about each of the 48 addicts who remained in treatment: (1) lifetime arrests by number and type; (2) crime committed during their last addiction period; (3) crime committed during the summer prior to admission; (4) crime during the admission period; (5) crime after 6 months of treatment; and (6) crime after 1 year in outpatient treatment. Because these data sets referred to different lengths of time, the figures were standardized to annual crime rates.

The 48 admissions who remained in treatment were similar to the larger admission cohort of 126 males in terms of their pretreatment criminality. The mean number of lifetime adult arrests for the 48 addicts was 6.2, and 40 of the addicts reported prior arrests (83.3 percent). The mean age of these 48 males at the time of first interview was 35.3 years.

The admission sample's involvement in crime during the five designated time periods is depicted in Table 10.6. During their last addiction period these 48 addicts were engaged in crime at the rate of 216.3 crime-days per year. At this time, 77.3 percent of the sample were committing crimes, and the mean crime-days per year was 279.9.

During the summer that preceded their admission to methadone maintenance treatment, 50.0 percent of the sample were engaged in crime, and the mean crime-days per year was 143.0 (for those involved in crime, it was 286.0 crime-days per year). There were two reasons for the lower participation rate during the summer pretreatment period than during their last addiction period. The first reason is that many of these patients were in other treatment programs or in jail during the summer that preceded their entry into the six methadone maintenance programs under study. Second, the last addiction period is a status rather than a specific calendar period. Therefore addiction-related variables such as crime are higher during such time "on the street."

After the 48 addicts entered methadone maintenance treatment during late 1985, their involvement in crime decreased substantially. Their mean crime-days per year decreased to 52.7, a 75.6 percent decrease from their last addiction period. Their participation in crime also declined; just over one-third (35.4 percent) were now engaged in crime. Admission to methadone maintenance treatment was thus a period of abrupt change that reduced criminal behavior for most patients.

The reduction in criminality that occurred following admission, however, was not consistent and continuous for these 48 patients. Indeed, an increase in their crime rate occurred after their admission period, from 53 to 94 crime-days per year. Apparently, the vagaries of adjusting to the daily routine of outpatient attendance at the six programs were considerable during this transition period. The finding that participation in crime did not continue to decline from the admission period to 6 months was unexpected. The finding that those involved in crime declined to 25.0 percent after 12 months in treatment was more in accord with expectations. A similar variation in mean crime-days per year for these 48 patients was observed: a slight rise at 6 months followed by a decline at 12 months.

When considering the effectiveness of the programs in reducing crime among newly admitted patients, it is important to note that it is the reduction in participation rates which was most evident. Thus after 1 year of outpatient methadone maintenance treatment, only 25.0 percent of the patients were engaged in crime. At the same time, those patients who were still involved in crime continued at a high level; the mean rate for those who were engaged in crime remained over 200 crime-days per year after 6 months or 12 months in treatment.

Reduction in Crime at the Six Programs

The extent to which crime was reduced among patients at each of the six programs (Table 10.7) was ascertained in order to determine whether the general reduction in crime was specific to particular programs or general among all six. It was found that a marked reduction in crime occurred after patients entered all six of the programs but that there also were important differences in the effectiveness of particular programs.

The extent to which patients at each of the six programs reduced their crime varied somewhat with respect to both aggregate crime-days per year and to participation rates (Table 10.7). With respect to the aggregate reduction in crime-days per year, this reduction varied from 94.4 percent to 86.8 percent (i.e., from 273.2 crime-days per year when addicted to 15.3 crime-days per year when in treatment at one program to a decline from 281.9 to 37.1 crime-days per year at another program). Although this re-

TABLE 10.7. Reduction in Crime Among 491 Patients at Six Methadone Maintenance Programs

		Last addiction period		Intreatment stable patients		Reduction in crime (%)	
Program	No. of patients	Mean CDs/year	Participation rate	Mean CDs/year	Participation rate	Crime-days	Participation
A	75	264.3	84.7	27.2	26.7	89.7	68.5
B	95	273.2	84.2	15.3	12.6	94.4	85.0
C	69	189.3	71.9	13.9	8.7	92.7	87.9
D	91	281.9	87.8	37.1	27.5	86.8	68.7
E	82	223.8	72.2	18.6	11.0	91.7	84.8
F	79	210.0	73.1	21.4	14.1	89.8	80.7
Total	491	243.8	79.5	22.5	16.9	90.8	78.7

CD, crime-days.

duction was somewhat affected by the variation in pretreatment crime rates, the similarity of the overall reduction at the six programs is notable (Fig. 10.2). At the same time, in-treatment crime is more than 2.5 times higher in one program than in another (i.e., 13.9 versus 37.1 crime-days per year).

Discussion

Pre-treatment Criminality

When considering the question of whether, or to what extent, methadone maintenance treatment reduces crime among heroin addicts, it is necessary to ascertain their prior rate of criminality. In the present study, it was found that the addicts from New York City, Philadelphia, and Baltimore (during their last addiction period) committed 484 mean offenses per year when addicted, and that, on average, they engaged in crime 238 days per year. This prior involvement in crime was surprisingly similar for the addicts from the three cities. Thus the types of offenses committed, the frequency of occurrence, and the participation rate during their last addiction periods[11] were quite similar for addicts from New York City, Philadelphia and Baltimore. These findings provide support for a commonality hypothesis about the structure and dynamics of the addict subculture in these cities.

The commonality thesis is substantiated by previous studies of addict populations in eastern U.S. cities that have employed comparable methodology (on-site data collection, face-to-face confidential interviews, determination of addiction versus nonaddiction periods, and crime-days

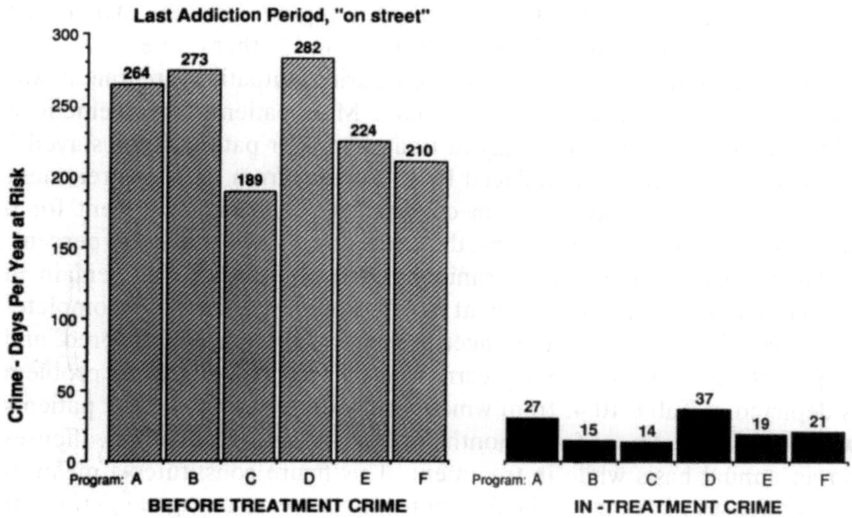

FIGURE 10.2. Crime among 491 patients before and during methadone maintenance treatment at six programs. Hatched bars = crime-days per year when addicted. Solid bars = crime-days per year after 6 months or more in treatment.

measures). These studies have consistently found that addicts as a group commit an inordinate amount of crime when engaged in the daily use of opiates and other drugs—some 220 to 260 crime-days per year. The present finding of a crime rate of 238 mean crime-days per year when addicted substantiates the previous research findings.[9,12,1,13,14]

When discussing the similarity of crime rates among various addict samples and populations, it is pertinent to note that the commonality observed refers to a similar *distribution* of crime rates rather than an overall uniformity of criminal behavior among the addicts studied. The frequency distribution of the number of offenses and crime-days amassed per year, the types of crimes committed, and the percentage of addicts engaged in crime are all similar in these studies.

Reduction in Crime During Methadone Maintenance Treatment

It was found that there was a marked reduction in criminal behavior during outpatient methadone maintenance treatment. For those 491 patients who remained in treatment for 6 months or longer, there was a 79 percent decline in the number of offenses committed on a yearly basis from their prior addiction status. This decline occurred with respect to all types of offenses: auto theft, store theft, other theft, burglary, robbery, prescription forgery,

forgery of checks, fencing stolen property, pimping, numbers racket, con games, loan sharking, assault, drug business, and "other crime."

The reduction in crime that occurred during outpatient treatment was related to the duration of this treatment. Most patients' involvement in crime decreased with longer stay in treatment. For patients who stayed 2 years, the crime rate was reduced by 91 percent from their pretreatment rate. For patients who stayed in continuous outpatient treatment for 6 years or longer at the six programs, the crime rate was reduced by 94 percent.

Although the reduction in criminality among patients who remain in methadone maintenance treatment is substantial, it is far from complete. This fact is important because lingering criminality cannot be ignored, and its persistence is a cause for concern. The scope of the remaining problem is depicted in Table 10.4, from which it may be seen that the 491 patients who were in treatment for 6 months or longer committed 50,103 offenses on an annual basis while in treatment. This figure constitutes a mean of 301.8 offenses per year for the 33.8 percent who were engaged in crime. It is evident, then, that a sizable number of patients persist in their criminal behavior after admittance to methadone maintenance treatment.

What is to be done? Two observations seem germane. First and foremost, it is imperative that the overall success in reducing crime be kept in mind. From Table 10.4, it can be seen that there was a reduction in annual offenses from 242,358 to 50,103—a reduction of more than 192,000 offenses per year! This remarkable reduction in criminality, 79 percent, occurred through outpatient methadone maintenance treatment. A reduction of this magnitude among addicts has commonly been accomplished previously only through residential stay or incarceration.

At the same time, there is reason to believe that patients' involvement in criminality can be further reduced, and efforts in this direction are in order. Supporting evidence for holding that criminal behavior among patients can be further reduced is provided by the length of stay in treatment findings and by the differences in outcome data among the six programs. With respect to length of stay, the association between years of outpatient treatment and lower crime rates demonstrates that prolonged treatment in a methadone maintenance program can further reduce crime. In addition, the finding that some programs are at least twice as effective as others in eliminating crime among their patients supports the contention that further reductions in crime are feasible. In this regard, it is relevant to note that methadone maintenance programs are not primarily organized to address the topic of patients' criminality. This issue is usually regarded as secondary after addressing the pressing problems of intravenous drug use, medical needs, counseling, and adherence to clinic rules. The question of which additional services—to effect crime reduction or other objectives—can efficaciously be provided at methadone maintenance programs remains to be answered.

References

1. Ball JC, Shaffer JW, Nurco DN (1983) The day-to-day criminality of heroin addicts in Baltimore—a study of the continuity of offence rates. Drug Alcohol Dependence 12:119–142
2. Nurco DN, Ball JC, Shaffer JW, Hanlon TE (1985) The criminality of narcotic addicts. J Nerv Ment Dis 173:94–102
3. The White House (1990) National Drug Control Strategy (January). Washington, DC: US Government Printing Office
4. Belenko, S (1990) The impact of drug offenders on the criminal justice system. In Weisheit, R: Drugs, Crime and the Criminal Justice System. Cincinnati: Anderson Publishing
5. Gerstein DR, Harwood HJ (eds) (1990) Treating Drug Problems, Vol. 1. Washington, DC: National Academy Press
6. Nurco DN, Cisin IH, Balter MB (1981) Addict careers. II. The first ten years. Int J Addict 16:1327–1356
7. Ball JC, Levine BK, Demaree RG, Newman JF (1975) Pretreatment criminalty of male and female drug abuse patients in the United States. Addict Dis 1:481–489
8. Inciardi JA, Chambers CE (1972) Unreported criminal activity of narcotic addicts. J Drug Issues 2:57–64
9. Ball JC, Rosen L, Flueck JA, Nurco DN (1981) The criminality of heroin addicts when addicted and when off opiates. In Inciardi JA (ed): The Drugs-Crime Connection. Vol. 5. Sage Annual Reviews of Drug and Alcohol Abuse. Beverly Hills: Sage Publications, pp. 39–65
10. Blumstein A, Cohen J, Roth JA, Visher CA (eds) (1986) Dimensions of active criminal careers. In: Criminal Careers and "Career Criminals." Washington, DC: National Academy Press, pp 55–95
11. Ball JC (1991) The similarity of crime rates among heroin addicts in New York City, Philadelphia and Baltimore. J Drug Issues. (in press)
12. Ball JC, Rosen L, Flueck JA, Nurco DN (1982) Lifetime criminality of heroin addicts in the United States. J Drug Issues 3:225–316
13. Nurco DN, Ball JC, Shaffer JW, et al (1986) A comparison by race/ethnicity of narcotic addict crime rates in Baltimore, New York and Philadelphia. Am J Drug Alcohol Abuse 12:297–307
14. Nurco DN, Shaffer JW, Ball JC, Kinlock TW (1984) Trends in the commission of crime among narcotic addicts over successive periods of addiction and nonaddiction. Am J Drug Alcohol Abuse 10:481–489

11
Treatment Success: Association With Patient Baseline, Program Elements, and In-treatment Process

After it had been found that the six methadone maintenance programs were effective in markedly reducing intravenous drug use, crime, and other deviant behavior among patients who remained in treatment, the question arose as to how this successful outcome came about. Was success due to particular patient baseline characteristics that antedated treatment? Was it due to general program characteristics or to specific treatment services provided? Was successful outcome primarily a function of patients' length of stay in treatment? Finding answers to these and related questions involved ascertaining why methadone maintenance treatment is effective. It was evident that these specific questions could be addressed only within a comprehensive evaluation framework and that the answers were likely to be interrelated. Thus it was necessary to determine the relative effect of both patient and treatment domain variables as well as such factors as retention in treatment and the effect of long-term stay.

When considering the analysis of treatment effectiveness of methadone maintenance programs, several general observations are relevant. First, we hypothesized that both program and patient characteristics are related to successful treatment outcome because treatment involves both programs and patients. Testing the hypothesis becomes a matter of determining which particular program and patient characteristics are conducive to successful outcome.

Second, successful patient outcome in methadone maintenance programs is a result of long-term treatment and rehabilitation. Opiate addiction is a chronic condition that requires long-term intervention (see Chapter 3). Therefore evaluation of treatment should consider successful outcome as a status patients realize after months or years of therapy. It is not a question of looking for the magic bullet that provides a quick cure. It is, rather, a question of investigating those conditions and factors that have, over the months and years, made rehabilitation possible.

Third, it is important to recognize that some methadone maintenance programs are markedly more effective than others. The analytical problem, then, is to identify and measure the program elements that make a difference with respect to successful patient outcome. This task is the focus of the chapter.

A fourth observation pertains to the selection of outcome measures. Although successful outcome of methadone maintenance treatment is a status that generally subsumes a common set of behavioral criteria (e.g., cessation of drug abuse and crime), it is not an all-encompassing status or criterion. There are other outcome dimensions that can and should be investigated, such as improvement in psychological status[1] or health.[2]

Finally, when approaching a statistical analysis of methadone maintenance treatment outcome in which the focus is on identifying *differentiating factors* among the programs and patients that are associated with success, it is important to recognize that common program features and necessary conditions may be overlooked. When ascertaining which program components or variables are most closely related to successful patient outcome, one can easily miss the reality that most programs require staffing 365 days a year, that a physical facility and patient records are indispensable to continued operation, and that, in sum, a treatment domain must be present. The point is that there are necessary conditions and variable factors associated with successful patient outcome; the necessary conditions are taken as givens, and attention is focused here on differentiating among variable factors in order to provide a rationale for improvement.

Research Questions Addressed

When considering the effectiveness of methadone maintenance treatment, analysis of the findings is organized around the following four questions.

1. Which pretreatment patient baseline characteristics are associated with successful patient outcome among methadone maintenance patients?
2. Which program elements are associated with successful patient outcome?
3. Which in-treatment process variables are associated with successful patient outcome?
4. Are patient, program, or process characteristics most closely related to successful patient outcome?

In the remainder of this chapter these research questions are addressed in some detail. First, pertinent patient preadmission baseline characteristics are described, followed by a discussion of key program measures and the derivation of five principal treatment domain components. The major content of each component is explained, and these summary measures are then named to facilitate interpretation.

A discussion of five process variables that measure patients' status or progress in methadone maintenance treatment is followed by consideration of the specific outcome variables used in this analysis. The sample of patients employed is described and the regression procedure set forth. Finally, findings pertaining to successful patient outcome are analyzed with respect to baseline patient characteristics, program components, and treatment process variables.

The Data

Patient Baseline Variables

Based on preliminary analysis and previous research findings, ten pretreatment baseline variables for each patient were included in the regression analyses, including basic demographic information, addiction history, previous experience in drug treatment programs, and criminal behavior. The manner in which the variables were entered into the regression calculations are indicated in Table 11.1. Race was reduced to a binary variable; the addiction history variables were transformed to suppress right skewness of these distributions; and the original nine-category employment variable was reduced to a simple three-point scale. The coding and transforming left

TABLE 11.1. Patient Baseline Variables (T_1)

Variable	Label	Code-transform	In-treatment cohort
Age at T_1 interview	AGE	Actual years	37.3 years[a]
Race	RACE	0 = white, caucasian 1 = all other	 58% nonwhite
Usual employment pattern during 3 years prior to this admission	EMPL	0 = unemployed or in controlled environment 1 = part time 2 = full time	30% unemployed 18% part time 52% full time
Age at onset of opiate addiction	ONSET	Actual years	18.9 years[a]
Years of regular heroin use—lifetime	HYEARS	log (1 + actual years)	10.6 years[a]
Years of regular use of other opiates—lifetime	OYEARS	log (1 + actual years)	2.3 years[a]
Years of regular cocaine use—lifetime	CYEARS	log (1 = actual years)	2.2 years[a]
Prior no. of treatments for drug abuse	TREAT	Actual number	3.3[a]
No. of arrests—lifetime	TOTARR	Actual number	7.4[a]
Crime-days rate, last addiction period, typical week	CRIME	Actual number	4.7[a]

[a] Mean.

race as the only categorical variable. Increasing values of the nine other variables indicate "older," "longer," or "more."

The mean values of the ten baseline variables for the in-treatment sample of 407 patients—the group that comprises the data set for this chapter—are also shown in Table 11.1. Their mean age was 37 years, 58 percent were nonwhite, 30 percent were unemployed prior to admission, age at onset of opiate addiction was 19 years, duration of heroin use was 11 years, other opiates were used 2.3 years, cocaine was used 2.2 years, the number of prior drug abuse treatments was 3.3, there were 7.4 mean lifetime arrests and they averaged 4.7 mean crime-days per week when addicted.

Treatment Domain Data: Five Principal Components

The comprehensive treatment domain data collected at the programs were summarized in 89 program variables (Appendix A). These variables measured the basic elements of the treatment domain: neighborhood–facility; patient census; staff characteristics and ratios; treatment and rehabilitation provided; treatment policy; and program management and administration.

To relate the treatment domain to patient outcomes, it was necessary to effect a data reduction that would permit the overall features of the treatment domain to be expressed in a few variables for statistical calculations. The end result of the data reduction was the derivation of five statistical variables (principal components) to depict the main aspects of the treatment domain. The data reduction was accomplished in three steps.

1. Setting aside variables. Variables that characterized patients individually and were averaged or combined as program descriptors were deleted as program variables for the regression analyses. Examples of such variables are percent of patients who were nonwhite, average methadone dose for all patients, and average duration of treatment. Variables that had practically the same value across all six programs were also set aside, e.g., full-time versus part-time directors (all but one program had a full-time director); years of operation (all six programs had been in operation at least 12 years); funding per patient (similar for five of six programs); descriptors of neighborhood situation, including parking at the program site; and extent of vocational and educational services. All of these program variables were either similar or had minimal values at the six programs.

2. *Combining variables.* To characterize the overall medical staff, the number of physicians, physicians' assistants (PAs), and nurse practitioners (NPs) were combined to provide a measure of full time equivalents (FTEs) per patient for the total medical staff. Likewise, years of experience at the program were combined for the three classes of medical staff; service rendered by medical staff was expressed simply as percent of patients seen per week by all classes of medical staff. Service delivered by the counseling staff was represented by percent of patients seen per week in both individual or group counseling sessions.

TABLE 11.2. Characteristic Vectors of Five Principal Components of 25 Key Variables in the Treatment Program Domain and Correlations of Variables with Principal Components

		Principal components and correlations									
Variable	Description	Prin 1	Corr	Prin 2	Corr	Prin 3	Corr	Prin 4	Corr	Prin 5	Corr
A. Services											
1 (55, 57)	% Pts. seen by counselors; indiv. and group sessions	.187	.59	−.246	−.69	.073	.19	−.153	−.26	.195	.28
2 (61)	Overall assessment of counseling services	.264	.88	−.011	.03	.074	.20	.225	.41	.089	.13
3 (34)	Missed medication rate (attendance)	.279	.87	.056	.15	.077	.19	.238	.40	−.118	−.17
4 (77)	% Patients treated by medical staff in week	.138	.41	−.292	−.77	−.068	−.16	.225	.37	.206	.28
5 (85)	Overall quality of medical services (82–84)	−.190	−.59	.119	.33	−.039	−.10	.430	.73	.044	.06
6 (87)	% Patients who provided urine in week	−.194	−.62	.253	.71	−.132	−.34	.025	.04	−.007	−.01
B. Counseling staff											
7 (52)	FTE counselors (per census)	.002	.00	−.085	−.21	.368	.83	.332	.51	.059	.07
8 (44)	Counselors' mean years at program	.106	.30	.297	.74	.173	.39	−.192	−.30	.269	.34
9 (51)	Turnover rate of counselors, per year	.187	.50	.206	.48	−.305	−.65	.074	.11	.236	.28
10 (63)	Morale of counselors, mean score	.171	.58	.205	.61	.190	.52	.017	.03	.118	.18
C. Medical staff											
11 (65, 66, 67)	FTE medical staff ratio (per census)	−.242	−.71	−.030	−.08	−.260	−.62	.159	.26	.153	.20
12 (74)	Years at program, MDs and PAs-NPs	−.101	−.29	.298	.76	.244	.57	.049	.08	−.054	−.07
13 (68, 69)	FTE dispensing staff ratio (per census)	−.001	−.00	−.048	.14	.353	.91	.149	.26	.190	.28
D. Director											
14 (36)	Years at this program	.337	.90	.074	.17	.020	.04	.084	.12	−.305	−.37
15 (37)	Years as director at this program	.194	.54	.187	.46	−.186	−.42	.255	.39	−.326	−.41
16 (40)	Direct involvement in patient care	.228	.64	.104	.26	.057	.13	−.453	−.69	−.134	−.17
17 (41)	Effectiveness, composite score	.204	.67	.119	.35	.217	.57	−.163	−.29	−.099	−.15

E. Administration–Management											
18 (6)	Rating of administration, effectiveness	.107	.30	.271	.68	−.257	−.59	.194	.30	.088	.11
19 (9)	Patients' records, assessment	−.025	−.07	.301	.73	−.261	−.58	−.127	−.19	.257	.32
20 (20)	Security at site–rating of patient flow	.088	.26	.301	.78	.183	.43	.194	.31	.151	.20
21 (10)	Coordination of treatment services	.209	.72	.164	.50	−.118	−.33	−.132	−.25	.162	.25
22 (19)	Composite rating of facility	−.065	−.19	.220	.57	.331	.79	.028	.04	.075	.10
G. Treatment policy											
23 (3)	Medical orientation	−.279	−.79	.149	.37	.073	.17	−.114	−.18	.325	.42
24 (4)	Rehabilitation orientation	.347	.73	−.275	−.51	−.065	−.11	.026	.03	.475	.45
25 (5)	Long-term maintenance orientation	.265	.86	.088	.25	−.166	−.43	.042	.07	−.047	−.07
Characteristic root		21.1		16.4		13.6		6.2		4.3	
Percent of total variance		34		27		22		10		7	

3. *Principal components*. Twenty-five key variables representing essential aspects of the treatment domain remained after sifting and combining treatment program variables as described above. See (Table 11.2). Among the 25 variables, the 17 that did not lie on the 1 = best/most to 5 = worst/least scale were normed to that 1 to 5 scale by a linear transformation that preserved relative distances between unscaled values. For example, the unscaled Years as Director of the Program (1, 10, 3, 0, 2, 13 years, respectively) were transformed to (4.69, 1.92, 4.08, 5.00, 4.38, 1.00). After transforming, all 25 variables conformed to the 1 to 5 scale.

Five principal components were then extracted for the 25 variables in each of the six programs (150 observations in total). A brief explanation of principal components is in order.[3] A principal component in the present context is an algebraic sum of the 25 program variables, each variable weighted by a coefficient (loading). Each of the five principal components is represented by its own specific set of 25 coefficients (Table 11.2.). The sets of coefficients (characteristic vectors or eigenvectors) are chosen to make the five components mutually uncorrelated. The five new variables (the principal components) are each a composite of the 25 original variables; each principal component represents a statistical dimension of the treatment domain. The statistical procedure employed to derive the five principal components from the 25 program variables was self-contained and not based on outcome findings.

Multiplying the 25 normed variables of program A by the corresponding elements of the characteristic vector of the first principal component results in a score for program A. That score is the first principal component for program A. Multiplying the same 25 variables times the elements of the second characteristic vector gives the second principal component for program A. Comparable calculations for each of the six programs gave five principal components for each program.

The six scores for each component (one component score for each program) were normed to lie in the range 1 to 5 (Table 11.3). The numbers in Table 11.3 are the independent variables for the regression analyses that represent the program domain.

TABLE 11.3. Principal Component Scores for the Six Treatment Programs

	Treatment program					
Principal component	A	B	C	D	E	F
Prin 1	5.00	1.00	2.20	4.25	3.72	3.44
Prin 2	2.32	1.00	5.00	1.64	3.78	1.55
Prin 3	1.00	2.27	1.83	2.31	5.00	4.79
Prin 4	1.00	2.24	2.82	5.00	2.54	1.82
Prin 5	2.52	1.89	4.09	3.02	1.00	5.00

TABLE 11.4. Principal Components of the Treatment Domain

Component	Description	Label
Prin 1	Counseling services, director, policy	COUNS-DIR-POL
Prin 2	Administration—management, staff experience	ADMIN-EXPER
Prin 3	Facility, staffing	FACIL-STAFF
Prin 4	Medical services	MED
Prin 5	Residual	RESID

The five principal components together "explain" the statistical properties of the 25 program variables among the six programs. The first principal component explains the most, in terms of variance among the programs, and the others explain less in descending order. Variance of each component (the characteristic root) and percent of total variance among the programs are given at the bottom of Table 11.2.

Interpretation of the Five Principal Components

The five principal components of the treatment program domain have the virtue of reducing 25 variables to five dimensions. The components, however, are mathematical artifacts until their features are interpreted in terms of the variables that are their primary constituent parts. The following remarks summarize the basis for attaching interpretive names to the components. The usual practice was followed in identifying individual program variables that were highly correlated, over all six programs, with the component score and then naming components according to those variables. The relevant correlations are shown in Table 11.2. Descriptions of the five components are summarized in Table 11.4.

COMPONENT I: COUNSELING SERVICES, DIRECTOR, AND POLICY

The first component (counseling services, director, and policy) was positively correlated with the provision of a high level of treatment services to patients. It included a high percent of patients regularly seen in individual counseling sessions and the overall adequacy of these services, and a high rate of attendance for medication (which is a measure of total services received). In addition to these 3 treatment service variables (Table 11.2, lines 1 to 3), this component was positively correlated with all four variables that refer to the director of the program (variables 14 to 17) as well as with variable 21, which refers to the effective coordination of treatment services. The third set of variables that "explain" this component refer to treatment policy; this component is associated with a strong rehabilitation and long-term maintenance policy. (This component is inversely correlated with the relative strength of the medical staff, as measured by FTEs; it is also inversely correlated with a medical orientation but not with the provision of medical services.)

Component 1, then, is composed of a dominant treatment emphasis, as four of the six provision-of-service variables have positive correlations. Second, this component reflects an effective program director, as measured by four variables. Third, the component subsumes a strong treatment policy orientation, so component 1 may be termed high in the provision of treatment services (especially counseling services), effective in leadership, and high in articulated treatment policy—or, in short, COUNS-DIR-POL.

Component 2: Administration and Experience

The second principal component (administration and experience) was found to be most highly correlated with two sets of variables: those measuring program administration and management and those measuring staff experience. All four of the administration variables (lines 18 to 21, Table 11.2) were positively correlated with this component. Also, there was a positive correlation with counselors' years of experience and that of the medical staff (variables 8 and 12). Negative correlations with percent of patients seen by counselors and percent of patients treated by medical staff were evident, indicating that Prin 2 did not represent delivery of services.

Component 2, then, primarily includes variables that have positive correlations with program administration and, to a lesser extent, those that denote staff experience. This component is not associated with a high level of provision of treatment services. For convenience, this component is termed: ADMIN-EXPER.

Component 3: Facility and Staff Ratio

Component 3 (facility and staff ratio) is most highly correlated with the adequacy of the physical facility and with the patient/staff ratio of the dispensing and counseling staff, as measured by FTE per patient (lines 7 and 13); conversely, the medical staff strength, as measured by FTE per patient, was correlated negatively. In addition, there is a negative correlation with three of the four administration (lines 18, 19, and 21).

Component 3, then, refers to the physical facility and includes a high ratio of dispensing and counseling staff to patients (i.e., FTE ratio). Concomitantly, this component has a negative association with adequate administration. Therefore the component includes indicators of less adequate program performance. Component 3 is designated as high in facility and staff ratio (FACIL-STAFF).

Component 4: Medical Services

Component 4 (medical services) was somewhat similar to component 1 with respect to having a correlation with treatment service variables. There was a positive correlation with four of the provision of service (lines 2 to 5), but especially the overall adequacy, or quality, of the medical services (line 5). Most of the remaining correlations with the 25 key treatment domain variables were minimal except for a negative association with the director's involvement with direct patient care.

This component is correlated with the provision of treatment services, especially the adequacy of medical services regularly provided to patients. The designation for this component is MED.

Component 5: Minimal Effect

None of the 25 key variables were highly correlated with component 5, minimal effect, or residual (RESID). This component seems to represent a weak combination of counselors' years of experience and a medical treatment orientation.

Review of the Five Components

To summarize the content of the five principal components and to comment on an overall interpretation of the correlations reviewed, it is noteworthy that two of the components (Prin 1 and Prin 4) are most evidently associated with the delivery of treatment services. Of these two, component 1 was also positively correlated with an effective program director and a strong rehabilitation and maintenance policy.

Component 4 (Prin 4) was similar to Prin 1 in its emphasis on services. Prin 4, however, stressed medical services rather than counseling services; the latter were more important in Prin 1. With regard to the provision of treatment services, Prin 4 complements Prin 1: together Prin 1 and Prin 4 loaded on five of the six service variables. Prin 4 is mainly quality of medical service with less involvement of the director, whereas Prin 1 represents counseling service, good performance by an experienced director, and a strong rehabilitation orientation.

Components 2 and 3 were not, for the most part, positively correlated with the provision-of-services variables; instead, these components were correlated with other aspects of the treatment domain, such as staff characteristics, the physical facility, and program administration.

Process Variables

Five variables that describe aspects of the treatment process as it impinges on individual patients were introduced as independent variables in the regression calculations for the in-treatment cohort (Table 11.5). The time reference point for treatment process variables is T_1, the date of the first interview. Four variables describe essential aspects of methadone maintenance treatment: dose, length of stay (how long the patient had been in continuous treatment during the current admission), missed methadone

TABLE 11.5. Treatment Process Variables

Variable	Label	Code-transform	In-treatment cohort
Length of stay for this admission up to T_1	LOS	log (1 + actual months)	47.2 months[a]
Missed methadone during 30 days prior to T_1	MISSMETH	0 = no days missed 1 = 1 or more days missed	22% missed doses
Take-home methadone doses per week at T_1	TAKEHOME	Actual number (0–6)	1.9 doses per week[a]
Methadone maintenance dose at T_1	DOSE	Actual milligrams	46.1 mg[a]
Terminated before T2	STATUS	0 = terminated 1 = continued in program at T_2	338/407 continued 69/407 terminated

[a] Mean

doses, and the number of take-home doses scheduled. A fifth variable, STATUS, indicates whether patients have been terminated or have otherwise left treatment by T_2. The five process variables are delineated in Table 11.5.

The methadone dose prescribed for patients in treatment is an indication of program policy (i.e., low dose versus high dose) as well as patients' treatment status. Lower doses may indicate recent admissions or those undergoing detoxification. Low doses may also be the result of treatment policy. High dose often is indicative of stable treatment status. In addition to these considerations, there is pharmacological interest in the relation of dose to treatment outcome. In this regard there is particular interest in the relation of methadone dose to the cessation or continuation of heroin use (see appendix B).

Length of stay in treatment is a common measurement of treatment process, as it is a gross measure of the amount of treatment received. The missed medication rate of patients has not commonly been studied, despite the established importance of attendance and compliance. The number of take-home doses of methadone is a clear measure of patients' progress in treatment because take-homes are scheduled or withheld on the basis of patients' performance while in treatment. Take-homes are commonly withheld because of positive urine tests; conversely, take-homes are permitted when a patient is complying with such behavioral criteria as good attendance, no "dirty" urine specimens, and regular employment.

The last process variable used in this analysis is stable versus terminated treatment. This variable denotes whether patients continued in their designated methadone maintenance treatment from T_1 to T_2, or left treatment during the year between the two interviews. As described in a prior chap-

TABLE 11.6. Patient Outcome Variables (T_2)

Outcome	Code-transform	In-treatment cohort
Days of HEROIN USE during last 30 days	$(\text{actual days})^{\frac{1}{2}}$	1.6 days[a] 18% used at least 1 day
Days of COCAINE USE during last 30 days	$(\text{actual days})^{\frac{1}{2}}$	2.5 days[a] 26% used at least 1 day
Use of ANY OPIATES OR COCAINE during last 30 days	0 = none 1 = 1 day or more	35% used at least 1 day
Months since LAST IV DRUG USE	$-\log(1 + \text{months})$	38 months[a] Median months = 16
No. of CRIMEDAYS during last 30 days	$(\text{actual days})^{\frac{1}{2}}$	2.5 days[a] 18% had at least 1 crime day

[a] Mean

ter, those who left treatment included dropouts, transfers, and cures. The purpose of including this variable in the analysis is to ascertain the effect of discontinuation versus continuation within this cohort.

Outcome Measures

Five outcomes were employed as dependent variables in the regression analyses. Three of them pertain to current use of opiates and cocaine, the fourth deals with intravenous drug use, and the fifth is current criminal behavior. All five outcomes referred to data obtained at the second interview (T_2). These five variables are displayed in Table 11.6.

The first outcome was the number of days during the 30 days prior to the T_2 interview that the patient reported heroin use. The information was obtained from a question in the Addiction Severity Index (ASI) that asked the patient to recount heroin use during the past month.

The second outcome was cocaine use during the past 30 days. The data were obtained from the ASI in the same manner as current heroin use.

The third outcome was use of any opiate drug or cocaine during the past 30 days. The outcome was reduced to binary form: no use or use of one or more drugs on 1 or more days. This variable combines heroin use, use of other opiates, and cocaine use into a single, composite outcome representing serious drug abuse. The variable was constructed by combining pertinent ASI items from the second interview. Information about current use of opiates other than heroin was especially relevant, as such use was common in this population.

The fourth outcome was intravenous drug use. The observation was the number of months since the patient had last used drugs intravenously, from the date of the second interview (T_2). This information was obtained from Part II of the second interview, which asked patients about their recent or past intravenous drug use.

The fifth outcome was criminal behavior. Specifically, each patient was asked to recount the number of days during the past 30 that he had engaged in illegal activities for profit. This item was also obtained from the ASI part of the interview.

All five outcomes were coded and transformed in such a way that large values of the variables indicate bad outcomes; small values indicate good outcomes. A zero value for HEROIN USE means no use, and a value of 30 means that the patient used heroin on all of the 30 days prior to T_2 interview. The negative sign for LAST IV DRUG USE forces large numbers of months (good outcomes) to become smaller (more negative) than small numbers of months (bad outcomes).

Patient Groups

There were 633 patients interviewed during late 1985 at the six methadone maintenance programs. One year later, a second face-to-face interview was completed with 506 of these patients. The two interviews are chronologically differentiated as time 1 or time 2 events (T_1 and T_2 interviews). Of the 506 patients who were reinterviewed at T_2, 488 had completed valid ASI interviews at both T_1 and T_2.

The 488 methadone maintenance patients who were interviewed twice fell into two cohorts on the basis of their T_1 treatment status and 2 groups on the basis of their T_2 status (Table 11.7). At T_1, the 488 patients included an admission cohort of 81 patients and an in-treatment cohort of 407 patients. The *admission cohort* consisted of 81 patients who were admitted to the six programs during the T_1 period; the *in-treatment cohort* consisted of 407 patients who had been in methadone maintenance treatment at the designated programs for 6 months or longer when first interviewed at T_1. The analyses of this chapter refer to the 407 patients of the in-treatment cohort, although a corollary analysis of the entire sample of 488 was also undertaken (see Appendix B). The reason for focusing on the in-treatment cohort was to include process variables from T_1 in the analysis. (These process variables would not apply to new admissions.)

With regard to treatment status at T_2, both in-treatment and admission cohorts consisted of patients who continued in treatment as well as those who had terminated treatment. There were four groups of patients in terms of their T_1 to T_2 treatment experience: (1) in-treatment patients at T_1 who remained in treatment at T_2 (n = 338); (2) in-treatment patients at T_1 who terminated before T_2 (n = 69); (3) admissions at T_1 who remained in treatment at T_2 (48); and (4) admissions at T_1 who terminated treatment before T_2 (n = 33). As noted, the analysis of this chapter is restricted to the in-treatment cohort of 407 patients. Therefore the terminated and stable samples in the statistical analysis refer to the 338 patients who were still in treatment at T_2 (the continuous cohort) and the 69 who terminated before

TABLE 11.7. Number of Patients According to Cohort (T1) and Status (T2)

Cohort	Stable (still in treatment)	Terminated (left before T_2)	Total
Admissions	48	33	81
In-treatment	338	69	407
Total	386	102	488

T_2 (the terminated sample). The T_2 STATUS of the in-treatment sample was therefore either terminated or still in treatment:

Statistical Procedures

The analysis has been structured in conventional statistical fashion by taking patient outcome as depending on patient baseline, program elements, and in-treatment process. The latter three are the independent variables of these analyses. For each quantitative outcome (e.g., months since last intravenous drug use), the relation between independent and dependent variables is the standard multiple linear regression model.

$$\text{Outcome} = \text{constant} + \boxed{\text{patient}} + \boxed{\text{program}} + \boxed{\text{process}} + \text{error} \quad (1)$$

The three boxes refer to weighted sums of the specific variables in each category of independent variables. The weights in each box are the regression coefficients (β-values), which measure the contribution of each variable to predicting the independent variable. The errors are assumed to be uncorrelated random variables; for statistical tests, the errors are assumed to be generated independently from the same Gaussian distribution. Application of least squares provides numerical estimates of the constant, the β-values, and an analysis of variance. The results give an estimate of the variance of the distribution of the errors. The error variance, in conjunction with factors depending on the independent variables, provides the ingredients of a standard error for each estimated β-value; from the standard errors the statistical uncertainty of the estimates may be judged. The hypothesis that $\beta = 0$ can be tested by Student's t, which is the estimated β-value divided by its standard error.

To evaluate the effect of a category of independent variables (i.e., patient baseline, program elements, or process), the regression computations were made for the full model as given above and then for the model with the category of interest omitted. For example, the overall effect of the variables contained in *patient baseline* is determined by comparing the calculations for the reduced model below (diagram 2) with the full model of diagram 1. The difference between the two sums of squares gives the effect of *patient baseline after program elements and process* have explained what they can.

$$\text{Outcome} = \text{constant} + \boxed{\text{program}} + \boxed{\text{process}} + \text{error} \qquad (2)$$

One of the patient outcomes is dichotomous. Current use of any opiate or cocaine (during the last 30 days) is expressed as no use = 0, and use on 1 day or more = 1. The outcome is binary, not a quantitative variable, such as days since last intravenous drug use. The probability of a "bad" outcome has been modeled as a logistic function in the same independent variables that were used for linear regression with quantitative outcomes. The logistic model is as follows.

$$\begin{aligned} &\Pr(\text{outcome} = 1) \\ &= [1 + \exp - \{\text{constant} + \boxed{\text{patient}} + \boxed{\text{program}} + \boxed{\text{process}}\}]^{-1} \qquad (3) \end{aligned}$$

Calculation of estimates of the parameters (β-values) followed routines that result in maximum likelihood estimates. Statistical tests for β-values of individual variables or β-values of an entire category of variables are made by comparing the likelihoods with the full model against the likelihood under the model that omits the parameters of interest. The value minus twice the logarithm of the ratio of the two likelihoods [$-2 \log(\text{LR})$] is distributed approximately like chi-squared. Large values of $-2 \log(\text{LR})$ provide evidence for rejecting the hypothesis that the β-values in question are zero.

Findings: Outcomes and Independent Variables

The aim of the regression analyses is to elucidate variation among patients in the average values of the outcomes in order to ascertain which independent variables, or categories of variables, correlate with these outcomes. Is variation among patient outcomes "explained" by the simple linear combinations of patient baseline, program components, and process variables? In the case of HEROIN USE, for example, does knowledge of an individual patient's baseline characteristics, the treatment program components associated with him, and his own process factors allow one to predict more or less than the average of 1.6 heroin days? The average values of the five outcome measures appear in Table 11.6.

A general answer is that modest portions of outcome variation *are* explained by the independent variables, and that the associations of independent variables and outcomes in this study are not the result of random fluctuations in the data. All three categories of independent variables played a statistically noticeable part in explaining one or more outcomes, and the program domain was consistently associated with all five outcomes.

Caution should be exercised when interpreting the findings. Although categories and many individual variables are highly significant in a statistical sense, prediction of outcome for individuals strictly on the basis of the regression equations would be uncertain, as indicated by relatively low multiple correlations.

The regression coefficients of Table 11.8 present some interesting patterns, but the coefficients in categories that were not found significant in Table 11.9 should be viewed as questionable. For example, the test for patient baseline (Pt) in the outcome HEROIN USE returned $F = 1.21$, which is far from the conventional 5 percent significance point of about 1.88. The indication from Table 11.9 is that patient baseline explained relatively little of the variation in HEROIN USE after program components (Pc) and process (Pr) were accounted for. Age of ONSET as a factor in HEROIN USE, which is footnoted in Table 11.8, may be judged plausible but is not conclusively established from these data.

Summaries of the variance analyses for each outcome are given in Table 11.9. Estimates of the regression coefficients and their standard errors (SE) are displayed in Table 11.8. Each horizontal block of Table 11.9 is the summary for one outcome; the arrangement of Table 11.8 puts the outcomes in five separate columns. The exact number of patients in the separate analyses that follow vary slightly due to missing data on specific variables. When discussing these results, attention is first directed toward the effect of patient baseline variables on treatment outcome, followed by a consideration of program components and then process variables.

Patient Baseline

As a category, patient baseline variables contributed to explaining current COCAINE USE of patients at T_2. Nonwhite patients and patients who had long histories of cocaine use tended to have greater current use of cocaine than other patients. In part, this fact reflects the longer histories of cocaine use among blacks and Hispanics in this study. Intravenous use of drugs was more likely for those with long histories of cocaine use.

The patient baseline was borderline significant for two outcomes. Age of ONSET of heroin use and CRIME during the last addiction period were noticeable as predictors of current use of ANY OPIATES OR COCAINE; ONSET (borderline) and years of cocaine use (CYEARS) were evidently associated with the outcome "Last IV drug use." The direction of the relation of age of onset was consistently toward better outcomes with an older age of onset and worse outcomes for those with younger age of onset.

Program Components

The program components were strikingly different from patient baseline. As a category, the program domain expressed by the principal components

TABLE 11.8. Patient Baseline, Program Components, Process Variables, and Patient Outcomes of In-treatment Sample: Regression Coefficients and Standard Errors

Independent variable	Patient outcome									
	Heroin use (n = 407)		Cocaine use (n = 407)		Any opiates or cocaine (n = 407)		Last IV drug use (n = 400)		Crime days (n = 406)	
	β	SE	β	SE	β	SE	β	SE	β	SE
Patient baseline										
AGE	−.004	.010	−.015	.012	.008	.024	−.015	.013	−.001	.013
RACE	−.199	.147	.481[b]	.173	.375	.330	−.188	.183	.007	.185
EMPL	.071	.068	.014	.080	.175	.152	.006	.084	−.013	.086
ONSET	−.030[a]	.015	−.008	.017	−.080[a]	.034	−.035	.018	−.037[a]	.019
HYEARS	.061	.088	−.099	.104	−.235	.195	.114	.110	.058	.112
OYEARS	−.050	.068	.029	.081	.081	.156	−.059	.086	.133	.086
CYEARS	.060	.070	.171[a]	.083	.073	.154	.180[a]	.087	.116	.089
TREAT	.002	.082	.056	.097	.125	.184	.057	.103	−.141	.104
TOTARR	−.004	.007	.003	.008	−.017	.014	−.011	.008	−.002	.008
CRIME	.010	.021	.037	.025	.122[a]	.048	.008	.026	.022	.026
Program components										
COUNS-DIR-POL	.121[a]	.054	.167[b]	.064	.483[b]	.125	.274[b]	.067	.144[a]	.069
ADMIN-EXPER	−.111[b]	.043	.002	.051	−.012	.099	−.020	.053	−.032	.054
FACIL-STAFF	−.132[b]	.044	−.093	.052	−.160	.095	−.225[b]	.055	−.019	.055
MED	.116[a]	.051	.181[b]	.061	.260[a]	.108	.233[b]	.064	.246[b]	.065
RESID	−.035	.045	−.007	.053	−.014	.101	−.073	.057	−.048	.057
Process variables										
LOS	−.072	.080	−.053	.095	−.240	.179	−.426[b]	.100	−.052	.101
MISSMETH	.073	.145	.380[a]	.171	.782[b]	.298	.436[a]	.180	.439[a]	.183
TAKEHOME	−.063	.037	−.090[a]	.044	−.289[b]	.094	−.185[b]	.046	−.076	.047
DOSE	−.008[a]	.003	.022	.004	−.004	.008	−.007	.004	.001	.004
STATUS	−.139	.157	−.051	.186	−.334	.331	−.264	.196	.263	.199

[a] $p < 0.05$.
[b] $p < 0.01$.

TABLE 11.9. Regressions of Outcomes on Patient Baseline, Program Components, and Process Variables: In-treatment Sample

Category	*df*	Mean square	*F*
Heroin use, past 30 days ($n = 407$, $R^2 = 0.18$)			
Patient baseline (Pt)	10	1.482	1.21
Program components (Pc)	5	5.849	4.79[b]
Process (Pr)	5	3.676	3.01[a]
Error	386	1.222	
Cocaine use, past 30 days ($n = 407$, $R^2 = 0.19$)			
Patient baseline	10	3.561	2.09[a]
Program components	5	6.001	3.52[b]
Process	5	4.409	2.58[a]
Error	386	1.707	
Any Opiates or Cocaine, past 30 days ($n = 407$, $R^2 = 0.15$)			
Patient baseline	10	Chi-square =	17.78
Program components	5	Chi-square =	23.76[b]
Process	5	Chi-square =	32.33[b]
Last IV drug use ($n = 400$, $R^2 = 0.39$)			
Patient baseline	10	3.357	1.79
Program components	5	15.784	8.40[a]
Process	5	28.483	15.16[a]
Error	379	1.879	
Crime days, past 30 days ($n = 406$, $R^2 = 0.13$)			
Patient baseline	10	3.126	1.60
Program components	5	7.218	3.69[a]
Process	5	4.293	2.19
Error	385	1.957	

Variance analyses were used for linear regressions and likelihood ratio statistics for logistic regressions. Conditional test for a category after accounting for the other two categories.

[a] $p < 0.05$.

[b] $p < 0.01$.

showed clear and consistent associations with all five outcomes (Table 11.9.). This finding of course was a reflection of different success rates among the six treatment programs that were investigated. Deriving principal components was an attempt to describe the programs in terms of many variables that catalogued operating characteristics and staff, rather than analyzing differences among the six programs per se. The latter would return the same *F* values as given in Table 11.9, but the nature of the differences would not be revealed in terms of dimensions that represent program characteristics.

All five outcomes showed strong statistical associations with the first and fourth program components. The first component COUNS-DIR-POL (which represents counseling service, an effective director, and an orientation toward maintenance and rehabilitation) was strongly associated with all outcomes. Patients in programs with strong COUNS-DIR-POL values (1 = best or most, 5 = worst or weakest) tended to have less current drug use, less current intravenous drug use, and less current crime.

The fourth component, MED, which was mainly a rating of adequacy of medical services, also was uniformly associated with less current drug use, longer periods without intravenous drugs, and less current crime.

The second and third components were inversely related to most outcomes; statistically strong inverse associations with current HEROIN USE were evident. Although the fifth principal component coefficients were negative for all outcomes, the statistical uncertainty of each coefficient indicates minimal explanatory influence of Prin 5 in terms of the outcomes investigated here. (Comparisons of the magnitudes of regression coefficients are appropriate among the five principal components, as they are scaled identically, but not between the components and patient baseline or treatment process variables.)

Process Variables

As a category, the five process variables attained statistical significance for four outcomes and were borderline significant for the fifth outcome (CRIME DAYS). HEROIN USE was the only outcome that showed a clear association (inverse) with methadone dose. Patients who were maintained on higher doses of methadone were less likely to be current heroin users than those on lower doses. There was no evidence that DOSE was associated with the other four outcomes.

The process variables MISSMETH and TAKEHOME, which indicate and recognize patient compliance and progress at T_1, were associated with current COCAINE USE, use of ANY OPIATES OR COCAINE, and LAST IV DRUG USE; and MISSMETH reached significance for the outcome CRIME DAYS. Patients who missed scheduled attendance were more likely to have bad outcomes; and patients who were granted more take-home methadone doses were the ones who were likely to have better outcomes.

Length of stay was strongly associated with LAST IV DRUG USE but did not attain nominal statistical significance for the other outcomes. The STATUS variable was not effective for predicting any outcome.

Discussion and Conclusion

To summarize results concerning patient baseline variables, it was found that race, age of onset of heroin use, history of cocaine use, and criminal behavior prior to admission were associated with treatment outcome to some degree. The association of race with cocaine use in these programs as well as the consistent association of younger age at onset of heroin use with unfavorable outcomes are perhaps the most interesting aspects of patient baseline findings. Although these findings are not surprising, it is notable that patient baseline, as measured by the ten variables used here, had relatively less impact on successful outcome than characteristics of the treatment program and what actually happened to the patient after he was admitted to a program.

Our interpretation of the regressions for the principal components of the treatment domain is that patients in programs with rehabilitation and long-term maintenance orientation, which also delivered more counseling services to patients and had more effective directors, tended to have better outcomes than patients in programs characterized by favorable staff/patient ratios in better facilities, where there was emphasis on administrative functioning rather than provision of services. That is not to say that understaffed, poor facilities produced good patient outcomes. Among the six programs, it happened that the ones with better staffing, facilities, and management were less successful in patient outcomes than programs that had less staffing and less adequate facilities but that delivered more services.

The two program components (COUNS-DIR-POL and MED, Table 11.8) that most clearly encompass the provision of treatment services to patients were uniformly, positively associated with successful patient outcomes. These findings support the contention that the actual provision of treatment and rehabilitation services differentiates between more and less successful programs.

It is somewhat surprising that length of stay (LOS) was not more closely associated with four of the five outcomes. At least two explanations for the absent or weak associations are plausible. Most of the patients had been in continuous treatment for several years at the time of first interview. Thus the generally long LOS at T_1 may have attenuated the influence of LOS at T_2. In this regard, studies using recent admissions, not long term stay patients, have found that length of stay is relatively short. In other words, long-term patients may pass a threshold beyond which LOS has relatively small differential effect.

On the other hand, effective treatment is undoubtedly an inducement to patients to continue in their treatment programs. Length of stay then becomes to some degree a proxy for effective treatment prior to T_1, rather than a distinct marker for success or failure at T_2.

Program staff are usually aware of the clinical importance of patients' attendance. Their conceptions were confirmed by the attendance variable MISSMETH, which was associated with four of the five outcomes. This variable refers to whether patients adhered to their weekly attendance schedule. Patients who missed scheduled attendance were more likely to have bad outcomes.

The number of take-home doses of methadone that patients were allowed per week (zero to six) was found to be an indicator of treatment success in about the same way as the attendance variable MISSMETH. This finding might well be expected, as program staff permit take-home privileges on the basis of patient compliance and evidence of progress toward rehabilitation. This result indicates that the line staff at the six programs were, to a considerable extent, correctly assessing the treatment status of patients. Not only were the staffs aware of which patients were progressing in their courses of treatment, but the clinical decisions on take-homes were in accord with outcome findings a year later.

In view of the continuing controversy concerning low dose versus high dose methadone, it is noteworthy that dose level was inversely related to the outcome HEROIN USE: the higher the dose, the less current use of heroin. Methadone dose as a predictor of outcome was limited, however, to the heroin use outcome. Dose per se gave no evidence of association with other outcomes.

Tests of statistical significance and *p*-values by themselves do not provide consistent measures of strength of evidence, nor do they give an indication of substantive importance. Rather than attempting to draw conclusions tied closely to the numerous statistical tests of Tables 11.8 and 11.9, attention is directed to the consistency of differences among programs (expressed as principal components), to the regular association of the process variables MISSMETH and TAKEHOME, and, except for age of onset of heroin use, the scattering of the few meaningful patient baseline variables across the patient outcome measures. It is concluded that differences among the programs, especially in the care delivered regularly to patients, overshadowed baseline differences among individual patients when accounting for the outcomes used in these analyses.

References

1. Chapter on treatment research. In: Drug Abuse Research (1987) The Second Triennial Report to Congress From the Secretary. DHHS Publication (ADM) 87–1486. Rockville: US Department of Health and Human Services, pp 59–75
2. Kreek MJ (1981) Medical management of methadone-maintained patients. In Lowinson JH, Ruiz P (eds): Substance Abuse: Clinical Problems and Perspectives. Baltimore: Williams & Wilkins, pp 660–673
3. Anderson TW (1984) An Introduction to Multivariate Statistical Analysis 2nd ed. New York: Wiley

12 Summation of Findings and Conclusion

This project to study the effectiveness of methadone maintenance treatment was jointly planned by the senior author and staff at the National Institute on Drug Abuse in 1984. In response to earlier expert reviews of the status of drug abuse treatment in the United States, it was held that large-scale intensive studies of particular types of treatment, or modalities, were warranted. The reasons advanced for supporting more intensive research about treatment effectiveness were various but emphasized such issues as matching drug abusing patients to appropriate treatment and determining the extent of psychiatric impairment in this population. At that time there was little or no interest in studying drug abuse treatment programs; the emphasis was on studying patients.

The reason for selecting methadone maintenance treatment as a focus of study was primarily practical. It was the modality of treatment that involved the largest population of drug abuse patients; moreover, considerable research had been undertaken that would provide a foundation for further research; and the senior author had had extensive experience studying opiate addicts.

The concept of the "black box" of drug abuse treatment was not generally current when the project was initiated. Articulation of drug abuse treatment as a "black box" about which little was known came slowly during the 1980s, although previously there was a research interest among practitioners in various specialized aspects of drug abuse treatment, such as group dynamics, psychotherapy, or new pharmacological interventions. Such specialized interest commonly involved only a few therapists at a single program, and it was different from planning a study of the effectiveness of numerous programs within a single treatment modality.

The plan that evolved to study the effectiveness of methadone maintenance treatment in New York City, Philadelphia, and Baltimore focused on both programs and patients. Six programs in these three cities were selected for intensive on-site study. Comprehensive data about the structure and operation of these methadone maintenance programs were collected by the EMMT staff during a 3-year period.

Obtaining Comprehensive Program Data

A new methodology of program evaluation was developed and implemented. This methodology involved the collection of comprehensive data about the entire treatment domain: neighborhood; physical facility; aggregate patient census; treatment and administrative staff; methadone-dispensing practices; counseling services provided and medical services delivered; treatment policy followed; administrative procedures and practices. These aspects of the programs were classified, described, and measured. The concept of program "output" was utilized to describe and measure the actual provision of treatment services to patients at the programs. This output was systematically measured at each of the programs in 1985 and then again in 1986.

Development of a methodology for on-site program evaluation involved preparation of a series of data collection instruments for staff interviews, facility surveys, record reviews, compilation of dispensing and urinalysis data, and similar tasks. This data collection at the programs by the project staff was confidential in that interview findings from the staff and data obtained about operations were not reported to program directors or anyone else. Although the findings were utilized in our research, these results were not linked to individuals or programs by name.

The plan for program data collection was predicated on a number of fundamental assumptions about intensive program evaluation. These assumptions included the distinction between in-house and outside data collection (e.g., between an in-house and an external audit), the requirement that a cooperative working relationship be established with the programs, that confidentiality of the research findings about individual programs be ensured, that data collection be undertaken by the project staff, and that the objective of the research would be to facilitate the improvement of methadone maintenance treatment.

Interviewing Patients at the Six Programs

The collection of detailed interview data from patients at the six programs was undertaken by the field staff of the Institute for Survey Research (ISR) in Philadelphia. Face-to-face interviews with 633 patients at the six programs were completed in 1985. Most of these patients were reinterviewed a year later while still in their respective methadone maintenance programs; if they had left treatment, they were located and reinterviewed in the community. The field work procedures for the patient interviews were developed by the EMMT staff in collaboration with the director and field staff of the Institute for Survey Research.

The plan for program data collection and the design for obtaining patient interviews were successfully completed. The two comprehensive on-site program data collection efforts were accomplished by the EMMT staff. This phase involved 287 man-days of work at these six programs during 1985–1986. The face-to-face patient interviews at the six programs were conducted by 12 professional interviewers from ISR who were specially trained for this project; 633 male addict patients were interviewed during late 1985, and 507 of these patients were reinterviewed a year later by the same interviewers.

The overall plan for obtaining data to determine the effectiveness of methadone maintenance treatment was found to be methodologically sound and feasible. The plan of collecting data about the four relevant domains—patients, programs, services, and outcome—was straightforward, although the treatment domain and the provision of services have generally been neglected as topics of study. The feasibility of implementing this comprehensive plan at active methadone programs in their neighborhood settings was unknown. How this data collection was accomplished at the six methadone maintenance programs in New York City, Philadelphia, and Baltimore is discussed in Chapter 2.

Candid Program Descriptions

Candid descriptions of the six programs were prepared to portray the operation of these outpatient clinics realistically and thereby to dispel various myths about methadone maintenance treatment. For reasons that are not apparent, the operation of methadone maintenance programs has seldom been described in detail since Dole's original delineation of this mode of treatment. As a consequence of this lack of knowledge as to what does and does not occur at methadone maintenance programs, various myths and unrealistic expectations have arisen.

A recitation of these myths would not contribute to our knowledge of how these programs operate. It is pertinent, however, to identify and lay to rest two common but contrary myths about methadone maintenance in order to indicate the gross lack of knowledge which exists about this mode of treatment.

Methadone maintenance treatment has been attacked as being merely "legalized addiction" that provides drugs to addicts without effecting their rehabilitation or cure. This myth—that the programs are ineffective and do not provide appropriate treatment—can best be dispelled by presentation of detailed descriptions of what occurs at the programs as well as by outcome studies of their effectiveness. These broadside attacks on methadone maintenance often seem to be motivated by unrealistic or idealistic notions about the life course of contemporary heroin addiction as well as the lack of knowledge about what occurs in the day-to-day treatment process. This "mere dispensing station" myth can best be dispelled by the dissemination of accurate information about what occurs during the treatment process and by providing findings about treatment effectiveness.

Surprisingly, a contrary myth about methadone maintenance has arisen in recent years, i.e., that these programs provide Cadillac services to select addict patients and that the extra, or frill, services are unnecessary. To anyone who has visited contemporary methadone maintenance programs in New York City, Philadelphia, Baltimore, and similar cities, this notion of excessive, or Cadillac, treatment services being provided would be ludicrous were it not pernicious in its effect. This notion is pernicious in that there is, in fact, a need for additional and improved services at most programs. Again, dispelling the myth of Cadillac services can best be accomplished by disseminating information about what does occur at the programs.

Two further observations about the candid program description are pertinent. First, the intent in presenting these portrayals is to open the black box of drug abuse treatment—to provide accurate detailed information about what occurs in outpatient methadone maintenance treatment in order to facilitate more systematic study, program evaluation, and subsequent improvement.

Second, it is pertinent to comment on the potential disadvantages inherent in the presentation of candid descriptions of individual treatment programs (the advantages of opening the black box are apparent). Two disadvantages or concerns are evident. The first is that some candid material from the descriptions may be selected and cast in a derogatory light to discredit methadone maintenance generally. Such selective use of the descriptions cannot be prevented, but the existence of the six complete descriptions should mitigate this danger of misrepresentation. The second concern is different. It pertains to readers concocting invidious comparisons among the programs to promote a favored treatment or rehabilitation policy about methadone therapy. Such use of the candid descriptions is inappropriate as it seems likely that several models of methadone maintenance treatment are viable and effective.

Treatment Domain

For reasons that are far from clear, the treatment domain in drug abuse research has never, until now, been comprehensively measured. In fact, it has generally been ignored as a research subject. As several reviewers have noted, "Treatment variables have not generally received attention by workers evaluating substance abuse treatments."[1] Interest in studying drug abuse treatment programs—the physical facility, community problems, staffing patterns and qualifications, treatment policy, administration, and funding—has been minimal. Conversely, attention has been focused on patients: their drug abuse history, deprived background, psychiatric status, need for education, and similar topics.

Although investigation of the reasons why the black box of drug abuse treatment has persisted is beyond the scope of this chapter, a few general observations are pertinent. It has been suggested[2] that comprehensive evaluation of drug abuse treatment programs (although highly desirable) is usually impractical because it is too costly and time-consuming. This viewpoint is prescient with respect to the difficulties and impediments that comprehensive evaluation entails. Furthermore, these practical considerations undoubtedly have been a major reason why such comprehensive evaluations have not been implemented.

In fairness to those researchers who have studied various discrete parts of the treatment domain, it should be emphasized that it is not that the cover of the black box has never been lifted—it has occasionally—but that the contents have not been sorted out and studied in toto. Separate studies have investigated parts of the treatment domain to address such questions as detoxification policy, medication dosage, methadone diversion, the role of ex-addict counselors, the efficacy of AIDS education, or the need for vocational counseling. These studies have made important contributions to our knowledge of particular areas. These disparate studies, however, have not provided us with knowledge about the overall structure and dynamics of the treatment domain. Furthermore, these separate ad hoc studies have been limited in their impact because they have not been articulated with one another, and an overall conceptual framework has been lacking.

Although this on-site evaluation of methadone maintenance treatment was planned to collect comprehensive data about how the designated programs are organized and function, it was not until the analysis of the program data had begun that the treatment domain conceptualization of Moos and Finney (see Chapter 1) was recognized as being a suitable theoretical framework for analysis and exposition. Adoption of the treatment domain conceptualization of drug abuse programs has proved to be efficacious for several reasons.

The treatment domain formulation prompts consideration of drug abuse programs from an institutional perspective. The focus is on the individual program and its environment, rather than on individual patients. In this sense, there is an analogy with the study of schools, hospitals or communities—these need to be studied in their own right as separate units and institutions.[3]

Two other observations about the treatment domain are relevant. The treatment domain conceptualization is both inclusive and neutral. It is inclusive in that it subsumes all aspects of the programs under study as within its scope of investigation. It is theoretically neutral in that it does not dictate the contents of the treatment domain or prejudge the relation among the elements studied. As a consequence, the treatment domain formulation proved to be especially valuable in providing a suitable framework for multivariate analysis.

Treatment Provided

The six methadone maintenance programs studied were found to be continuously preoccupied with providing various services to some 1900 male and female patients. Four of the six programs were open 365 days a year, and two were open all days except Sundays. With regard to attendance, 77 percent of these patients were scheduled to attend 5 days or more per week; 54 percent of the patients were scheduled to attend every day of the week the clinic was open. The programs were, then, actively engaged in providing oral methadone and other services to ex-addict patients who travel to these outpatient clinics every day.

The attendance rate of patients at the clinics was surprisingly high. Only 4.9 percent of the scheduled doses were missed, so daily attendance was 95.1 percent. Among the six programs, the daily attendance rate varied from 99.7 to 92.2 percent. This high attendance rate is noteworthy because it indicates patients' commitment to treatment as well as the fact that specific services are continually provided.

When studying the dispensing practices, it was found that the six programs varied considerably in the methadone dosage prescribed. There were two low dose programs, three average dose programs, and one higher dosage program. The mean methadone doses at the programs were 26.4, 37.1, 47.2, 49.2, 51.0, and 65.5 mg, respectively.

With respect to dispensing methadone at the clinic versus providing take-home doses, it was found that three-fourths of the doses dispensed per week were for on-site consumption under direct observation. Only 23.2 percent of the doses prepared were prescribed as take-home methadone.

Although a patient's enrollment at a specific methadone maintenance program involved daily attendance as well as supervisory contact with the security and dispensing staff, the principal rehabilitation function was performed by counselors. Each patient was assigned to a designated counselor whose job it was to plan, supervise, and, hopefully, effect his rehabilitation from "street life." Each patient's counselor was, then, his supervisor, foster parent, and guardian.

The main service provided by counselors was face-to-face individual sessions with patients to discuss treatment progress and rehabilitation plans. These individual counseling sessions were commonly held twice a month. In addition, counselors often met briefly with the patients on their caseload for brief conversations or contacts on an "as-needed" basis. This direct patient care was based upon each patient's needs as well as the resources available. With regard to organizing the delivery of various services to patients, this was undertaken by the counselors as part of their case management and referral function.

In addition to the regular services provided by counselors to all methadone maintenance patients (individual sessions, brief contacts, case management, and referral), some programs offered such services as group counseling sessions, family therapy, psychological assessment, vocational training, and education classes. The provision of these additional services was, however, usually restricted to a few patients or not consistently available at most programs. At the same time, it should be noted that most programs made strenuous efforts to provide as many services as possible, given their budgetary and staffing constraints.

Medical coverage at the programs was provided by physicians, physicians' assistants (PAs), nurse practitioners (NPs), and to a lesser extent the dispensing nurses. Each of the six programs employed one or more part-time physicians, four had some coverage by a PA or an NP, and all but one had dispensing nurses. The amount of medical care provided to these 1900 patients varied considerably among the six programs, depending in large part on the medical staff available. Overall, one-third of the patients received some treatment from the medical staff on a weekly basis. This figure (one-third), however, tends to overemphasize the medical care provided while underestimating patients' needs, as the one-third count includes all types of medical contacts and care. Furthermore, this figure does not convey the considerable unmet medical needs of these patients.

Determination of Effectiveness

One of the principal criteria for evaluating the effectiveness of methadone maintenance is the extent to which patients' drug abuse is reduced or eliminated as a consequence of treatment. It was found that a reduction in drug abuse commonly occurs after admission and continues for as long as patients remain in outpatient treatment. When patients leave methadone maintenance programs, however, relapse to prior drug abuse patterns is the predominant outcome.

When reviewing the findings about the reduction of drug abuse that occurs as a consequence of methadone maintenance treatment, it is relevant to use several baseline periods for comparison: the patient's lifetime preadmission history of regular drug abuse, the prevalence of drug abuse during the last addiction period, and the change in drug abuse that occurs during treatment.

The 617 male methadone maintenance patients selected for study had a long history of opiate addiction as well as years of regular use of other illicit drugs. These patients had 11.2 years of regular heroin use, 8.9 years of other opiate use (for the 30 percent who regularly abused this class of drugs), and 5.8 years of cocaine abuse (for the 47 percent who regularly abused this drug). Almost all of these patients (98 percent) were regular intravenous drug users prior to admission for treatment.

To recapitulate the main findings about the reduction in drug abuse that occurred during methadone maintenance treatment, it was found that opiate use markedly declined after admission. After 6 months in treatment 77 percent of the patients had ceased heroin use, and 92 percent had ceased such use after 4.5 years. Similarly, use of other opiates declined to the extent that 92 percent were not using other opiates after 6 months, and 96 percent had ceased after 4.5 years in treatment.

The abuse of nonopiate drugs was also found to decline during methadone maintenance treatment, but the prevalence of use of a few drugs remained above that of the opiates. Thus, sedative use declined after 6 months in treatment to use by 22 percent of the patients, but it only declined further to use by 17 percent of the patients after 4.5 years in treatment. Comparable figures for the decline in cocaine use were a 28 percent prevalence after 6 months and a 17 percent prevalence after patients had been in treatment 4.5 years or longer. Declines in the use of barbiturates and amphetamines were also found, but the prevalence rates of such use were low at admission (4 and 5 percent), so the declines were minimal.

The prevalence of regular cannabis use and alcohol use to intoxification remained comparatively high during methadone maintenance treatment, although there was a significant reduction in use of the former. Cannabis use at admission was reported by 48 percent of the patients; at 6 months and 4.5 years or longer the prevalences were 48 and 37 percent, respectively. The admission, 6-month, and 4.5-year prevalence rates for alcohol intoxification were 39, 33, and 30 percent, respectively. There was, then, little or no change in alcohol use to intoxication among these patients.

The extent to which drug abuse was reduced during methadone maintenance treatment was also analyzed with respect to the decline in intravenous drug use. It was found that 71 percent of the patients at the six programs had ceased intravenous drug use after several years of treatment. Unexpectedly, it was found that there were marked differences among the programs' success rates in controlling intravenous drug use: Whereas 90.2 percent of the patients at one program were no longer intravenous drug users, only 42.9 percent at another program had given up such drug use. These findings indicate considerable variation in program effectiveness. The question arises as to whether this differential effectiveness is due to patient or program factors. Investigation of this question led to a multivariate analysis in which it was found that certain program and process factors were more closely related to successful outcome than baseline patient characteristics.

The follow-up findings about the 105 patients who left methadone maintenance treatment were unequivocal. Most of those who left rapidly relapsed to destructive drug abuse: 82 percent relapsed to intravenous drug abuse within 1 year. Although a few ex-patients were able to abstain from drug abuse (7 of 23 who left with treatment completed had not relapsed by the time of follow-up), most relapsed and some had already returned to treatment.

Reduction in Crime

A marked reduction in crime occurred after the addicts entered methadone maintenance treatment. It was found that there was a 79 percent decline in the number of offenses committed for those in treatment for 6 months or longer from the number committed during their last addiction period. The annual reduction was from 242,358 offenses to 50,103 offenses. This overall 79.3 percent reduction in offenses included declines of over 80 percent in 11 of 15 types of crime.

A reduction in crime was also found to occur by patients' length of stay in treatment: 37 percent of admissions reported current criminal behavior, and criminality declined to 22 percent of the patients after 1 year in treatment and to 11 percent after 6 years in treatment. A substantial reduction in crime occurred among patients at all six programs.

When reviewing these findings about the reduction in criminality that occurs during methadone maintenance treatment, several observations are pertinent. First, it is worth noting that there is a greater reduction in drug-related crime than in more professional types of crime: Drug business offenses declined by 81 percent, whereas numbers racket offenses declined by only 47 percent. The point is that the decline in crime that occurs varies somewhat depending on the type of offense. At the same time, it should be emphasized that there is a substantial reduction in all types of crime from pretreatment levels.

A second observation pertains to the lesser emphasis placed on the reduction of criminal behavior in methadone maintenance treatment than on the reduction of drug abuse. The programs were not established to control criminal behavior, and this focus is secondary to that of controlling illicit drug use. Regular urinalysis is required to monitor patients' drug abuse, but no comparable information is obtained about patients' current criminality. Therefore the reduction in criminality that occurs among patients in methadone maintenance programs is to a considerable extent a secondary or unplanned consequence of treatment. The point here is not to denigrate the considerable rehabilitative efforts made in this regard by counselors and other staff, as these efforts are commendable and worthy of full support, but to note that active and consistent efforts to control criminal behavior outside of the clinic is not a core part of treatment policy. This second point leads to the last one.

The third point refers to realistic expectations about the reduction of crime in methadone maintenance treatment. It seems important to recognize that the goal of complete elimination of criminal behavior among patients in methadone maintenance programs is unrealistic. Such an absolute goal is utopian for this population. Rather, a realistic approach to controlling patients' criminal behavior is to strive toward a continual reduction in the participation rate and the frequency of commission.[4] From this perspective, methadone maintenance is effective in reducing crime. As with other aspects of treatment, however, improvement is indicated.

Multivariate Analysis

With respect to the multivariate analysis presented in Chapter 11, three summary observations seem appropriate. First and foremost, this procedure demonstrates that a statistical outcome analysis based on baseline patient characteristics, treatment domain elements, and process variables is viable—that a multivariate analysis of the treatment domain is feasible. Undoubtedly, additional sources of program data can be obtained and alternative analytical procedures employed—and these efforts need to be made. The main point, however, is that a viable procedure for such a comprehensive analysis is available once the requisite data have been amassed.

Second, the results of the multivariate analysis indicate that treatment success in these methadone maintenance programs is related to specific patient characteristics, identifiable program elements, and definite process variables. Although the findings reveal that treatment domain factors and process variables are more evidently related to successful patient outcome than baseline preadmission characteristics of patients, the fact that all three areas contribute to successful outcome is a major finding.

Finally, the rationale of this multivariate analysis should not be confused with the results of a particular study. It seems likely that others will find different combinations of variables in the three areas (patients, programs, and process) to be related to successful outcome in methadone maintenance treatment as diverse programs and populations are investigated. These additional findings, however, will not contravene the rationale of comprehensive drug abuse treatment evaluation. Indeed, it is precisely in this manner that an appropriate body of knowledge will be accumulated.

Local Environment and City

The decision to evaluate methadone maintenance programs in three cities, rather than one, was fortuitous despite the extra difficulties imposed on the research staff by this far-flung data collection undertaking. The decision was fortuitous because the dozens of trips to programs in New York City, Philadelphia, and Baltimore resulted in a new perspective about the operation and effectiveness of programs in each of these cities. Two observations are germane in this regard. The first refers to the local environment of each program and the second to the city.

In the process of interviewing staff and otherwise collecting data at the six programs, it became apparent that each program had its own unique neighborhood, facility, patients, and staff. One, then, could not evaluate effectiveness without considering this local environment. For example, if most patients at a program are long-term unemployed residents of deteriorating inner city areas, they are different from a patient population composed of steadily employed males from residential neighborhoods. Similarly, if the medical needs of patients are extensive and their principal source of care is a methadone program, this program is different from one in which these medical needs are addressed elsewhere. The point is that separate programs cannot be realistically appraised without regard to the local environment and patient census.

In addition to the fact that each program operates in its own local environment—each treatment domain is unique—methadone maintenance programs are also part of city and state bureaucracies, which commonly impose their own parameters on the treatment policy, staffing, and services to be provided. Programs within a city, then, should be evaluated against this institutional background because the city and state not only allot funds they also mandate how programs should operate. Marked variations among methadone maintenance programs in the US have been documented in a recent (1990) General Accounting Office field study.[5]

This observation about the role of the city or state in the operation of methadone maintenance programs is not meant to imply that uniform national standards should be implemented because, as noted above, programs have their local environments, special problems, and support groups. Rather, the point to be emphasized is that a more meaningful evaluation framework can only be implemented on a citywide or statewide level after an appropriate database infrastructure has been established. At present, given the limited state of our knowledge about methadone maintenance programs in our major cities (baseline patient and treatment domain data are lacking), it is not possible to determine the relative effectiveness of particular programs controlling for local environment. This determination can be made only after appropriate citywide databases are established and operational. In this last regard, it is pertinent to note that the establishment of a citywide drug abuse treatment database would require continuous operation for several years before it became efficacious for evaluation.

The need to establish a national data system pertaining to drug abuse treatment programs has been noted in three state of the art assessments published in 1990. The White House's *National Drug Control Strategy* stated, "We still lack basic demographic and statistical information about drug treatment patients and the programs they enter."[6] An Office of Technology Assessment report, "The Effectiveness of Drug Abuse Treatment: Implications For Controlling AIDS/HIV Infection," found that "The *number* of treatment facilities for drug abuse in the United States is not well documented," (italics added).[7] The Institute of Medicine concluded after a major investigation, *Treating Drug Problems*, that "as perhaps the most important and immediately needed utilization management requirement, the committee recommends that all drug treatment programs receiving public support be required to participate in a client-oriented data system."[8]

A final point to be made about the evaluation of drug abuse treatment programs in the 1990s is that both intensive on-site studies of specific programs and large-scale citywide or national databases are needed. The intensive studies will replicate and extend the present findings about treatment effectiveness; the larger databases will provide a framework for comparative analysis of the treatment domain. These two types of evaluation studies are complementary in that each enhances the findings of the other.

Conclusion

This study and previous findings have established that methadone maintenance treatment is effective in reducing drug abuse, crime, and other deviant behavior among patients who stay in treatment. But much remains to be done. The programs need to be improved, expanded, and forged into a treatment and rehabilitation system. This improvement is now supportable because it has been ascertained that increased effectiveness is a consequence of improvement in the treatment and rehabilitative services provided to patients. In sum, then, the effectiveness reported by Dole and Nyswander during the 1960s still obtains provided appropriate treatment is forthcoming.

References

1. McLellan AT, Alterman AI, Woody GE (1991) A quantitative measure of substance abuse treatment programs: the treatment services review. J Nerv Ment Dis
2. Des Jarlais DC, Deren S, Lipton DS (1981) Cost effectiveness studies in the evaluation of substance abuse treatment. In Lowinson JH, Ruiz P (eds): Substance Abuse: Clinical Problems and Perspectives. Baltimore: Williams & Wilkins, pp 806–816
3. Reiss AJ, Tonry M (eds) (1986) Communities and Crime, Vol. 8. Chicago: University of Chicago Press
4. Anglin MD, Hser YI (1990) Treatment of drug abuse. In Tonry M, Wilson JQ (eds): Drugs and Crime. Chicago: University of Chicago Press, pp 393–460
5. United States General Accounting Office (1990) Methadone Maintenance: Some Treatment Programs are not Effective; Greater Federal Oversight Needed. Washington, DC: US Government Printing Office

Appendix A. 89 Measures of the Treatment Domain (As in Chapters 5 and 6)

A. Neighborhood and Facility

1. The type of neighborhood in which the program is located (middle class residential, working class residential, average commercial area, run down commercial area or slum area)
2. Staff involvement with the local community—extent of
3. Community relations problems
4. Parking space available
5. The overall adequacy of the building
6. Repair of the building
7. Cleanliness of the rooms and interior
8. Composite score of facility adequacy (average of 5–7)
9. Adequacy of security provided with regard to patient flow in the building

B. Aggregate Patient Characteristics at Each Program

10. Census of methadone maintenance patients
11. The percent of patients in treatment less than one year
12. The percent of patients in treatment 5 years or longer
13. The percent of patients who are non-white
14. The number of patients on the waiting list

C. Director

15. Director's years of experience at this program
16. Years of experience as director
17. Director's years of education
18. Director's percent of time employed at the program
19. Director's involvement with patient care
20. Director's treatment effectiveness: composite score

D. Counselors

21. Number of counselors employed at each program
22. Number of full-time counselors (by FTE)

23. Mean years of experience of counselors at this program
24. Mean years of education of counselors
25. Percent of counselors with advanced degrees
26. Mean salary of full-time counselors
27. Percent of counselors who are ex-addicts
28. Percent of counselors who are minority group members
29. Annual turnover rate of counselors at each program

E. Medical Staff

30. Number of physicians employed at the program (by FTE)
31. Number of physicians' assistants employed (by FTE)
32. Number of nurse practitioners (by FTE)
33. Number of dispensing nurses (by FTE)
34. Number of pharmacists employed (by FTE)
35. Total medical staff employed (by FTE)
36. Mean years of experience at program of physicians
37. Mean years of experience of physicians' assistants or nurse practitioners

F. Program Administration and Treatment Policy at Each Program

38. Identification of program—(unique ID)
39. Years of operation of program
40. Annual per patient cost for the treatment provided
41. Adequacy of funding—comparative assessment
42. Status of patient records
43. General administration of program
44. Management and coordination of treatment services
45. Medical orientation of program
46. Social rehabilitation orientation of program
47. Long-term maintenance policy

G. Additional Areas of Program Measurement

48. The number of counselors (by FTE) per 250 patients
49. The number of medical staff (by FTE) per 250 patients
50. The number of physicians (by FTE) per 250 patients
51. The total number of treatment staff (by FTE) per 250 patients
52. Staff-Patient minority group concordance, 1985
53. The mean counselors' rating of their program's effectiveness
54. Counselors' high morale

H. Methadone Dispensing at Each Program

55. Days per week clinic open
56. Hours per week clinic open
57. Mean methadone dose (mg.) 1985
58. Mean methadone dose (mg.) 1986

59. Percent change in mean dose, 85–86
60. Percent patients on less than 30 mg. methadone
61. Percent of patients with takehomes, 1985
62. Percent of patients with takehomes, 1986
63. Change in percent of patients with takehomes, 85/86
64. Missed medication rate, per week
65. Patient dose satisfaction

I. Services Provided by Counselors

66. Mean caseload of counselors (1986)
67. Mean minutes of individual sessions
68. Percent of patients seen (per week) in individual session
69. Stability of individual counseling sessions—1985 vs. 1986
70. Percent of patients in group sessions
71. Stability of group sessions—1985 vs. 1986
72. Vocational services provided
73. Educational services provided
74. Number of secondary counseling services consistently provided at each program

J. Medical Services at Each Program

75. Number of patients seen by total medical staff in week
76. Number of patients seen by total medical staff per FTE in week
77. Percent of patients seen by total medical staff in week
78. Percent medical coverage by MDs
79. Number of patients treated by physicians in week
80. Number of patients treated in week per FTE physician
81. Percent of patients treated by physicians in week

K. Urinalysis

82. Percent of patients who provided urine per week
83. Number of urines provided per patient in week
84. Number of urinalysis tests used by program

L. Quality of Care Provided at Each Program

85. Assessment of the overall adequacy or quality of counseling services provided
86. Assessment of the adequacy or quality of medical care provided
87. Assessment of the psychiatric coverage provided
88. Assessment of the referral services provided
89. Composite score: Quality of medical care (from 86, 87 and 88)

Appendix B. Heroin Use in Past 30 Days (T_1) For 407 Methadone Maintenance Patients by Current Methadone Dose

Methadone Dose	Heroin Days in Past 30: 0	1–5	6–10	11–15	16–20	21–25	26–30	Total	Heroin Use, Percent
0	0	1	0	0	0	0	0	1	100
1–10	14	3	3	0	1	0	2	23	39
11–20	30	13	6	3	0	0	2	54	44
21–30	35	10	3	2	1	0	0	51	31
31–40	54	4	0	1	0	0	1	60	10
41–50	55	5	1	2	0	0	0	63	13
51–60	58	2	0	0	0	0	0	60	3
61–70	44	2	0	0	0	0	0	46	4
71–80	43	0	0	0	0	0	0	43	0
81–90	2	0	0	0	0	0	0	2	0
90+	4	0	0	0	0	0	0	4	0
Total	339	40	13	8	2	0	5	407	16.7

Median dose = 45 mg

Dose	Used Heroin
"Low" (0–45 mg)	57/204 = 27.9%
"High" (46 mg+)	11/203 = 5.4%

Relative risk of heroin use for "low" dose = 5.16

Appendix C. Further Analysis With Regard to Chapter 11: Regression Analyses of Total Patient Sample (n = 488)

The admission cohort (81 patients who had been in their treatment programs for less than 3 months at T_1) were combined with the in-treatment cohort of 407 patients. The definitions of patient baseline variables and principal components of the treatment domain remain as stated in Chapter 11. Four of the treatment process variables were not applicable to the admission cohort and were not used in the analyses of the total sample. Instead, cohort, status, and interaction of cohort and status were used as process variables for the total sample (Table C2).

Inclusion of the 81 new admissions did not change the patient baseline profile in any important way (compare Tables 11.1 and C1). Outcomes for the admission cohort were generally somewhat worse, on average, than for the in-treatment cohort. Combining the two cohorts produced slightly worse outcomes for the total sample than for the in-treatment cohort alone (compare Tables 11.6 and C3).

The regression analyses for the total sample are summarized in Tables C4 and C5. The results for the principal components of the treatment domain are similar to the findings reported in Chapter 11 for the in-treatment cohort. Patients in programs that delivered a high level of services tended to have better outcomes than those in programs that delivered lower levels of service. Among the six programs in this study, the ones that delivered high levels of service were also the ones whose directors performed well, and these programs were oriented toward maintenance and rehabilitation.

Among patient baseline variables, years of regular cocaine use was clearly associated with current cocaine use, months since last intravenous drug use, and current criminal activities.

Patients in the admission cohort had worse outcomes than those in the in-treatment cohort. Patients who terminated treatment during the follow-up year also tended to have worse outcomes than those who continued in their programs. The cohort and status variables were most evident for the heroin use outcome.

TABLE C.1. Patient Baseline Variables (T_1)

Variable	Label	Code-transform	Total sample (n = 488)
Age at T_1 interview	AGE	Actual years	36.8 years[a]
Race	RACE	0 = white, caucasian 1 = all other	59% Nonwhite
Usual employment pattern during 3 years prior to this admission	EMPL	0 = unemployed or in controlled environment 1 = part time 2 = full time	30% unemployed 18% part time 52% full time
Age at onset of opiate addiction	ONSET	Actual years	18.8[a]
Years of regular heroin use—lifetime	HYEARS	log (1 + actual years)	10.8[a]
Years of regular use of other opiates—lifetime	OYEARS	log (1 + actual years)	2.4[a]
Years of regular cocaine use—lifetime	CYEARS	log (1 + actual years)	2.6[a]
Prior treatments for drug abuse (no.)	TREAT	Actual number	3.4[a]
No. of arrests—lifetime	TOTARR	Actual number	7.3[a]
Crime-days rate, last addiction period, typical week	CRIME	Actual number	4.7[a]

[a] Mean.

TABLE C.2. Process Variables (Patient Groups)

Variable	Label	Code	Total sample
Patient cohort	COHORT	0 = admission 1 = in treatment	81/488 407/488
Terminated before T_2	STATUS	0 = terminated 1 = continued in program at T_2	102/488 386/488
Interaction	COHSTA	COHORT × STATUS	

TABLE C.3. Patient Outcome Variables (T_2)

Outcome	Code-transform	Total sample (n = 488)
Days of HEROIN USE during last 30 days	$(\text{actual days})^{\frac{1}{2}}$	2.1 days[a] 20% used at least 1 day
Days of COCAINE USE during last 30 days	$(\text{actual days})^{\frac{1}{2}}$	2.8 days[a] 28% used at least 1 day
Use of ANY OPIATES OR COCAINE during last 30 days	0 = none 1 = 1 day or more	38% used at least 1 day
Months since LAST IV DRUG USE	−log (1 + months)	34 months[a] median months = 12
No. of CRIMEDAYS during last 30 days	$(\text{actual days})^{\frac{1}{2}}$	2.9 days[a] 20% had at least 1 crime day

[a] Mean

TABLE C.4. Patient Baseline, Program Components, Process Variables, and Patient Outcomes: Regression Coefficients and Standard Errors for the Total Sample

Independent variable	Heroin use (n = 488)		Cocaine use (n = 488)		Any opiates or cocaine (n = 488)		Last IV drug use (n = 480)		Crime days (n = 487)	
	β	SE	β	SE	β	SE	β	SE	β	SE
Patient baseline										
AGE	−.004	.010	−.019	.011	−.005	.020	−.037[b]	.012	−.010	.012
RACE	−.181	.142	.608[b]	.160	.630[a]	.279	.135	.172	.109	.177
EMPL	.099	.067	−.002	.075	.167	.132	.042	.081	−.061	.083
ONSET	−.025	.015	−.004	.016	−.050	.029	−.005	.018	−.025	.018
HYEARS	.145	.088	−.035	.099	−.181	.173	.193	.106	.192	.110
OYEARS	−.131	.068	.003	.076	−.009	.134	−.061	.082	.162	.084
CYEARS	.077	.067	.244[b]	.075	.158	.127	.205[a]	.080	.180[a]	.083
TREAT	−.027	.079	.015	.089	.078	.151	.136	.096	−.019	.098
TOTARR	−.004	.007	.003	.008	−.011	.013	−.002	.008	−.002	.008
CRIME	.009	.021	.034	.023	.111[b]	.041	.002	.025	.010	.026
Program components										
COUNS-DIR-POL	.234[b]	.044	.188[b]	.050	.592[b]	.093	.400[b]	.053	.166[b]	.055
ADMIN-EXPER	−.113[b]	.042	.013	.047	.033	.083	−.006	.051	−.009	.052
FACIL-STAFF	−.202[b]	.041	−.141[b]	.046	−.284[b]	.078	−303[b]	.050	−.042	.051
MED	.123[a]	.050	.148[b]	.057	.159	.093	.156[a]	.061	.183[b]	.063
RESID	−.037	.044	.006	.049	.037	.084	−.046	.053	−.036	.054
Process variables										
COHORT	− .967[b]	.264	−.263	.297	−.272	.485	−.526	.316	−.041	.328
STATUS	−1.004[b]	.282	−.280	.318	−.510	.514	−.631	.340	.083	.351
COHSTA	.712[a]	.324	.084	.365	−.294	.594	−.092	.390	.060	.407

[a] $p < 0.05$.
[b] $p < 0.01$.

TABLE C.5. Regressions of Outcomes on Patient Baseline, Program Components, and Process Variables for Total Sample (n = 488)

Category	Due to	*df*	Mean square	*F*
Heroin in use, past 30 days				
(n = 488, $R^2 = 0.20$)				
Patient baseline (Pt)	Pt | Pr, Pc	10	2.447	1.67
Program components (Pc)	Pc | Pt, Pr	5	18.085	12.36[b]
Process (Pr)	Pr | Pt, Pc	3	14.759	10.09[b]
Error		469	1.463	
Cocaine use, past 30 days				
(n = 488, $R^2 = 0.17$)				
Patient baseline	Pt | Pr, Pc	10	7.544	4.06[b]
Program components	Pc | Pt, Pr	5	11.927	6.43[b]
Process	Pr | Pt, Pc	3	2.438	1.31
Error		469	1.856	
Any Opiates or Cocaine,				
past 30 days (n = 488, $R^2 = 0.12$)				
Patient baseline	Pt | Pr, Pc	10	Chi-square =	24.41[b]
Program components	Pc | Pt, Pr	5		68.12[b]
Process	Pr | Pt, Pc	3		12.15[b]
Last IV drug use				
(n = 480, $R^2 = 0.29$)				
Patient baseline	Pt | Pr, Pc	10	6.049	2.88[b]
Program components	Pc | Pt, Pr	5	41.410	19.69[b]
Process	Pr | Pt, Pc	3	22.252	10.58[b]
Error		461	2.103	
Crime days, past 30 days				
(n = 487, $R^2 = 0.10$)				
Patient baseline	Pt | Pr, Pc	10	5.891	2.61[b]
Program components	Pc | Pt, Pr	5	8.695	3.85[b]
Process	Pr | Pt, Pc	3	2.865	1.25
Error		468	2.258	

Variance analyses were used for linear regressions and likelihood ratio statistics were used for logistic regressions. Conditional test for a category after accounting for the other two categories.

[a] $p < 0.05$.
[b] $p < 0.01$.

Bibliography

Abdul-Quader AS, Friedman SR, Des Jarlais D, et al (1987) Methadone maintenance and behavior by intravenous drug users that can transmit HIV. Contemp Drug Probl 14:425–434.

Agar MH, Stephens RC (1975) The methadone street scene: the addict's view. Psychiatry 38:381–387.

Aiken LS, LoSciuto LS, Ausetts MA, Brown BS (1984) Paraprofessionals versus professional drug counselors: The progress of clients in treatment. Int J Addict 19:383–401.

Allison M, Hubbard RL (1985) Drug abuse treatment process: a review of the literature. Int J Addict 20:1321–1345.

Allison M, Hubbard RL, Rachal JV (1985) In: Treatment Process in Methadone, Residential, and Outpatient Drug Free Programs. Rockville: NIDA Research Monograph.

Altman F, Schnoll SH (1983) Discussion summary. In Cooper JR, Altman F, Brown B, Czechowicz D (eds): NIDA Treatment Research Monograph Series: Research on the Treatment of Narcotic Addiction: State of the Art. (ADM) 83–1281. Rockville: US Department of Health and Human Services, pp 573–574.

Anderson TW (1984) An Introduction to Multivariate Statistical Analysis 2nd ed. New York: Wiley.

Anglin MD, Almog IJ, Fisher DG, Peters KR (1989) Alcohol use by heroin addicts: evidence for an inverse relationship. A study of methadone maintenance and drug-free treatment samples. Am J Drug Alcohol Abuse 15:191–207.

Anglin MD, Booth MW, Ryan TM, Hser YI (1988) Ethnic differences in narcotics addiction. II. Chicano and Anglo addiction career patterns. Int J Addict 23:1011–1027.

Anglin MD, Fisher DG (1987) Survival analysis in drug program evaluation. Part II. Partitioning treatment effects. Int J Addict 24:377–387.

Anglin MD, Hser YI (1990) Treatment of drug abuse. In Tonry M, Wilson JQ (eds): Drugs and Crime. Chicago: University of Chicago Press, pp 393–460.

Anglin MD, Hser YI, Booth MW (1987) Sex differences in addict careers: treatment. Am J Drug Alcohol Abuse 13:253–280.

Anglin MD, McGlothlin WH (1984) Outcome of narcotic addict treatment in California. In Tims FM, Ludford JP (eds): NIDA Research Monograph Series 51: RAUS Drug Abuse Treatment Evaluation: Strategies, Progress, and Prospects.

(ADM)84–1329. Rockville: US Department of Health and Human Services, pp 106–128.

Anglin MD, Speckart G (1986) Narcotic use, property crime and dealing: structural dynamics across the addiction career. J Quant Criminol 2:355–375.

Appel P (1984) Model clinic evaluation: final report. In: Treatment Issues, Report 38. New York: New York State Division of Substance Abuse Services, Bureau of Research Evaluation and Planning.

Arif A, Westermeyer J (1990) Methadone in the Management of Opioid Dependence: Programs and Policies Around the World. New York: Praeger.

Austin GA, Johnson BD, Carroll EE, Lettieri DJ (eds) (1977) Drugs and Minorities. Rockville: US Department of Health and Human Services, pp 78–507.

Aylett P (1982) Methadone dose assessment in heroin addiction. Int J Addict 17:1329–1336.

Babst DV, Chambers CD, Warner A (1971) Patients' characteristics associated with retention in a methadone maintenance program. Br J Addict 66:195–204.

Bale RN, Van Stone WW, Kuldau JM, et al (1980) Therapeutic communities vs. methadone maintenance: a prospective controlled study of narcotic addiction treatment: design and one year followup results. Arch Gen Psychiatry 37:179–193.

Ball JC (1967) The reliability and validity of interview data obtained from narcotic drug addicts. Am J Sociol 72:650–654.

Ball JC (1969) Marijuana smoking and the onset of heroin use. In Cole JO, Wittenborn JR (eds): Drug Abuse: Social and Psychopharmacological Aspects. Springfield: Charles C Thomas, pp 117–128.

Ball JC (1972) On the treatment of drug dependence. Am J Psychiatry 128:107–108 (editorial).

Ball JC (1975) Sample selection in American follow-up studies of drug abusers. In Boström H, Larsson T, Ljungstedt N (eds): Skandia International Symposia: Drug Dependence-Treatment and Treatment Evaluation. Stockholm: Almqvist & Wiksell, pp 221–231.

Ball JC The similarity of crime rates among heroin addicts in New York City, Philadelphia and Baltimore. J Drug Issues (Spring) 21:2 (in press).

Ball JC, Chambers CD (eds) (1970) Epidemiology of Opiate Addiction in the U.S. Springfield: Charles C Thomas.

Ball JC, Corty E (1988) Basic issues pertaining to the effectiveness of methadone maintenance treatment. In Leukefeld CG, Tims FM (eds): NIDA Research Monograph Series 86: Compulsory Treatment of Drug Abuse: Research and Clinical Practice. (ADM)88–1578. Rockville: US Department of Health and Human Services, pp 178–191.

Ball JC, Corty E, Bond H, et al (1987) The reduction of intravenous heroin use, non-opiate abuse and crime during methadone maintenance treatment. In Harris LS (ed): NIDA Research Monograph Series 81: Problems of Drug Dependence 1987. (ADM)88–1564. Rockville: US Department of Health and Human Services, pp 224–230.

Ball JC, Corty E, Erdlen DL, Nurco DN (1986) Major patterns of polydrug abuse among heroin addicts. In Harris LS (ed): NIDA Research Monograph Series 67: Problems of Drug Dependence, 1985. (ADM)86–1448. Rockville: US Department of Health and Human Services, pp 256–262.

Ball JC, Corty E, Petroski SP, et al (1986) Medical services to 2,394 patients at

methadone programs in three states. J Subst Abuse Treat 3:203–209.
Ball JC, Cottrell ES (1965) Admission of narcotic drug addicts to public health service hospitals, 1935–1963. Public Health Rep 80:471–475.
Ball JC, Graff H (1974) Phase I evaluation of drug treatment programs in Pennsylvania. In Fisher S, Freedman AM (eds): Opiate Addiction. Washington, DC: Winston & Sons, pp 175–183.
Ball JC, Graff H (1975) Drug treatment programs in Pennsylvania: a statewide evaluation. Am J Public Health 65:592–598.
Ball JC, Lange WR, Myers CP, Friedman SR (1988) Reducing the risk of AIDS through methadone maintenance treatment. J Health Soc Behav 28:214–226.
Ball JC, Levine BK, Demaree RG, Newman JF (1975) Pretreatment criminality of male and female drug abuse patients in the United States. Addict Dis 1:481–489.
Ball JC, Nurco DN (1983) Criminality during the life course of heroin addiction. In Harris LS (ed): NIDA Research Monograph Series 49: Problems of Drug Dependence 1983. (ADM)84–1316. Rockville: US Department of Health and Human Services, pp 305–312.
Ball JC, Pabon DO (1965) Locating and interviewing narcotic addicts in Puerto Rico. Sociol Soc Res 49:401–411.
Ball JC, Rosen L, Flueck J, Nurco DN (1981) The criminality of heroin addicts when addicted and when off opiates. In Inciardi JA (ed): The Drug-Crime Connection, Vol. 5. Beverly Hills: Sage Publications, pp 39–65.
Ball JC, Rosen L, Flueck JA, Nurco DN (1982) Lifetime criminality of heroin addicts in the United States. J Drug Issues 3:225–316.
Ball JC, Shaffer JW, Nurco DN (1983) The day-to-day criminality of heroin addicts in Baltimore—a study in the continuity of offence rates. Drug Alcohol Depend 12:119–142.
Batki SL (1988) Treatment of intravenous drug users with AIDS: the role of methadone maintenance. J Psychoactive Drugs 20:213–216.
Battjes RJ, Pickens RW (eds) (1988) NIDA Research Monograph 80: Needle sharing among intravenous drug abusers: national and international perspectives. (ADM)88–1567. Rockville: US Department of Health and Human Services.
Bayer R, Koenigsberg L (1981) Retention rates among methadone patients: an analysis of the New York experience 1964–1976. Int J Addict 16:33–41.
Bazell R (1973) Drug abuse: methadone becomes the solution and the problem. Science 179:772–775.
Belenko, S (1990) The impact of drug offenders on the criminal justice system. In Weisheit R: Drugs, Crime and the Criminal Justice System. Cincinnati: Anderson Publishing.
Bespalec, DA (1974) Relapse rates after treatment for heroin addiction. J Comm Psychiatry 2, pp 85–87.
Bickel WK, Rizzuto P, Zielony RD, et al (1989) Combined behavioral and pharmacological treatment of alcoholic methadone patients. J Subst Abuse 1:161–171.
Bickel WK, Stitzer ML, Bigelow GE, et al (1988) A clinical trial of buprenorphine: comparison with methadone in the detoxification of heroin addicts. Clin Pharmacol Ther 43:72–78.
Blumstein A, Cohen J, Roth JA, Visher CA (eds) (1986) Dimensions of active criminal careers. In: Criminal Careers and "Career Criminals." Washington, DC: National Academy Press, pp 55–95.

Bonito AM, Nurco DN, Shaffer JW (1976) The veridicality of addicts' self-reports in social research. Int J Addict 11:719–724.
Bourne P (1975) Methadone: Benefits and Shortcomings. Washington, DC: Drug Abuse Council, pp 1–25.
Bourne PG (1981) A 10-year perspective on the addiction problem. In Lowinson JH, Ruiz P (eds): Substance Abuse: Clinical Problems and Perspectives. Baltimore: Williams & Wilkins, pp 35–42.
Bowden CL, Maddux JF, Esquivel M (1978) Arrest before and during methadone maintenance. Int J Addict 13:921–931.
Bowden CL, Maddux JF, Esquivel M (1980) Outpatient methadone withdrawal for heroin dependence. Am J Drug Alcohol Abuse 7:323–333.
Bracy SA, Simpson DD (1982–1983) Status of opioid addicts 5 years after admission to drug abuse treatment. Am J Drug Alcohol Abuse 9:115–127.
Brewington V, Arella L, Deren S, Randell J (1987) Obstacles to the utilization of vocational services: an analysis of the literature. Int J Addict 22:1091–1118.
Brill L, Chambers CD (1971) A multi-modality approach to methadone treatment of narcotic addicts. Soc Work 16:39–51.
Bromet EJ, Moos RH, Bliss F (1976) The social climate of alcoholism treatment programs. Arch Gen Psychiatry 33:910–916.
Brown BS (ed) (1979) Addicts and Aftercare: Community Integration of the Former Drug User. Sage Annual Reviews of Drug and Alcohol Abuse. Vol 3. Beverly Hills: Sage Publications.
Brown BS, Ashery RS (1979) Aftercare in drug abuse programming. In DuPont RL, Goldstein A, O'Donnell J (eds): Handbook on Drug Abuse. Washington, DC: US Government Printing Office, pp 165–173.
Brown BS, Brewster GW (1973) A comparison of addict-clients retained and lost to treatment. Int J Addict 8:421–426.
Brown BS, Gfroerer J, Thompson P, Bardine A (1985) Setting and counselor type as related to program retention. Int J Addict 20:723–736.
Brown BS, Guavey SK, Meyers MB, Stark SD (1971) In their own words: addicts' reasons for initiating and withdrawing from heroin. Int J Addict 6:635–645.
Brown BS, Jansen DR, Benn GL (1975). Changes in attitudes towards methadone. Arch Gen Psychiatry 32:214–218.
Brown BS, Joe GW, Thompson P (1985) Minority group status and treatment retention. Int J Addict 20:319–335.
Brown BS, Thompson RF (1973) Impact of straight and formerly addicted counselors on client functioning. In: Proceedings of the Fifth National Conference on Methadone Treatment, Vol 1. New York: National Association for the Prevention of Addiction to Narcotics, pp 228–234.
Brown BS, Watters JK, Inglehart AS, Akins C (1982–1983) Methadone maintenance dosage levels and program retention. Am J Drug Alcohol Abuse 9:129–139.
Butynski W, Canova D (1988) State Resources and Services Related to Alcohol and Drug Abuse Problems—Fiscal Year 1987: an analysis of state alcohol and drug abuse profile data. Washington, DC: National Association of State Alcohol and Drug Abuse Directors.
Cacciola J, Griffith J, McLellan AT (eds) (1988) Addiction Severity Index: Instruction Manual, 4th ed. Washington, DC: NIDA Research Project DA02559 and the Veterans Administration.

Carlson G, Westermeyer J (1990) Minneapolis-St. Paul. In Arif A, Westermeyer J (eds): Methadone in the Management of Opioid Dependence: Programs and Policies Around the World. New York: Praeger.

Centers for Disease Control (1987) Update: acquired immunodeficiency syndrome (AIDS)—United States. MMWR CDC Surveill Summ Aug 14:522–526.

Chabalko J, La Rosa JC, DuPont RL (1973) Death of methadone users in the District of Columbia. Int J Addict 8:897–908.

Chaiken JM, Chaiken MR (1982) Varieties of Criminal Behavior. Santa Monica: Rand.

Chaiken JM, Chaiken MR (1983) Crime rates and the active criminal. In Wilson JQ (ed): Crime and Public Policy. San Francisco: Institute for Contemporary Studies.

Chambers CD, Brill L (1973) Methadone: Experiences and Issues. New York: Behavioral Publications.

Chambers CD, Russel WJ, Mofett AD (1972) The incidence of cocaine abuse among methadone maintenance patients. Int J Addict 7:427–441.

Chapple PAL, Gray G (1968) One year's work at a centre for the treatment of addicted patients. The Lancet 1:908–911.

Chien I, Rosenfeld E (1957) Juvenile narcotics use. In: Law Contemporary Problems. Durham: Duke University of Law 22:52–68.

Chein I, Gerard DL, Lee RS, Rosenfeld E (1964) The Road to H: Narcotics, Delinquency, and Social Policy. New York: Basic Books.

Childress AR, McLellan AT, Woody GE, O'Brien CP (1990) Are there minimum conditions necessary for methadone maintenance? In Leukefeld C, Pickens R (eds): Review of Drug Abuse Treatment Research. Rockville: US Government Printing Office.

Clayton RR (1986) A note from the deputy editor: AIDS and drug abuse—crises and challenges. J Health Soc Behav 27:vi–vii.

Clayton RR (1987) The nature and extent of drug abuse. In: Drug Abuse and Drug Abuse Research: The Second Triennial Report to Congress from the Secretary, Department of Health and Human Services. Rockville: National Institute on Drug Abuse, pp 13–31.

Cohen J (1986) Research on criminal careers: individual frequency rates and offense seriousness. In Blumstein A, Cohen J, Roth JA, Visher CA (eds): Criminal Careers and Career Criminals. Washington, DC: National Academy Press, pp 292–418.

Cohen M, Howard A, Klien DF, Newfield K (1976) Evaluating outcome criteria used in methadone maintenance programs. Int J Addict 11:283–294.

Cohen S (1981) The Substance Problems. New York: Haworth Press.

Collins JJ, Rachal JV, Hubbard RL, et al (1982) Criminality in a Drug Treatment Sample: Measurement Issues and Initial Findings. Research Triangle Park: Research Triangle Institute.

Connell PH (1975) Review of methadone maintenance schemes. In Boström H, Larsson T, Ljungstedt N (eds): Skandia International Symposia: Drug Dependence-Treatment and Treatment Evaluation. Stockholm: Almqvist & Wiksell, pp 133–146.

Connor T, Kremen E (1971) Methadone maintenance—is it enough? Int J Addict 6:279–298.

Conover WJ (1980) Practical Nonparametric Statistics, 2nd ed. New York: Wiley.
Coombs RH, Fry LJ, Lewis PG (eds) (1976) Socialization in Drug Abuse. Cambridge: Schenkman Publishing.
Cooper JR (1989) Methadone treatment and acquired immunodeficiency syndrome. JAMA 262:1664–1668.
Cooper JR, Altman F, Brown B, Czechowicz D (eds) (1983) NIDA Treatment Research Monograph Series: Research on the Treatment of Narcotic Addiction: State of the Art. (ADM)83-1281. Rockville: US Department of Health and Human Services.
Corty E, Ball JC (1987) Admissions to methadone maintenance: comparisons between programs and implications for treatment. J Subst Abuse Treat 4:181–187.
Corty E, Ball JC (1986) What can we know about addiction from the addicts we treat? Int J Addict 21:1139–1144.
Corty E, Ball JC, Myers CP (1988) Psychiatric symptomatology in methadone maintenance patients. J Consult Clin Psychol 56:776–777.
Courtwright D, Joseph H, Des Jarlais D (1989) Addicts Who Survived: An Oral History of Narcotic Use in America, 1923–1965. Knoxville: University of Tennessee Press.
Courtwright DT, Joseph H, Des Jarlais DC (1981) Memories from the street: oral history of elderly methadone patients. Oral Hist Rev 9:47–64.
Cox TJ, Longwell B (1974) Reliability of interview data concerning current heroin use from heroin addicts on methadone. Int J Addict 9:161–165.
Cushman P (1977) Ten years of methadone maintenance treatment: some clinical observations. Am J Drug Alcohol Abuse 4:543–553.
Cushman P, Trussell R, Gollance H, et al (1976) Methadone maintenance treatment of narcotic addiction: a unit of medical care based on over 50,000 patient treatment years. Am J Drug Alcohol Abuse 3:221–233.
D'Amanda C (1983) Program policies and procedures associated with treatment outcome. In Cooper JR, Altman F, Brown BS, Czechowicz D (eds): NIDA Treatment Research Monograph Series: Research on the Treatment of Narcotic Addiction: State of the Art. (ADM)83-1281. Rockville: US Department of Health and Human Services, pp 637–679.
Deleon G (1974) Phoenix House: psychopathological signs among male and female drug-free residents. Addict Dis 1:135–151.
Deleon G, Rosenthal M (1979) Therapeutic communities. In DuPont RI, Goldstein A, O'Donnell J (eds): Handbook on Drug Abuse. Washington, DC: US Government Printing Office, pp 39–47.
Des Jarlais DC (1990) Stages in the response of the drug abuse treatment system to the AIDS epidemic in New York City. J Drug Issues 20:335–347.
Des Jarlais DC, Deren S, Lipton DS (1981) Cost effectiveness studies in the evaluation of substance abuse treatment. In Lowinson JH, Ruiz P (eds): Substance Abuse Clinical Problems and Perspectives. Baltimore: Williams & Wilkins, pp 806–816.
Des Jarlais DC, Friedman SR (1989) AIDS and the IV drug user. Science 245:578.
Des Jarlais DC, Friedman SR (1987) HIV infection among intravenous drug users: epidemiology and risk reduction. AIDS 1:67–76.
Des Jarlais DC, Friedman SR (1987) Target groups for preventing AIDS among intravenous drug users. J Appl Soc Psychol 17:251–268.

Des Jarlais DC, Friedman SR, Hopkins W (1985) Risk reduction for the acquired immunodeficiency syndrome among intravenous drug users. Ann Intern Med 103:755–759.

Des Jarlais DC, Friedman SR, Novick DM, et al (1989) HIV-1 infection among intravenous drug users in Manhattan, New York City, from 1977 through 1987. JAMA 261:1008–1012.

Des Jarlais DC, Friedman SR, Strug D (1986) AIDS and needle sharing within the IV-drug use subculture. In Feldman D, Johnson T (eds): The Social Dimensions of AIDS: Methods and Theory. New York: Praeger, pp 111–125.

Des Jarlais DC, Joseph H, Courtwright DT (1985) Old age and addiction: a study of elderly patients in methadone maintenance treatment. In Gottheil E, et al (eds): The Combined Problems of Alcoholism, Drug Addiction and Aging. Springfield: Charles C Thomas, pp 201–209.

Des Jarlais DC, Joseph H, Dole VP (1981) Long-term outcomes after termination from methadone maintenance treatment. Ann NY Acad Sci 362:231–238.

Dietch RF (1979) Program management: magical expectations and harsh realities. In DuPont RI, Goldstein A, O'Donnell J (eds): Handbook on Drug Abuse. Washington, DC: US Government Printing Office, pp 409–414.

Dobbs WH (1971) Methadone treatment for heroin addicts: early results provide more questions than answers. JAMA 218:1536–1541.

Dole VP (1988) Implications of methadone maintenance for theories of narcotic addiction. JAMA 260:3025–3029.

Dole VP (1989) Methadone maintenance. In Courtwright D, Joseph H, Des Jarlais D: Addicts Who Survived: An Oral History of Narcotic Use in America, 1923–1965. Knoxville: University of Tennessee Press, pp 331–343.

Dole VP (1971) Methadone maintenance treatment for 25,000 heroin addicts. JAMA 215:1131–1134.

Dole VP, Joseph H (1978) Long-term outcome of patients treated with methadone maintenance. Ann NY Acad Sci 311:181–189.

Dole VP, Nyswander M (1965) A medical treatment for diacetylmorphine (heroin) addiction: a clinical trial with methadone hydrochloride. JAMA 193:80–84.

Dole VP, Nyswander ME (1983) Behavioral pharmacology and treatment of human drug abuse-methadone maintenance of narcotic addicts. In: Smith J, Lane JD (eds) The Neurobiology of Opiate Reward Processes. New York: Elsevier Biomedical Press, pp 211–233.

Dole VP, Nyswander ME (1976) Methadone maintenance treatment: a ten-year perspective. JAMA 235:2117–2119.

Dole VP, Nyswander ME, Des Jarlais DC, Joseph H (1982) Sounding board: performance-based rating of methadone maintenance programs. N Engl J Med 306:169–172.

Dole VP, Nyswander ME, Kreek MJ (1966) Narcotic blockade. Arch Intern Med 118:304–309.

Dole VP, Nyswander ME, Warner A (1968) Successful treatment of 750 criminal addicts. JAMA 206:2708–2711.

Dole VP, Singer B (1979) On the evaluation of treatments for narcotics addiction. J Drug Issues 2:205–211.

D'Orban PT (1974) A follow-up study of female narcotic addicts: variables related to outcome. Br J Psychiatry 124:28–33.

Drotman DP (1987) Now is the time to prevent AIDS. Am J Public Health 77:143.

Drug Abuse Council (1973) Methadone Maintenance: The Experience of Four Programs. Washington, DC: The Drug Abuse Council.

DuPont RI, Goldstein A, O'Donnell J, Brown BS (eds) (1979) Handbook on Drug Abuse. Washington, DC: US Government Printing Office.

Edelin KC, Gurganious L, Golar K, Oellerich D, et al (1988) Methadone maintenance in pregnancy: consequences to care and outcome. Obstet Gynecol 71:399–404.

Edwards, G (1979) British policies on opiate addiction: ten years working of the revised response, and options for the future. Brit. J. Psychiat. 134:1–13.

Edwards JG, Goldie A (1987) A ten-year follow-up study of Southampton opiate addicts. Br J Psychiatry 151:679–683.

El-Guebaly N, O'Riordan J (1988) Manitoba's methadone program: the first 15 years. Can Med Assoc J 138:407–408.

Federal Register (1980) September 19 (Part 21CFR291505), pp 1–12.

Fisher DG, Anglin MD (1987) Survival analysis in drug problem evaluation. Part I. Overall program effectiveness. Int J Addict 22:115–134.

Friedman SR, Des Jarlais DC (1988) Five common misconceptions about intravenous drug users. Med Aspects Hum Sex 1:90–101.

Friedman SR, Des Jarlais DC, Sotheran JL, et al (1987) AIDS and self-organization among intravenous drug users. Int J Addict 22:201–219.

Galea RP, Lewis BF, Baker LA (eds) (1988) AIDS and IV Drug Abusers: Current Perspectives. Owings Mills: National Health Publishing, Exhibit I-1, I-2, pp xxvii, xxx–xxxi.

Gandossy RP, Williams JR, Cohen J, Harwood HJ (1980) Drugs and crime: a survey and analysis of the literature. Washington, DC: US Government Printing Office.

Gawin FH, Kleber HD (1985) Cocaine use in a treatment population: patterns and diagnostic distinctions. In Kozel NJ, Adams EH (eds): NIDA Research Monograph Series 61: Cocaine Use in America: Epidemiological and Clinical Perspectives. (ADM)85–1414. Rockville: US Department of Health and Human Services, pp 182–192.

Gearing FR (1972) Methadone maintenance: six years later. Contemp Drug Prob 1:191–206.

Gearing FR (1971) Evaluation of methadone maintenance treatment programs. In Einstein S (ed): Methadone Maintenance. New York: Marcel Dekker.

Gearing FR (1970) Successes and failures in methadone maintenance treatment of heroin addiction in New York City. In: Proceedings of the Third National Conference on Methadone Treatment. Rockville: US Public Health Service, Pub. No. 2172, pp 2–16.

Gearing FR, Schweitzer MD (1974) An epidemiologic evaluation of long-term methadone maintenance treatment for heroin addiction. Am J Epidemiol 100:101–112.

Gerstein DR, Harwood HJ (eds) (1990) Treating Drug Problems. Vol. 1. Washington, DC: National Academy Press.

Giles W, Pattern T, Sanders F, et al (1989) Outpatient methadone programme for pregnant heroin using women. Aust NZ J Obstet Gynaecol 3:225–229.

Ginzburg HM, Mhairi GM, Glass JW (1987) AIDS, HTLV-III diseases, minorities and intravenous drug abuse. Adv Alcohol Subst Abuse 6:7–21.

Glasscote RM, Sussex JN, Jaffe JH, et al (1972) The Treatment of Drug Abuse:

Programs, Problems, Prospects. Washington, DC: American Psychiatric Association.

Gold ML, Sorensen JL, Mc Canlies TM, et al (1988) Tapering from methadone maintenance: attitudes of clients and staff. J Subst Abuse Treat 5:37–44.

Goldstein A (1972) Heroin addiction and the role of methadone in its treatment. Arch Gen Psychiatry 26:291–297.

Goldstein A, Horns WA, Hansteen RW (1977) Is on-site urine testing of therapeutic value in a methadone treatment program? Int J Addict 12:717–728.

Goldstein A, Judson BA (1983) Critique of William A. Hargreaves: methadone dose and duration for maintenance treatment. In Cooper JR, Altman F, Brown BS, Czechowicz D (eds): Research on the Treatment of Narcotic Addiction: State of the Art. (ADM)83–1281. Rockville: US Department of Health and Human Services, pp 80–91.

Gorsuch RL, Abbamonte M, Sells SB (1976) Evaluation of treatments for drug users in the DARP: 1971–1972 admissions. In Sells SB, Simpson DD (eds): The Effectiveness of Drug Abuse Treatment. Vol 4. Evaluation of Treatment Outcomes for 1971–1972 Admission Cohort. Cambridge: Ballinger, pp 10–251.

Gottheil E (1977) Common questions about methadone treatment. J Med Soc NJ 74:667–671.

Gottheil E, McLellan AT, Druley KA (eds) (1981) Matching Patient Needs and Treatment Methods in Alcoholism and Drug Abuse. Springfield: Charles C Thomas.

Gottheil E, McLellan AT, Druley KA (eds) (1981) Reasonable and unreasonable methodological standards for the evaluation of alcoholism treatment. In: Matching Patient Needs and Treatment Methods in Alcoholism and Drug Abuse. Springfield: Charles C Thomas, pp 371–389.

Graff H, Ball JC (1976) The methadone clinic: function and philosophy. Int J Soc Psychiatry 22:140–146.

Griffiths P, Wells B, Strang J, Gossop M (1988) Changes in methadone withdrawal doses over a five year period: 1982–1986. Br J Addict 83:189–191.

Gust SW, Walsh JM (1989) NIDA Research Monograph Series 91: Drugs in the Workplace: Research and Evaluation Data. (ADM)89–1612. Rockville: US Department of Health and Human Services.

Hall SM (1983) Methadone treatment: a review of the research findings. In Cooper JR, Altman F, Brown B, Czechowicz D (eds): NIDA Treatment Research Monograph Series: Research on the Treatment of Narcotic Addiction: State of the Art. (ADM)83–1281. Rockville: US Department of Health and Human Services, pp 575–632.

Hall SM, Loeb P, Coyne K, Cooper J (1981) Increasing employment in ex-heroin addicts I. Criminal justice sample. Behav Ther 12:443–452.

Hall SM, Loeb P, Coyne K, Cooper J (1981) Increasing employment in ex-heroin addicts II. Methadone maintenance sample. Behav Ther 12:453–460.

Hall SM, Loeb P, Norton J (1977) Improving vocational placement in drug treatment clients: a pilot study. Addict Behav 2:227–234.

Hammersley R, Forsyth A, Morrison V, Davies JB (1989) The relationship between crime and opioid use. Br J Addict 84:1029–1043.

Hammersley R, Morrison V (1988) Crime amongst heroin, alcohol and cannabis users. Med Law 7:185–193.

Hardy AM, Allen JR, Morgan WM, Curran JW (1985) The incidence rate of acquired immunodeficiency syndrome in selected populations. JAMA 253:215–220.

Hargreaves WA (1983) Methadone dosage and duration for maintenance treatment. In Cooper JR, Altman F, Brown B, Czechowicz D (eds): NIDA Treatment Research Monograph Series: Research on the Treatment of Narcotic Addiction: State of the Art. (ADM)83–1281. Rockville: US Department of Health and Human Services, pp 19–79.

Harwood HJ, Hubbard RL, Collins JJ, Rachal JV (1988) The costs of crime and the benefits of drug abuse treatment: a cost-benefit analysis using TOPS data. In Leukefeld CG, Tims FM (eds): NIDA Research Monograph Series 86: Compulsory Treatment of Drug Abuse: Research and Clinical Practice. (ADM)88–1578. Rockville: US Department of Health and Human Services.

Havassy B, Hall S (1981) Efficacy of urine monitoring in methadone maintenance. Am J Psychiatry 138:1497–1500.

Haverkos HW (1988) Overview: HIV infection among intravenous drug abusers in the United States and Europe. In Battjes RJ, Pickens RW (eds): NIDA Research Monograph Series 80: Needle Sharing Among Intravenous Drug Abusers. (ADM)88–1567. Rockville: US Department of Health and Human Services, pp 7–17.

Hayford SM, Epps RP, Dahl-Regis M (1988) Behavior and development patterns in children born to heroin-addicted and methadone-addicted mothers. J Nat Med Assoc 80:1197–1200.

Henningfield JE, Clayton R, Pollin W (1990) Involvement of tobacco in alcoholism and illicit drug use. Br J Addict 85:279–292.

Heyman F (1972) Methadone maintenance as law and order. Society June:15–25.

Higgins ST, Stitzer ML, Bigelow GE, Liebson IA (1986) Contingent methadone delivery: effects on illicit-opiate use. Drug Alcohol Depend 17:311–322.

Higgins ST, Stitzer ML, Bigelow GE, Liebson IA (1984) Contingent methadone dose increases as a method for reducing illicit opiate use in detoxification patients. In Harris LS (ed): NIDA Research Monograph Series 55: Problems of Drug Dependence, 1984. (ADM)85–1393. Rockville: US Department of Health and Human Services, pp 178–184.

Holland S (1986) Measuring process in drug abuse treatment research. In DeLeon G, Ziegenfuss JT (eds): Therapeutic Communities for Addictions: Readings in Theory, Research and Practice. Springfield: Charles C Thomas, pp 169–181.

Holmstrand J, Anggard E, Gunne L (1978) Methadone maintenance: plasma levels and therapeutic outcome. Clin Pharmacol Ther 23:175–180.

Hubbard RL, Marsden ME, Rachal JV, et al (1989) Drug Abuse Treatment: A National Study Of Effectiveness. Chapel Hill: University of North Carolina Press.

Hubbard RL, Rachal JV, Craddock SG, Cavanaugh ER (1984) Treatment outcome prospective study (TOPS): client characteristics and behaviors before, during, and after treatment. In Tims FM, Ludford JP (eds): NIDA Research Monograph Series 51: RAUS Drug Abuse Treatment Evaluation: Strategies, Progress, and Prospects. (ADM)84–1329. Rockville: US Department of Health and Human Services, pp 42–68.

Hunt DE, Lipton DS, Goldsmith DS, Strug DL, et al (1985–1986) It takes your heart: the image of methadone maintenance in the addict world and its effect on recruitment. Int J Addict 20:1751–1771.

Hunt DE, Strug DL, Goldsmith DS, Lipton DS, et al (1984) An instant shot of 'aah': cocaine use among methadone clients. J Psychoactive Drugs 16:217–227.

Iguchi MY, Stitzer ML, Bigelow BE, Liebson IA (1988) Contingency management in methadone maintenance: efforts of reinforcing and aversive consequences on illicit polydrug use. Drug Alcohol Depend 22:1–7.

Inciardi JA (1977) Methadone diversion: experiences and issues. In: NIDA Research Monograph Series. (ADM)77–488. Rockville: US Department of Health and Human Services.

Inciardi JA (ed) (1981) The Drugs-Crime Connection. Vol 5. Beverly Hills: Sage Publications.

Inciardi JA, Chambers CD (1972) Unreported criminal activities of narcotic addicts. J Drug Issues 2:57–64.

Jackson Binion V (1982) Sex differences in socialization and family dynamics of female and male heroin users. J Soc Issues 38:43–57.

Jaffe JH (1979) The swinging pendulum: the treatment of drug abusers in America. In Dupont RI, Goldstein A, O'Donnell J (eds): Handbook on Drug Abuse. Washington, DC: US Government Printing Office, pp 3–16.

Jaffe JH (1984) Evaluating drug abuse treatment: a comment on the state of the art. In Tims FM, Ludford JP (eds): NIDA Research Monograph Series 51: RAUS Drug Abuse Treatment Evaluation: Strategies, Progress, and Prospects. (ADM)84–1329. Rockville: US Department of Health and Human Services, pp 13–28.

Jaffe JH (1987) Footnotes in the evolution of the American national response: some little known aspects of the first American strategy for drug abuse and drug traffick prevention: the inaugural Thomas Okey memorial lecture. Br J Addict 82:587–600.

Jaffe JH, Senay EC (1971) Methadone and 1-methadyl acetate. JAMA 216:1303–1305.

Johns AR, Gossop M (1985) Prescribing methadone for the opiate addict: a problem of dosage conversion. Drug Alcohol Depend 16:61–66.

Johnson BD, Goldstein PJ, Preble E, et al (1985) Taking Care of Business: The Economics of Crime by Heroin Users. Lexington: Lexington Books.

Johnson BD, Kaplan MA, Schmeidler J (1990) Days with drug distribution: which drugs?: how many transactions?: with what returns. In Weisheit R (ed): Drugs, Crime and the Criminal Justice System. Kentucky: Anderson Publishing.

Johnston LD, Nurco DN, Robins LN (eds) (1977) Conducting follow-up research on drug treatment programs. Rockville: US Department of Health and Human Services.

Joseph H (1988) The criminal justice system and opiate addiction: a historical perspective. In: Leukefeld CG, Tims FM (eds): Compulsory Treatment of Drug Abuse: Research and Clinical Practice. (ADM)88–1578. Rockville: US Department of Health and Human Services, pp 106–125.

Joseph H, Appel P (1985) Alcoholism and methadone treatment: consequences for the patient and program. Am J Drug Alcohol Abuse 11:37–53.

Joseph H, Dole VP (1970) Methadone patients on probation and parole. Federal Probation 34:42–48.

Judson BA, Ortiz S, Crouse, et al (1980) A follow-up study of heroin addicts five years after first admissions to a methadone treatment program. Drug Alcohol Depend 6:295–313.

Kaplan HB, Johnson RJ, Bailey CA, Simon W (1987) The sociological study of AIDS: a critical review of the literature and suggested research agenda. J Health Soc Behav 28:140–157.

Kirn TF (1988) Methadone maintenance treatment remains controversial even after 23 years of experience. JAMA 260:2970–2975.

Kissin B, Lowinson JH, Millman RB (eds) (1978) Recent developments in chemotherapy of narcotic addiction. Ann NY Acad Sci 311:1–315

Kleber HD, Gold MS (1978) Use of psychotropic drugs in treatment of methadone maintained narcotic addicts. In Kissin B, Lowinson JH, Millman RB (eds): Ann NY Acad Sci 311:81–98.

Kleber HD, Slobetz F (1979) Outpatient drug free treatment. In DuPont RI, Goldstein A, O'Donnell J (eds): Handbook on Drug Abuse. Washington, DC: US Government Printing Office, pp. 31–38.

Klein JM, Miller SI (1986) Three approaches to the treatment of drug addiction. Hos Community Psychiatry 37:1083–1085.

Klepak D (1978) Evaluation of treatment effectiveness: the New York State experience. Ann NY Acad Sci 311:248–252.

Knowles R, Anderson G (1971) Setting up a methadone maintenance program. Hos Community Psychiatry 22:38–43.

Kolar AF, Brown BS, Weddington WW, Ball JC (1990) A treatment crisis: cocaine use by clients in methadone maintenance programs. J Subst Abuse Treat 7:101–107.

Kosten TR, Rounsaville BJ, Kleber HD (1987) A 2.5-year follow-up of cocaine use among treated opioid addicts: have our treatments helped? Arch Gen Psychiatry 44:281–284.

Kosten TR, Rounsaville BJ, Kleber HD (1988) Antecedents and consequences of cocaine abuse among opioid addicts: a 2.5-year follow-up. J Nerv Ment Dis 176:176–181.

Kosten TR, Gawin FH, Rounsaville BJ, Kleber HD (1986) Cocaine abuse among opioid addicts: demographic and diagnostic factors in treatment. Am J Drug Alcohol Abuse 12:1–16.

Kosten TR, Rounsaville BJ, Kleber HD (1983) Concurrent validity of the addiction severity index. J Nerv Ment Dis 171:606–610.

Kosten TR, Rounsaville BJ, Kleber HD (1987) Multidimensionality and prediction of treatment outcome in opioid addicts: a 2.5-year follow-up. Compr Psychiatry 28:3–13.

Kozel NJ, Adams EH (1986) Epidemiology of drug abuse: an overview. Science 234:970–974.

Kreek MJ (1983) Health consequences associated with the use of methadone. In Cooper JR, Altman F, Brown BS, Czechowicz D (eds): NIDA Research Monograph Series: Research on the Treatment of Narcotic Addiction: State of the Art. (ADM)83–1281. Rockville: US Government Printing Office, pp 456–491.

Kreek MJ (1981) Medical management of methadone-maintained patients. In Lowinson JH, Ruiz P (eds): Substance Abuse: Clinical Problems and Perspectives. Baltimore: Williams & Wilkins, pp 660–673.

Kreek MJ (1979) Methadone in treatment: physiological and pharmacological issues. In DuPont RI, Goldstein A, O'Donnell J (eds): Handbook on Drug Abuse. Washington, DC: US Government Printing Office, pp 57–86.

Kreek MJ (1987) Multiple drug abuse patterns and medical consequences. In Meltzer HY: Psychopharmacology: The Third Generation of Progress. New York: Raven Press.

Kremen E, Bayer R (1983) Some issues in group therapy with methadone patients. In Cooper JR, Altman F, Brown BS, Czechowicz D (eds): NIDA Research Monograph Series: Research on the Treatment of Narcotic Addiction: State of the Art. (ADM)83–1281. Rockville: US Department of Health and Human Services, pp 456–491.

Lambert EY (ed) (1990) NIDA Research Monograph Series 98: The Collection and Interpretation of Data from Hidden Populations. (ADM)90–1678. Rockville: US Department of Health and Human Services.

Lange WR, Ball JC, Pfeiffer MB, et al (1989) The Lexington addicts, 1971–1972: demographic characteristics, drug use patterns, and selected infectious disease experience. Int J Addict 24:609–626.

Lange WR, Snyder FR, Lozovsky D, et al (1987) HIV infection in Baltimore: antibody seroprevalence rates among parenteral drug abusers and prostitutes. Md Med J 35:757–761.

Lehman AF, Myers CP, Corty E (1989) Assessment and classification of patients with psychiatric and substance abuse syndromes. Hosp Community Psychiatry 40:1019–1025.

Lennard HL, Epstein LJ, Rosenthal MS (1972) The methadone illusion. Science 176:881–884.

Lettieri DJ, Sayers M, Wallenstein Pearson H (1980) NIDA Research Monograph Series 30: Theories on Drug Abuse: Selected Contemporary Perspectives. (ADM)80–967. Rockville: US Department of Health and Human Services.

Leukefeld CG, Tims FM (eds) (1988) NIDA Research Monograph Series: Compulsory Treatment of Drug Abuse: Research and Clinical Practice. (ADM)88–1578. Rockville: US Department of Health and Human Services.

Liappas JA, Jenner FA, Vicente B (1988) Literature on methadone maintenance clinics. Int J Addict 23:927–940.

Lindman, HR (1974) Analysis of Variance in Complex Experimental Designs. San Francisco: W.H. Freeman.

Lipton DS, Appel P (1984) The state perspective. In Tims FM, Ludford JP (eds): NIDA Research Monograph Series 51: RAUS Drug Abuse Treatment Evaluation: Strategies, Progress, and Prospects. (ADM)84–1329. Rockville: US Department of Health and Human Services, pp 151–166.

Longwell B, Miller J, Nicholas AW (1978) Counselor effectiveness in a methadone maintenance program. Int J Addict 13:307–315.

LoScuito LA, Aiken LS, Ausetts MA (1979) Professional and paraprofessional drug abuse counselors: three reports. Rockville: US Department of Health and Human Services.

LoScuito LA, Aiken LS, Ausetts MA, Brown BS (1984) Paraprofessional versus professional drug abuse counselors: attitudes and expectations of counselors and their clients. Int J Addict 19:232–252.

Lowinson JH, Millman RB (1979) Clinical aspects of methadone maintenance treatment. In DuPont RI, Goldstein A, O'Donnell J (eds): Handbook on Drug Abuse. Washington, DC: US Government Printing Office, pp. 49–56.

Lowinson JH, Ruiz P (eds) (1981) Methadone maintenance in perspective. In Lowinson JH, Ruiz P (eds): Substance Abuse Clinical Problems and Perspectives. Baltimore: Williams & Wilkins, pp. 344–354.

Luborsky L, McLellan AT, Woody GE, O'Brien CP, Auerbach A (1985) Therapist success and its determinants. Arch Gen Psychiatry 42:602–611.

Luborsky L, Woody GE, McLellan AT, O'Brien CP (1982) Can independent judges recognize different psychotherapies? An experience with manual-guided therapies. J Consult Clin Psychol 50:49–62.

Lukoff IF, Kleinman PH (1977) The addict life cycle and problems in treatment evaluation. In Schecter A, Mule SJ (eds): Rehabilitation Aspects of Drug Dependence. Cleveland: CRC Press.

Maddux JF (1988) History of drug abuse treatment in Texas. Tex Med 84:57–61.

Maddux JF, Bowden CL (1972) Critique of success with methadone maintenance. Am J Psychiatry 129:100–106.

Maddux JF, Desmond DP (1981) Careers of Opioid Users. New York: Praeger.

Maddux JF, Desmond DP (1975) Reliability and validity of information from chronic heroin users. J Psychiatr Res 12:87–95.

Maddux JF, Desmond DP (1990) San Antonio. In Arif A, Westermeyer J (eds): Methadone in the Management of Opioid Dependence: Programs and Policies Around the World. New York: Praeger.

Maddux JF, Desmond DP, Esquivel M (1980) Outpatient methadone withdrawal for heroin dependence. Am J Drug Alcohol Abuse 7:323–333.

Maddux JF, McDonald LK (1973) Status of 100 San Antonio addicts one year after admission to methadone maintenance. Drug Forum 2:239–252.

Marmor M, Des Jarlais DC, Cohen H (1987) Risk factors for infection with human immunodeficiency virus among intravenous drug abusers in New York City. AIDS 1:39–44.

Martin E (1987) Managing drug addiction in general practice—the reality behind the guidelines: discussion paper. J R Soc Med 80:305–307.

Martin W (1970) Commentary on the second national conference on methadone treatment. Int J Addict 5:545–552.

Martin WR, Isbell H (1978) Drug Addiction and the U.S. Public Health Service. Washington, DC: US Government Printing Office.

McCarthy JJ, Borders OT (1985) Limit setting on drug abuse in methadone maintenance patients. Am J Psychiatry 142:1419–1423.

McGahan PL, Griffith JA, Parente R, Mclellan AT (1982) Composite Scores from the Addiction Severity Index. Washington, DC: NIDA Project DA02554 and the Veteran's Administration.

McGlothlin WH (1979) Criminal justice clients. In DuPont RI, Goldstein A, O'Donnell J (eds): Handbook on Drug Abuse. Washington, DC: US Government Printing Office, pp 203–209.

McGlothlin WH (1979) Drugs and Crime. In DuPont RI, Goldstein A, O'Donnell J (eds): Handbook on Drug Abuse. Washington, DC: US Government Printing Office, pp 357–364.

McGlothlin WH, Anglin MD (1981) Long-term follow-up of clients of high and low dose methadone programs. Arch Gen Psychiatry 38:1055–1063.

McGlothlin WH, Anglin MD, Wilson BD (1977) An evaluation of the California civil addict program. In Services Research Monograph Series. Rockville: US Department of Health and Human Services.

McGlothlin WH, Anglin MD, Wilson BD (1977) A follow-up of admissions to the

California civil addict program. Am J Drug Alcohol Abuse 4:197–199.

McGlothlin WH, Anglin MD, Wilson BD (1978) Narcotic addiction and crime. Criminology 16:293–316.

McLellan AT, Alterman AI, Woody GE. A quantitative measure of substance abuse treatment programs: the treatment services review. J Nerv Ment Dis (in press).

McLellan AT, Childress AR, Griffith J, Woody GE (1984) The psychiatrically severe drug abuse patient: methadone maintenance or therapeutic community? Am J Drug Alcohol Abuse 10:77–95.

McLellan AT, Luborsky L, Cacciola J, et al (1985) Guide to the addiction severity index: background, administration and field testing results. Washington, DC: US Government Printing Office.

McLellan AT, Luborsky L, Cacciola J, et al (1985) New data from the addictions severity index: reliability and validity in three centers. J Nerv Ment Dis 173:412–423.

McLellan AT, Luborsky L, O'Brien CP, et al (1986) Alcohol and drug treatment in three different populations: Is there improvement and is it predictable? Am J Drug Alcohol Abuse 12:101–120.

McLellan AT, Luborsky L, O'Brien CP, et al (1982) Is treatment for substance abuse effective? JAMA 247:1423–1427.

McLellan AT, Luborsky L, O'Brien CP, Woody GE (1980) An improved diagnostic evaluation instrument for substance abuse patients: the addiction severity index. J Nerv Ment Dis 168:26–33.

McLellan AT, Luborsky L, Woody GE, et al (1981) Are the addiction- related problems of substance abusers really related? J Nerv Ment Dis 169:232–239.

McLellan AT, Luborsky L, Woody GE, et al (1983) Predicting response to alcohol and drug abuse treatments: Role of psychiatric severity. Arch Gen Psychiatry 40:620–625.

McLellan AT, MacGahan JA, Druley KA (1979) Changes in drug abuse clients—1972–1978: Implications for revised treatment. Am J Drug Alcohol Abuse 6:151–162.

McLellan AT, O'Brien CP, Alterman AI, Druley KA (1980) Matching substance abuse patients to appropriate treatments: A conceptual and methodological approach. Drug Alcohol Depend 5:189–195.

McLellan AT, Woody GE, Luborsky L, et al (1983) Increased effectiveness of substance abuse treatment: A prospective study of patient-treatment matching. J Nerv Ment Dis 171:597–605.

McLellan AT, Woody GE, Luborsky L, Goehl L (1988) Is the counselor an "active ingredient" in substance abuse rehabilitation: An examination of treatment success among four counselors. J Nerv Ment Dis 176:423–430.

Metzger D, Platt JJ (1987) Methadone dose levels and client characteristics in heroin addicts. Int J Addict 22:187–194.

Meyer R (1983) Introduction to part III factors affecting the outcome of methadone treatment. In Cooper J, Altman F, Brown B, Czechowicz D (eds): NIDA Treatment Research Monograph Series: Research on the Treatment of Narcotic Addiction: State of the Art. Rockville: US Department of Health and Human Services, pp 495–499.

Mieczkowski T (1990) The accuracy of self-reported drug use: An evaluation and analysis of new data. In Weisheit R (ed): Drugs, Crime and the Criminal Justice

System. Cincinnati: Anderson Publishing.
Milby JB (1981) Addictive Behavior and Its Treatment. New York: Springer Publishing.
Milby JB (1988) Methadone maintenance to abstinence: How many make it? Int J Addict 176:409–422.
Miller D (1971) Methadone maintenance-toward a rational approach. J Am Pharm Assoc NS11:364–368.
Moos RH (1974) Evaluating Treatment Environments. New York: Wiley.
Moos RH, Finney JW (1987–1988) Alcoholism program evaluation: the treatment domain. Drugs Society 2:31–51.
Moos RH, Finney JW, Cronkite RC (eds) (1990) Alcoholism Treatment: Context, Process, and Outcome. New York: Oxford University Press.
Murphy SB, Reinarman C, Waldorf D (1989) An 11-year follow-up of a network of cocaine users. Br J Addict 84:427–436.
Murphy S, Rosenbaum M (1988) Money for methadone II. Unintended consequences of limited-duration methadone maintenance. J Psychoactive Drugs 20:397–402.
Nash G (1976) An analysis of twelve studies of the impact of drug abuse treatment upon criminality. In Drug Use and Crime: Report of the Panel on Drug Use and Criminal Behavior. Research Triangle Park: Research Triangle Institute.
National Drug Control Strategy (1989) The White House (September). Washington, DC: Superintendent of Documents.
National Drug Control Strategy (1990) The White House (January). Washington, DC: Superintendent of Documents.
Newman RG (1977) The role of social and psychiatric services. In Cates M (ed): Methadone Treatment in Narcotic Addiction: Program Management, Findings and Prospects for the Future. New York: Academic Press, pp 64–68.
Newman RG (1987) Methadone treatment: defining and evaluating success. N Engl J Med 317:447–450.
Newman RG (1990) New York City. In Arif A, Westermeyer J (eds): Methadone in the Management of Opiod Dependence: Programs and Policies Around the World. New York: Praeger.
Novick DM, Joseph H, Croxson TS, et al (1990) Absence of antibody to human immunodeficiency virus in long-term, socially rehabilitated methadone maintenance patients. Arch Intern Med 150:97–99.
Novick DM, Klan I, Kreek MJ (1986) Acquired immunodeficiency syndrome and infection with hepatitis viruses in individuals abusing drugs by injection. Bull Narcotics 38:15–25.
Novick DM, Pascarelli EF, Joseph H, et al (1988) Methadone maintenance patients in general medical practice: a preliminary report. JAMA 259:3299–3302.
Nurco DN, Ball JC, Shaffer JW, Hanlon TE (1985) The criminality of narcotic addicts. J Nerv Ment Dis 173: 94–102.
Nurco DN, Ball JC, Shaffer JW, et al (1986) A comparison by race/ethnicity of narcotic addict crime rates in Baltimore, New York and Philadelphia. Am J Drug Alcohol Abuse 12:297–307.
Nurco DN, Cisin IH, Balter MB (1981) Addict careers. II. The first ten years. Int J Addict 16:1327–1356.
Nurco DN, Shaffer JW, Ball JC, Kinlock TW (1984) Trends in the commission of

crime among narcotic addicts over successive periods of addiction and nonaddiction. Am J Drug Alcohol Abuse 10:481–489.

Nurco DN, Shaffer JW, Hanlon TE, et al (1987) Attitudes towards narcotic addiction. J Nerv Ment Dis 175:653–660.

Nurco DN, Shaffer JW, Hanlon TE, et al (1988) Relationships between client/counselor congruence and treatment outcome among narcotic addicts. Compr Psychiatry 29:48–54.

Nurco DN, Wegner N, Baum H, Makotsky A (1979) A case study: narcotic addiction over a quarter of a century in a major American city, 1950–1977. NIDA Service Research Report. Rockville: US Department of Health and Human Services.

Nurco DN, Wegner N, Stephenson P, et al (1983) Ex-Addicts' Self-Help Groups: Potentials and Pitfalls. New York: Praeger.

Nyswander ME (1967) The methadone treatment of heroin addiction. Hospital Practice 2:27–33.

O'Donnell JA, Jones JP (1968) Diffusion of the intravenous technique among narcotic addicts. J Health Soc Behav 9:120–30.

O'Donnell JA, Voss HL, Clayton RR, et al (1976) Young Men and Drugs: A Nationwide Survey. Washington, DC: US Government Printing Office.

Parrino MW (1987) A review of Hong Kong's methadone treatment system recommendations for New York State, pp 1–9.

Paulus I (1968) A comparative study of long-term and short-term withdrawal of narcotic addicts voluntarily seeking comprehensive treatment. Br J Addict 63:129–141.

Paulus I, Halliday R (1967) Rehabilitation and the narcotic addict: results of a comparative methadone withdrawal program. Cana Medi Associ J 96:655–659.

Peachey JE, Franklin T (1988) Methadone treatment in Canada: the clinical questions continue. Cana Medi Associ Journal 138:17–19.

Pescor MJ (1943) A statistical analysis of the clinical records of hospitalized drug addicts. Public Health Rep, Supple 143. Washington, DC: US Government Printing Office, pp 1–30.

Pescor MJ (1943) Follow-up study of treated narcotic drug addicts. Public Health Rep, Supple 170. Washington, DC: US Government Printing Office.

Pickens RW, Fletcher BW. Overview of treatment issues. In: Improving Drug Abuse Treatment, NIDA Monograph (In press).

Pickens RW, Heston LL (eds) (1979) Psychiatric Factors in Drug Abuse. New York: Grune & Stratton.

Plair W, Jackson L (1970) Narcotic Use and Crime: A Report on Interviews with 50 Addicts Under Treatment. Research Report 33. Washington, DC: District of Columbia, Department of Corrections.

Platt JJ (1986) Heroin Addiction: Theory, Research and Treatment. Florida: Robert E. Krieger Publishing.

Powers K, Hanssens DM, Hser Y-I, Anglin MD (1990) Measuring the long-term effects of public policy: the case of narcotics use and property crime. Management Science (In press).

Preble E, Casey JJ (1969) Taking care of business—the heroin users' life on the street. Int J Addict 4:1–24.

Price RK, Cottler LB, Robins LN. Patterns of drug abuse treatment utilization in a general population. NIDA Research Monograph Series: Proceedings of the

Committee on Problems of Drug Dependence, 1990. Rockville: US Department of Health and Human Services. (In press).

Primm BJ, Cook DR, Drew J (1981) The problem of addiction in the black community. In Lowinson H, Ruiz P (eds): Substance Abuse: Clinical Problems and Perspectives. Baltimore: Williams & Wilkins, pp 703, 705, 711.

Pyun KH, Ochs HD, Dufford MTW, Wedgwood, RJ (1987) Perinatal infection with human immunodeficiency virus. N Engl J Med 317:611–14.

Quinones MA, Doyle KM, Sheffet A, Louria DB (1979) Evaluation of drug abuse rehabilitation efforts: a review. Am J Public Health 69:1164–1169.

Reiss AJ, Tonry M (1986) Communities and Crime. Chicago: University of Chicago Press.

Robins LN (1973) A Follow-up of Vietnam Drug Users: Interim Final Report 1973. Special Action Office for Drug Abuse Prevention, No. HSM–42–72–75.

Robins LN (1974) A follow-up of Vietnam veteran's drug use. J of Drug Issues, 4:61–63.

Robins LN (1979) Addicts careers. In DuPont RI, Goldstein A, O'Donnell J (eds): Handbook on Drug Abuse. Washington, DC: US Government Printing Office, pp 325–336.

Rosenbaum M, Murphy 5 (1984) Always a junkie?: the arduous task of getting off methadone maintenance. J Drug Uses 14:527–552.

Rosenthal MS (1989) The therapeutic community: exploring the boundaries. Br J Addict 84:141–150.

Roszell DK, Calsyn DA (1986) Methadone dosage: patient characteristics and clinical correlates. Int J Addict 21:1233–1246.

Rounsaville BJ, Kleber HD (1985) Untreated opiate addicts: how do they differ from those seeking treatment. Arch Gen Psychiatry 42:1072–1077.

Rounsaville BJ, Kosten TR, Weissman MM, Kleber HD (1986). Prognostic significance of psychopathology in treated opiate addicts: a 2.5 year follow-up study. Arch Gen Psychiatry 43:739–745.

Rounsaville BJ, Weissman MM, Kleber HD, Wilber C (1982). Heterogeneity of psychiatric diagnosis in treated opiate addicts. Arch Gen Psychiatry 39:161–166.

Saxon AJ, Calsyn DA, Haver VM, Erickson L (1990) A nationwide survey of urinalysis practices of methadone maintenance clinics. Arch Pathol Lab Med 114:94–100.

Schwartzman J (1977) Methadone maintenance and addict abstinence. Int J Addict 12:497–507.

Sells SB (ed) (1974) Effectiveness of Drug Abuse Treatment. Vols 1 and 2. Cambridge: Ballinger.

Sells SB (1977) Methadone maintenance in perspective. J Drug Issues 7:13–22.

Sells SB (1979) Treatment effectiveness. In DuPont RI, Goldstein A, O'Donnell J (eds): Handbook on Drug Abuse. Washington, DC: US Government Printing Office, pp 105–118.

Sells SB, Demaree RG, Hornick CW (1979) Comparative Effectiveness of Drug Abuse Treatment Modalities. Services Research Administrative Report. Rockville: US Department of Health and Human Services.

Sells SB, Simpson DD (eds) (1976) Effectiveness of Drug Abuse Treatment. Vol. 3-5. Cambridge, Massachusetts: Ballinger.

Senay EC (1990) Drug abuse treatment in Illinois: 1966–1984. In Arif A, Wlestermeyer J (eds): Methadone in the Management of Opioid Dependence: Programs

and Policies Around the World. New York: Praeger.
Senay EC (1988) Methadone and public policy. Br J Addict 83:257–263.
Senay EC (1985) Methadone maintenance treatment. Int J Addict 20:803–821.
Senay EC (1989) Methadone maintenance. In: Treatments of Psychiatric Disorders. A Task Force Report of the American Psychiatric Association. Washington DC: APA 2:1342–1430.
Siddall JW, Conway GL (1988) Interactional variables associated with retention and success in residential drug treatment. Int J Addict 23:1241–1254.
Simpson DD (1984) National treatment system evaluation based on drug abuse reporting program (DARP): follow-up research. In Tims FM, Ludford JP (eds): Drug Abuse Treatment Evaluation: Strategies, Progress and Prospects. (ADM)84–1329. Rockville: US Department of Health and Human Services.
Simpson DD (1979) The relation of time spent in drug abuse treatment to post-treatment outcome. Am J Psychiatry 136:1449–1453.
Simpson DD, Joe GW, Lehman WEK, Sells SB (1986) Addiction careers: etiology, treatment and 12-year follow-up outcomes. J Drug Issues 16:107–122.
Simpson DD, Lloyd MR (1977) Alcohol and illicit drug use: national follow-up study of admissions to drug abuse treatment in the DARP during 1969–1971. (ADM)77–496. Rockville: US Department of Health and Human Services.
Simpson DD, Lloyd MR, Gent MJ (1976) Reliability and Validity of Data: National Follow-up Study of Admissions to Drug Abuse Treatment in the DARP During 1969–1971. Fort Worth: Texas Christian University, Institute of Behavioral Research.
Simpson DD, Savage LJ (1980) Drug abuse treatment readmissions and outcomes. Arch Gen Psychiatry 37:896–901.
Simpson DD, Sells SB (1982) Effectiveness of treatment for drug abuse: An overview of the DARP research program. Adv Alcohol Subst Abuse 2:7–29.
Simpson DD, Sells SB (eds) (1990) Opioid Addiction and Treatment: a 12-Year Follow-up. Malabar: Robert E. Krieger Publishing.
Singer B (1986) Self-selection and performance-based ratings: a case study in program evaluation. In Warner H (ed): Drawing Inferences from Self-Selected Samples. New York: Springer-Verlag, pp 29–49.
Singleton EG, Sherman MF, Bigelow GE (1984) The index of choice: indications of methadone patients' selection of naltrexone treatment. Amer J Drug Alcohol Abuse 10:209–221.
Siquel EN, Spillane WH (1978) The effect of prior treatment on treatment success. Int J Addict 13:797–805.
Sisk JE, Hatziandreu EJ, Hughes R, et al (1990) The Effectiveness of Drug Abuse Treatment: Implications for Controlling AIDS/HIV Infection. Washington, DC: Congress of the United States, Office of Technology Assessment.
Sorenson JL, Hall SM, Loeb P, et al (1988) Dissemination of a job seekers' workshop to drug treatment programs. Behav Ther 19:143–155.
Speckhart G, Anglin MD (1985) Narcotics and crime: an analysis of existing evidence for a causal relationship. Behav Sci Law 3:259–282.
Speckhart G, Anglin MD (1986) Narcotics and crime: a causal modeling approach. J Quant Criminol 2:3–28.
Stephens RC (1972) The truthfulness of addict respondents in research projects. Int J Addict 7:549–558.
Stephens RC, Ellis RD (1975) Narcotic addicts and crime: analysis of recent trends. Criminology 12:474–488.

Stimmel B (1987) AIDS, alcohol and heroin: a particularly deadly combination. Adv Alcohol Subst Abuse 6:1–5.

Stimmel B, Cohen M, Sturiano V, et al (1983) Is treatment for alcoholism effective in persons on methadone maintenance? Am J Psychiatry 140:862–866.

Stimson GV (1987) British drug policies in the 1980s: a preliminary analysis and suggestions for research. Br J Addict 82:477–488.

Stimson GV, Oppenheimer E, Thorley A (1978) Seven-year follow-up of heroin addicts: drug use and outcome. Br Med J 1:1190–1192.

Stitzer ML, Bickel WK, Bigelow GE, Liebson IA (1986) Effect of methadone dose contingencies on urinalysis test results of polydrug-abusing methadone-maintenance patients. Drug Alcohol Depend 18:341–348.

Stitzer ML, McCaul ME, Bigelow GE, Liebson IA (1983) Oral methadone self-administration: effects of dose and alternative reinforcers. Clin Pharmacol Ther 34:29–35.

Stitzer ML, McCaul ME, Bigelow GE, Liebson IA (1984) Chronic opiate use during methadone detoxification: effects of a dose increase treatment. Drug Alcohol Depend 14:37–44.

Strategy Council on Drug Abuse (1979) Federal Strategy for Drug Abuse and Drug Traffic Prevention. Washington, DC: US Government Printing Office.

Strug DL, Hunt DE, Goldsmith DS, et al (1985) Patterns of cocaine use among methadone clients. Inter J Addict 20:1163–1175.

Tennant FS, Rawson RA, Cohen A, et al (1983) Methadone plasma levels and persistent drug abuse in high dose maintenance patients. Subst Alcohol Actions Misuse 4:369–374.

Terry CE, Pellens M (1928) The Opium Problem. New York: Bureau of Social Hygiene. (1970) Reprinted by Montclair: Patterson Smith.

Tims FM (1981) Effectiveness of drug abuse treatment programs. NIDA Research Monograph Series. (ADM)84–1143. Rockville: US Department of Health and Human Services.

Tims FM (1982) Assessing treatment: the conduct of evaluation within drug abuse treatment programs. (ADM)82–1218. Rockville: US Department of Health and Human Services.

Tims FM, Leukefeld CG (eds) (1986) Relapse and recovery in drug abuse. NIDA Research Monograph Series 72. Rockville: Department of Health and Human Services.

Tims FM, Ludford JP (eds) (1984) NIDA Research Monograph Series 51: RAUS: Drug Abuse Treatment Evaluation: Strategies, Progress, and Prospects. (ADM) 84–1329. Rockville: US Department of Health and Human Services.

Tonry M (1990) Research on drugs and crime. In Tonry M, Wilson JQ (eds): Drugs and Crime. Vol. 13. Chicago: University of Chicago Press, pp 1–8.

Treatment research (1987). In: Drug Abuse and Drug Abuse Research: The Second Triennial Report to Congress. (ADM)87–1486. Rockville: US Department of Health and Humans Services, pp 59–75.

Trebach AS (1982) The Heroin Solution New Haven. Yale University Press.

Treece C, Nicholson B (1980) DSM-III personality type and dose levels in methadone maintenance patients. J Nerv Ment Dis 168:621–628.

United States General Accounting Office (1980) Action Needed to Improve Management and Effectiveness of Drug Abuse Treatment. Washington, DC: US Department of Commerce. Publication NTIS PB80-167299.

United States General Accounting Office (1985) Reported Federal Drug Abuse

Expenditures—Fiscal Years 1981 to 1985. Washington, DC: US Government Printing Office.
United States General Accounting Office (1990) Methadone Maintenance: Some Treatment Programs are not Effective; Greater Federal Oversight Needed. Washington, DC: US Government Printing Office.
Vaillant GE (1966) A twelve-year follow-up of New York narcotic addicts. I. The relation of treatment to outcome. Am J Psychiatry 22:727–737.
Vaillant GE (1966) A twelve-year follow-up of New York narcotic addicts. III. Some social and psychiatric characteristics. Arch Gen Psychiatry 15:559–609.
Vaillant GE (1973) A 20-year follow-up of New York narcotic addicts. Arch Gen Psychiatry 29:237–241.
Voss HL, Stephens RC (1973) Criminal history of narcotic addicts. Drug Forum 2:1–202.
Waldorf D (1973) Careers in Dope. Englewood Cliffs: Prentice-Hall.
Wang RIH, Kochar C, Hasegawa AT, Roh BL (1982) Initial methadone dose in treating opiate addiction. Inter J Addict 17:357–363.
Weddington WW. Towards a rehabilitation of methadone maintenance: integration of relapse prevention and aftercare. Inter J Addict (In press).
Weiland WF, Chambers CD (1970) Methadone maintenance: A comparison of two stabilization techniques. Inter J Addict 5:645–659.
Wells EA, Hawkins JD, Catalano RF (1988) Choosing drug use measures for treatment outcome studies. I. The influences of measurement approach on treatment results. Inter J Addict 23:851–873.
Wesson DR (1988) Revival of medical maintenance in the treatment of heroin dependence. JAMA 259:3314–3315.
Westermeyer J (1989) National and international strategies to control drug abuse. Adv Alcohol Subst Abuse 8:1–35.
Westermeyer J (1989) Nontreatment factors affecting treatment outcome in substance abuse. Am J Drug Alcohol Abuse 15:13–29.
White House Meeting (1988) Behavioral regulation of illicit drug abuse within the treatment setting. May 16.
Wilmarth SS, Goldstein A (1974) Therapeutic Effectiveness of Methadone Maintenance Programs in the USA. Geneva: World Health Organization.
Wolkstein E, Hastings-Black D (1979) Vocational rehabilitation. In DuPont RI, Goldstein A, O'Donnell J (eds): Handbook on Drug Abuse. Washington, DC: US Government Printing Office, pp 159–164.
Woody GE (1983) Treatment characteristics associated with outcome. NIDA Treatment Research Monograph Series: Research on the Treatment of Narcotic Addiction: State of the Art. (ADM) 83–1281, pp 541–564.
Woody GE, Luborsky L, McLellan AT, O'Brien CP (1983) Psychotherapy for opiate addicts: does it help? Arch Gen Psychiatry 40:639–645.
Zacune J, Mitcheson M, Malone S (1969) Heroin use in a provincial town—one year later. Int J Addict 4:557–570.
Zahn MA, Bencivengo M (1974) Violent death: a comparison between drug users and non-drug users. Addict Dis 1:283.
Zweben JE, Payte JT (1990) Methadone maintenance in the treatment of opioid dependence—a current perspective. In: Addiction Medicine (Special Issue). West J Med 152:588–599.

Index

MIX
Papier aus verantwortungsvollen Quellen
Paper from responsible sources
FSC® C105338

If you have any concerns about our products,
you can contact us on
ProductSafety@springernature.com

In case Publisher is established outside the EU,
the EU authorized representative is:
Springer Nature Customer Service Center GmbH
Europaplatz 3, 69115 Heidelberg, Germany

Printed by Libri Plureos GmbH
in Hamburg, Germany